Because I Knew You is courageous, intimate, and revealing, at turns excruciating and exhilarating. Dr. Macauley honestly explores his own emotional wounds, enabling us to witness how his personal healing becomes a well of compassion and a source of therapeutic prowess.

IRA BYOCK, MD
author of *The Four Things That Matter Most,*
Dying Well, and *The Best Care Possible*

Because I Knew You is an extraordinary memoir—a tender, raw, personal, and deeply sophisticated inquiry into life and loss. The exquisite beauty of these essays expresses an intense striving to understand humanity at its most vulnerable, and it succeeds brilliantly. Stunning in its scope, searing in its vision, this book assumes a humility before all the questions of the eternal. Dr. Robert Macauley writes with feeling about mortality, immortality, pain, love, despair, and hope. I do not have enough superlatives to describe this profound narrative. Macauley's incisive interrogations into life and death echo those of Dr. Atul Guwande. Even if life spares you the need to face the deepest challenges presented in *Because I Knew You*, to read it is to heal from any pain. It is a work for the ages.

Robin Oliveira
author of *My Name Is Mary Sutter*,
I Always Loved You, and *Winter Sisters*

A profound and totally engrossing exploration of the painful yet beautiful world of children facing serious illness. To their remarkable courage, Bob Macauley adds his own fascinating journey, not only as the doctor who cares for them but someone in need of healing, too. Pick up this book to be inspired, but rest assured that the human stories and life lessons will remain with you long after you put it down.

Elisha Waldman, MD
author of *This Narrow Space: A pediatric oncologist, his Jewish,*
Muslim, and Christian parents, and a hospital in Jerusalem

By reminding us what really matters and inspiring us to make a difference when we are most needed, *Because I Knew You* turns grief into courage and hardship into hope.

Stephen P. Kiernan
author of *Last Rights: Rescuing the end of life*
from the medical system and *The Baker's Secret*

With tenderness, grace, and hard-won insight, Dr. Macauley shares with us his painful yet life-celebrating journey with terminally ill children. Amid tragedy, he insists on each patient's humanity, uncovering what they love, what they dream to be, discovering with them ways in which to fit their dreams into their brief yet abundant lives. The core of this mesmerizing and unexpectedly uplifting book is what these children teach him. Their courage, their insistence on life lived with joy, changes the good doctor who possesses a painful past, indeed heals the good doctor. *Because I Knew You* is an instant classic and a book especially suited to our times.

CONNIE MAY FOWLER
author of *Before Women had Wings*
and *A Million Fragile Bones*

We must remember that, behind all the data and electronic record that is driving medical care today, there is a patient, their family, and their provider, each with their own story. In this memoir of his evolution as doctor and human being, Dr. Macauley exquisitely relates the stories of captivating children who are living with serious illness and their courageous parents, and shows what the care experience can look like and become when a doctor accompanies them open-heartedly in their joy and suffering. Certainly, this is a must-read for anyone considering becoming a clinician; but really, it is for anyone who seeks inspiration for what it means to be a loving witness to the struggles of others and how we can be transformed by such presence.

BLYTH LORD
Executive Director, Courageous Parents Network

Part memoir, part manual, Bob's beautiful book will take you all sorts of places that are otherwise very hard to get to. Go! Learn, as the author himself did, how brave, honest, wise, and generous humans can be.

BJ MILLER
author of *A Beginner's Guide to the End* and
the TED Talk "What Really Matters at the End of Life"

because i knew you

*How some remarkable sick kids
healed a doctor's soul*

by Robert Macauley

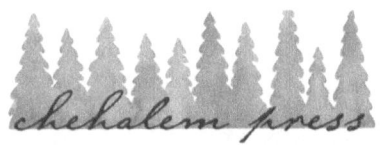

because i knew you

How some remarkable sick kids healed a doctor's soul

©2024 by Robert Macauley

Chehalem Press
Newberg, Oregon
www.chehalempress.com

All rights reserved. No part may be reproduced
for any commercial purpose by any method without
permission in writing from the copyright holder.

Printed in the United States of America

Interior and cover design: Mareesa Fawver Moss

Cover image: Heather Green

Author photo: QO Photography

ISBN 978-1-59498-151-7

For my patients, who showed me what it means to be a kid,
for Canolucha, who gave me the best job in the world,
and for Pam, who left her true north to go west with this not-so-young man.

Contents

Fifteen years ago 1
Chapter 1: In the beginning...5
Chapter 2: A very good life 23
Chapter 3: Why is this so important to you? 41
Chapter 4: When hello means goodbye................................59
Chapter 5: When the "right" answer isn't 79
Chapter 6: The finite miracle of modern medicine 95
Chapter 7: Never, never giving you up 115
Chapter 8: Return of sensation...139
Chapter 9: Battalions of sorrows...163
Chapter 10: Back when I was in medical school 183
Chapter 11: The very best of friends 203
Chapter 12: Doing to and doing for 227
Chapter 13: My people 247
Chapter 14: Irrigation and debridement..................................265
Chapter 15: Redemption 289
References 315
Abbreviations and medical terms 345
Acknowledgments 347
If you want to help 353
Author biography..355

I've heard it said
That people come into our lives
For a reason
And we are led to those
Who help us most to grow if we let them
And we help them in return
Well, I don't know if I believe that's true
But I know I'm who I am today
Because I knew you.

"For Good,"
from the musical *Wicked*,
by Stephen Lawrence Schwartz

Fifteen years ago

I was on my second glass of wine when Dave cornered me.

"So why palliative care?" he asked.

I usually need to define that term for people, but since Dave and I were mingling at the welcome reception for a program to train "tomorrow's leaders in palliative care"—which he was co-directing—he was well aware that it's a medical specialty focused on reducing suffering for patients with serious illness, who are often approaching the end of their lives. I assumed he was asking because I was one of only a handful of pediatricians selected for the program since, thankfully, most patients who need palliative care are adults.

As I had many times before, I explained how I loved taking care of kids and also wanted to be involved in crucial moments of my patients' lives. My early work as a primary care pediatrician had offered the first but rarely the second, and medical ethics—which I subsequently came to focus on—the reverse. Pediatric palliative care let me do both.

"You could have been a pediatric oncologist," Dave observed.

"Or an ICU doc."

I glanced over his shoulder to see what was on the nearest hors d'oeuvre tray. "My hospital already had enough of those."

"So find another place to work."

"I like my hospital," I replied, wondering if Dave had missed the memo about cocktail parties being designed for nibbles and chit-chat. "And what we didn't have was a pediatric palliative care team, so a few years ago, I started one."

His cobalt eyes bored through me. "That's the hospital's problem, not a why."

Maybe you could chill out, Dave, I thought as I scanned the room, catching a glimpse of Susan, the other co-director, who looked to be having an enviably lighthearted conversation with another program participant. Like me, she had also changed specialties, leaving a successful career as a psychiatrist to start all over in palliative care. When someone had asked her why, she explained her shift in simple terms: "I felt like I'd finally found my people." People who dedicated their lives to something that the rest of the world prefers not to think about because they understand that palliative care is more about living than dying.

"True," I said, turning back to Dave, "but kids deserve the same care that adults are getting."

"Granted. And someone else could have provided it."

I took another sip of wine, wondering if I was emotionally prepared for the rest of the program if the opening reception was this intense.

"Which brings me back to my initial question," Dave said, leaning in a little too close. "Why palliative care?"

"Because I don't want anyone else to hurt the way I did when I was a kid!"

Around the crowded room, people's lips were still moving, but it felt like the world had gone silent. I'd never made that connection, let alone admitted that to anybody else. Maybe it was two glasses of wine on an empty stomach or being surrounded by what were starting to feel like "my people," many of whom would go on to become close friends. But mostly it was Dave, who wasn't going to let up until he understood my hopes and fears, which I would come to learn is the mark of a great palliative care doctor.

Dave eventually wandered off in search of someone else to interrogate, leaving me to ponder what I'd just said. It's taken fifteen years—during which time I treated the patients described in this book, who taught me all I know about courage, honesty, and what it really means to be a kid—but I think I finally figured it out.

Chapter 1

In the beginning

— Firsts —

Physicians never forget their first patient. For me, it was a baby in the Neonatal Intensive Care Unit (NICU) who weighed less than a pound. To this third-year medical student—finally allowed to see patients after spending two years in the classroom and lab—the NICU felt like a science fiction movie. Everywhere you looked, there were creatures in incubators with disproportionately large heads and bodies that seemed too tiny to be human. Intravenous lines infiltrated their hand or elbow or even scalp or belly button, as feeding tubes snaked up through their nose and down into their stomach, doing what most people take for granted and what these babies were not yet (and might never be) able to do for themselves: breathe, eat, drink.

So green I practically had chlorophyll coursing through my veins, my primary goal was to not touch anything I wasn't supposed to touch, since even the common cold can be deadly to premature babies. And in the NICU, there are a *lot* of things you're not supposed to touch.

As the youngest child of older parents, I just assumed that all babies looked like the patients there. That's why I became deeply concerned one Sunday during my NICU rotation about the infant who was being baptized at my church. Tipping the scale at eight pounds or more, he must, I felt certain, be suffering from some form of gigantism, which surely carried a dire prognosis. Fortunately, just as I was about to fulfill my ethical obligation by breaking this bad news to his parents, a classmate noticed my concern and assured me that all was well. Except, that is, for my distorted perception of normal babies.

— Hannah —

I never learned what happened to my very first patient, who was stable and growing well when I finished my NICU rotation three weeks later. My next stop was the general pediatric ward, where the first patient who could actually talk to me—although she probably doesn't realize it—was largely responsible for my career choice. Hannah was a five-year-old girl with pigtails, coke-bottle glasses, and spina bifida, who needed to have complex surgery on her back. The operation went smoothly, but she still had to spend another week in the hospital in a prone position to keep pressure off her back.

There wasn't much to do for her "medically," and since I was reasonably efficient and able to get my clinical work done before it was acceptable for a medical student to leave for the day, I had some free time on my hands. Most of it I spent wheeling Hannah around the ward on her tummy in a little red wagon before returning to her hospital room where we'd pretend to call each other on a matching pair of plastic Fisher-Price phones. We spent so much time together, in fact, that the nurses started coming to me with questions about her medications, at which point I'd refer them to a real doctor who actually knew the answers.

My surprise at how much I enjoyed hanging out with Hannah and the other kids on the ward reflects a basic fact about pediatricians: we're either kids who never grew up—think Robin Williams in *Patch Adams*—or we grew up way too fast and never got the chance to be kids ourselves. I'm definitely the latter, expected from a very early age to be invariably polite and disproportionately mature. I would "dress for dinner" at parties my parents hosted for celebrities and foreign dignitaries, where my father would present me as Exhibit A: the epitome of how an upstanding young man—or, in my case, elementary schooler—ought to behave. Hannah helped me realize not only that I still had a bit of kid left in me but also how much I enjoyed taking care of children, who are more honest and real than adults.

There were other firsts along the way: the first patient I was actually in charge of caring for as a doctor, the first life I helped save, the first death I declared. They all had one very important thing in common: standing next to me—or at most a phone call away—was a senior physician who was ready to step in if I went astray, ensuring that the patient got the best care and I received appropriate feedback so as not to repeat any mistakes I might have made.

That wasn't the case with my first palliative care patient. Fifteen years after wheeling Hannah's little red wagon around the pediatric ward—during which time I'd done my pediatric residency, worked for a few years as primary care doc, and thought I'd found my calling as a medical ethicist—I decided to start a pediatric palliative care program at the hospital where I worked, for all the reasons I listed for Dave. Unable to take an entire year off to do a formal fellowship, I instead read lots of textbooks, sought out every educational experience I could find, and compiled copious notes. When I hit *Send* on the email announcing the University of Vermont Medical Center's newly christened Pediatric Advanced Care Team (PACT)—the modern version of hanging out one's shingle—I was as prepared as any self-taught doctor could be. And since my hospital wasn't doing any pediatric palliative care up to that point, I figured that something had to be better than nothing.

— Nicky —

In medicine, there's a well-known phrase used to describe clinical training: *See one, do one, teach one.* It refers to the "trickle down" approach to medical education where fully trained attending physicians teach fellows who teach residents who teach interns who teach medical students. Pretty much everyone is simultaneously learning and teaching, often something they may have just learned from somebody else.

Those also happen to be the six scariest words in medicine. Just think how you would feel if, as you're being wheeled into the operating room, your surgeon leaned over and said through their mask, "Relax! I saw someone do this operation yesterday, and I paid really close attention. I've totally got this."

Of course, trainees perform only the most mundane interventions after witnessing them once. There's usually a well-defined progression of observing many times, gradually being granted greater responsibility under direct supervision, and only much later performing the procedure independently.

Except in my case, because I didn't have the luxury of seeing a palliative care consult before I did my first. Beyond book learning, all I had was some experience in ethics consultation, which also deals with complex situations where the stakes are high. But whereas ethics is about eliminating morally impermissible options—and perhaps offering some guidance about how to select from the ones that remain—palliative care is more about entering into the suffering of the patient and family and helping them navigate through it. Luckily for me, my ethics mentor was an intensely compassionate physician, and I could only hope that some of what Dr. Orr had taught me would translate to palliative care.

That first consult came on Christmas Eve, which is a light day for clinical ethics because the hospital is skeleton-staffed and the doctors on duty are more concerned with keeping their patients alive than with exploring moral nuance. Except in the Pediatric Intensive Care Unit (PICU), where a boy whom I'll call Nicky* was going to die no matter what we did. In retrospect, I wonder if the PICU docs figured that things couldn't get any worse, so how much harm could a consult from the new PACT team do?

---

* While I'm still in touch with the parents of the patients described in Chapters 6–15—who all gave their permission to tell their child's story, affording a wonderful opportunity for reconnection and reminiscence—many years have passed since I treated the patients described in Chapters 1–5. Unable to reach out to them for permission, I've avoided using their real names (signified by "whom I'll call...") and, out of respect for their privacy, also changed certain noncritical details.

Nicky had mucopolysaccharidosis type II, more commonly referred to as Hunter syndrome. It's caused by a genetic absence of a crucial enzyme, which causes harmful cellular byproducts to build up in internal organs. This leads to developmental delays as well as a characteristic appearance: enlarged lips and tongue, coarse skin, and a forehead big enough to make the eyes perpetually squint. Contrary to appearances, though, Nicky wasn't a tough guy. He was a sweet kid who loved watching TV and going to the store with his mom. He was also fifteen years old, which happens to be the median life expectancy for patients with Hunter syndrome.

Despite his serious condition, Nicky's life had been remarkably unmedicalized, with only a few hospitalizations on top of the routine physician visits. That was all thanks to his mother, Lorraine, since Nicky's dad had left them years earlier. (Whatever he'd thought he was signing up for as a parent, the real thing turned out to be way more demanding.) Lorraine wore thick glasses, and behind them, her eyes had a fierce light, especially when she was talking about her son. She'd fought for him throughout his life, not only to attend school but to be in the same classroom with all the other kids his age. Nicky was going to have the experiences that every kid dreams about, like going to baseball games and Disney World, even if he couldn't appreciate every nuance and even if some people wouldn't meet his gaze because they were afraid of staring. Medical professionals could recognize instantly what Nicky had—if not Hunter's specifically, then one of the other mucopolysaccharidoses—but laypeople just knew that he had *something* and that it was probably bad.

Lorraine was responsible (genetically speaking) for that, too. Unlike more common diseases like cystic fibrosis—which is autosomal recessive, meaning that both parents have to provide a defective copy of the gene for a child to be affected—Hunter's is X-linked recessive, meaning that it's caused by a defect in one of the sex chromosomes. As long as you have one normal X gene, you'll be fine. Girls (whose sex chromosomes are XX) are rarely affected because they get one X from Mom and another from Dad, so the worst that usually happens is that they're carriers. Boys, though, are XY, so their only X comes from Mom. If she's a carrier, then her son has a fifty-fifty chance of getting her "bad X" and going on to develop an incurable and untreatable disease.

Of course, no parent would ever intentionally pass along a genetic mutation, and many don't even realize they're harboring one until their child is diagnosed. But that doesn't mean parents don't feel responsible—or that they don't rage at God or the universe or whatever metaphysical dice came up snake eyes—because there was also a fifty-fifty chance that Nicky would inherit Lorraine's "good X," in which case he would have been perfectly healthy. Not even a carrier. His Hunter's story wouldn't have ended at that point because there wouldn't have been a story to begin with.

That was all lurking in the background when I introduced myself—for the first time as a palliative care physician—to Lorraine. She probably suspected (rightly) that one of the reasons I was consulted was to make sure she understood the gravity of the situation, so she decided to save me the trouble.

"I probably know more about Hunter's than you do, Doctor," she said (again rightly), going on to explain how she'd noticed immediately after Nicky was born that he wasn't like all the other babies. The diagnosis didn't take long, and over the past fifteen years, she'd joined support groups for Hunter's parents and attended medical conferences promising novel therapies. "And I'm well aware of how long patients with this condition tend to live."

She stressed the word *tend* because "median life expectancy" simply means that half of kids won't make it that far while the other half will live longer. And since Nicky had exceeded textbook expectations so many times before, it made perfect sense to her that he might do so again. That was why, a week earlier, when he could no longer breathe on his own, she'd agreed to put him on a ventilator, hoping that, with treatment, he would recover. Since then, she'd barely left his side as the PICU team did everything they could to help his lungs improve: antibiotics, breathing treatments, chest physical therapy. Her extended family and their whole Catholic parish—not to mention random folks she happened to bump into at the supermarket and anyone else willing to listen—were all praying for Nicky.

Lorraine was going through something that no parent should ever experience, but that didn't change the fact that many had before her. Enough for textbooks to have been written about how to care for parents trying to navigate the impossible, which I'd read and whose advice I now followed line by line. Instead of telling her what she already knew—or trying to convince her not to follow her heart—I just observed what a remarkable kid Nicky clearly was. I empathized with the situation she found herself in and validated (as I would have in an ethics consult) her right to make decisions in his best interests. I asked her what she hoped for, although that was pretty obvious: recovery and going home. I also asked what she was afraid of, which was equally clear.

"We're not there yet," she said firmly.

I could practically see her remembering joyous moments over the past fifteen years—Nicky finally starting to walk, his first day of school—when she dared to dream that this day would never come, the day when she might really have to let him go.

She seemed to wait for me to try to talk her into (or out of) something, and when I didn't, she asked in a softer voice, "But how will I know when we are?"

"I think Nicky will tell you."

Not in words, I explained, but in how he looked. If he seemed to be in pain or fading away, she might consider redirecting his care and focusing on comfort. But as long as he still had a chance of being able to do what made life worth living for him, it made perfect sense to keep going.

Lorraine looked like she needed some time alone with Nicky, so I headed for the PICU office to update the director, whom I'll call Dr. Williamson. But before I could describe the conversation with Lorraine, he asked, "Did she change the code status?"

I shook my head, finally recognizing what should have been obvious from the start. Dr. Williamson wasn't looking for palliative care to provide emotional support or manage symptoms or companion a family through complex decision-making. He wanted me to get the DNR (for Do Not Resuscitate Order) because he believed the focus should be more on keeping Nicky comfortable than alive, which was becoming increasingly hard to achieve. A lot of people think that's all palliative care is, which is why we're often consulted at the very, very end of a patient's life.

It was a truly inauspicious beginning for the PACT team. I hadn't been able to deliver a DNR to Dr. Williamson, leaving him dissatisfied—and perhaps reluctant to consult palliative care again in the future—and me feeling like I hadn't really done much of anything. I'd just listened to Lorraine for over an hour with seemingly nothing to show for it.

Maybe I wasn't cut out for palliative care. Just because you're drawn to a line of work, after all, doesn't mean you'll be good at it. And the University of Vermont Medical Center had made do for a long time without a pediatric palliative care team, so who was I to think that my contribution would make any difference?

Looking back now, with many years of experience, I shouldn't have been surprised by Lorraine's reaction. Palliative care takes a lot of time, both in getting to know a family and then walking with them down a difficult road. We help families come to terms with a diagnosis and make agonizing treatment decisions to ensure their child doesn't suffer. Saying goodbye to your child is such a profoundly unnatural thing for a parent to do; it takes even the most reflective of parents a long while to be able to let go, if they ever can.

This palliative care thing was so new to me that I had no clue what to do next. We doctors are fix-it people, trained to prevent death, not to prepare patients and families for it. Yet despite all the wonders of modern medicine, patients may still be "overmastered by their diseases," to use Hippocrates's phrase. With no more medical interventions to deploy—and confronted by our own fallibility and self-doubt—it's tempting to shift our attention to patients who are still "salvageable," leaving the social worker or chaplain to companion the family in the final moments of their loved one's life.

I couldn't stop Nicky from dying or spare Lorraine the anguish that would follow, but even though I didn't know what to do, at least I knew what not to do: leave. Those palliative care textbooks I'd read had been absolutely clear: when a patient is dying, our job is to remain present amid suffering and sorrow. No matter how much you just want to get the hell out of there, as far away from suffering as you can.

So I did something that felt almost undoctorly: I grabbed an empty seat in the middle of the PICU and waited. All around me, co-workers rushed to complete their work in order to get home for Christmas Eve with their families. Lights blinked, and alarms occasionally went off, each monitoring one facet—breathing, heartbeat, blood pressure—of a child clinging to life. I breathed and listened, overwhelmed by a feeling of helplessness, imagining what Lorraine must be experiencing behind the closed door to Nicky's room.

Medical school didn't train me for that. Fortunately, my other vocation did.

— Medicine or ministry? —

People who knew me as a kid aren't surprised that I went on to become an ordained minister. I grew up with a mother who learned the piano so she could play "How Great Thou Art" and who would recite psalms from memory as she ferried me to sports practices. As my family moved around a great deal, she often enrolled me in evangelical Christian schools. It was at one of those, in response to an invitation of faith from my wonderful teacher, Miss Neal, that I asked forgiveness for my sins (which seemed heinous in the moment but quite modest in retrospect, seeing as I was only in sixth grade). Afterward, Miss Neal joyfully completed my Spiritual Birth Certificate, noting the date of my being born again, which I proudly tacked on my bedroom door.

My outward life didn't really change much after that since I'd always been the kind of kid who did what he was told, as long as it didn't involve cursing, drinking, or dancing (although the latter was due more to lack of rhythm than principled objection). But I did feel a deep sense of acceptance and belonging, having found a place where it was actually cool to be a goody-goody like me.

It wasn't surprising, then, that I ended up attending Wheaton College, the so-called "Harvard of Christian colleges" (which is surely a unidirectional comparison, as it's hard to imagine Harvard boasting that it's the "Wheaton of secular schools"). Like most students heading off to university, I envisioned the next four years as an opportunity to question assumptions and explore new ideas. Unfortunately, Wheaton isn't like most colleges, and it was a far cry from my mother's welcoming, socially conscious Methodism. The range of permissible inquiry is narrow: it's fine to debate whether the rapture will occur before or after the seven years of tribulation prophesied in the book of Revelation, but God forbid—and I mean that literally—you begin to wonder why the gender of the person you love matters so much or whether people who don't self-identify as Christian can be "saved."

I graduated lost and bruised, plagued by questions that felt honest and profound to me but which my peers decried as signs of insufficient faith, with potentially eternal consequences. (In case it's not clear, I'm talking about hell.) After having spent the previous four years trying to decide between a career in medicine or ministry, I opted for the former, partly because—as my classmates would often warn me—it was bad enough that my own soul was in peril without dragging others down with me.

I did love theology, though, so I deferred medical school in order to pursue a graduate degree at Oxford. My year in England was transformative in many ways, including experiencing an Anglican church for the first time. Accustomed to hour-long sermons about the consequences of sin, at first I didn't know what to do with meditative reflections followed by everyone kneeling together at the altar rail, reaching out for something missing in their lives. Having slogged through both volumes of Calvin's *Institutes of the Christian Religion* to learn what Presbyterians believe, I wasn't prepared for the comparatively succinct prayed theology of the *Book of Common Prayer*, which focuses more on how you live than what you proclaim (and certainly who you cast judgment on). Daring to share my nagging doubts with fellow parishioners, I was touched by their reassurance that questioning was a sign of seeking rather than unbelief, even if not everyone agreed with the answers I was coming up with.

Upon returning to the States, I discovered that my top choice for medical school (Yale) also had a divinity school, which happened to be one of only ten Episcopal seminaries in the country. Some might attribute that to providence and others to serendipity, but I was simply grateful for the opportunity to pursue both things I loved. So, after completing a combined MD-MDiv program, I was ordained as an Episcopal priest just before I started my residency in pediatrics at Johns Hopkins.

Once my medical training was completed, I initially tried to split time between hospital and parish jobs. It didn't take long to realize that this was an impossible task (especially with a growing family), since there really isn't such thing as a part-time physician or priest. So I settled into full-time work as a medical ethicist, which was the best way I'd yet found to combine my medical knowledge and pastoral sensibilities. But I never forgot those early years as a parish priest, visiting hospitals and nursing homes and the living rooms of people who were dying, offering silent prayers and remaining available if anyone needed me. I got used to not being able to fix things—because, as a priest, I was never expected to—which proved helpful that afternoon in the PICU.

— Nicky: Part two —

While Lorraine sat beside Nicky's bed, holding his hand, I reverted to a more pastoral stance, waiting for an opportunity to offer comfort or guidance. In some ways, though, it was harder than what I'd experienced in parish ministry since I didn't have any priestly things to do. Lorraine wasn't asking me for spiritual counsel—her parish priest had that covered—and even if she had been, it wasn't my place to offer it. All I had to provide was presence, bringing to mind the old pastoral care maxim that turns a common aphorism (and all my medical training) on its ear: "Don't just do something, stand there."

Which isn't easy, because retreat is the normal response to intense suffering. The classic biblical example of that occurred in the Garden of Gethsemane, where Jesus wrestled with his impending death on the eve of the crucifixion. He asked his three closest friends to stay awake with him and pray, yet they kept dozing off. Not because they didn't care but because the emotional pain was so intense that they would do anything to escape it.

So I tried my best to stay awake for Nicky and Lorraine. I checked in on them frequently, offering her a listening ear or simply a gentle touch on the shoulder. Along the way, I heard a lot of "Nicky stories," as Lorraine described the wonder in his eyes the first time they wheeled him through the turnstiles at Fenway Park or how he'd tear the wrapping paper off his presents on Christmas morning, breathless to discover what lay inside. Occasionally I'd sprinkle in some palliative care sayings that I'd picked up from all those books I'd read and presentations I'd attended, such as, "We're trying everything, and it's not working," or, "His body is telling us something," or, "I worry that we're starting to do things to him, not for him."

I still wasn't brave enough, though, to say the D-word: death.

By evening, something had begun to change in Lorraine. It was probably less what I or the other doctors said and more what Nicky showed her, lying motionless with a slightly pained expression on his increasingly puffy face, the result of his kidneys failing to eliminate the IV fluid required to prop up his blood pressure. The less he looked like the boy she'd loved from the moment of his birth, the clearer it became that she'd never get her son back.

"Okay," she whispered to me across Nicky's bed, as darkness fell. "It's time."

She'd never done this before—and no parent should ever have to do this—so she wasn't sure what came next. I reassured her she didn't have to sign any legal documents and also that we'd never do anything to hasten Nicky's death. We would, though, make absolutely sure that he didn't suffer as he died. Then I described exactly what would happen: we would start a low-dose morphine drip to prevent any pain or difficulty breathing, and after she and others who loved Nicky had a chance to say goodbye, we would stop the ventilator.

Before doing so, Dr. Williamson switched off the respiratory and heart rate monitors—which I'd totally forgotten about—so that the family wouldn't focus on the dwindling numbers on the screens but rather on the boy whose life was coming to an end. Then he removed the breathing tube and quietly exited the room, leaving only Nicky, the extended family, and me. We all bowed our heads as their parish priest prayed—as I had, in that role, many times before—for consolation for the family.

Except he didn't stop there. He went on to ask God to help Nicky breathe on his own, and the murmuring in the room left no doubt that this was everyone else's hope, too. The physician in me knew that wouldn't happen, and the pastor in me questioned the focus on bodily survival rather than spiritual comfort—I guess priests can also be fix-it people—but I wasn't tempted to correct him. In that moment, I too yearned for the impossible. Maybe all of us doctors were wrong. Maybe Nicky would beat the odds once again.

Stopping the ventilator had been an inhumanly difficult decision for Lorraine to make; relinquishing the last shred of hope would be even worse.

She leaned over and rested her forehead on her son's, which was already becoming dusky. Without a monitor to track his respiration rate, though, it was difficult to tell how often (or even if) he was actually breathing. At first the family seemed grateful for every extra moment they had with him, especially now that he was finally free of the machines and monitors. But as the minutes piled up, they grew more resigned that the miracle we'd prayed for would not be happening.

Wondering how long this could go on, eventually they glanced back at me, standing against the rear wall of Nicky's room. Following textbook advice, I'd warned them that he might not die immediately, but even I wasn't prepared for how time slowed down. Each second felt like an eternity, as a part of us couldn't bear to say goodbye, while another yearned for the pain—Nicky's as well as our own—to finally be over.

I stepped forward and reached for the stethoscope hanging on the IV pole. Placing it on Nicky's chest, I heard only a vast silence where a loud, steady rhythm should have been. I didn't say anything yet, though, having been fooled in the past by heartbeats separated by seemingly too great a distance. I not only needed to be sure he was dead; I also needed a moment to muster the courage to tell his family that he was gone.

After a solid thirty seconds of hearing nothing, I removed the stethoscope from my ears and turned to Lorraine, searching for the right words—any words—even as I thought back to the other times I'd informed a family that their loved one had died, either as priest or physician. Sometimes the reaction is raw, as if the family have themselves been mortally wounded. I've seen parents literally writhe on the floor or wail so loudly that security came running.

It was different with Nicky's family, maybe because they'd had fifteen years to prepare for the day they hoped would never come, which no one is ever really prepared for. Even if I'd found the right words, they weren't needed. Lorraine saw the look on my face, the almost imperceptible tilt of my head. She knew.

Around the room there was silent weeping as the entire family encircled Lorraine, ready to catch her if she fell. I stepped back to honor their grief, unsure if they even wanted me to stay. Unsure, too, whether I'd actually helped them at all.

Dr. Williamson may have consulted the brand new PACT team in the belief that at least palliative care wouldn't make anything worse, but that's a pretty low bar to clear. I hadn't cured the patient's disease—which medical school taught me was my job as a doctor—or even made Nicky more comfortable since the PICU team already had that covered. For all I knew, Lorraine might have decided to focus on comfort without my involvement, with everything turning out exactly the same way without "palliative care." (I put that in quotation marks because, at the time, I wasn't even sure that was what I was providing. Basically, I was taking my experience as a pediatrician, adding in a few tablespoons of ethics and a dash of pastoral care in the hope that the end result would be worth something.)

I felt that I should be doing something for someone, but with Nicky now gone, I had no clue what that was. If medical school didn't spend much time on caring for patients at the end of life, it didn't devote *any* to caring for families after a patient dies. So I edged closer to the door, assuming that if anyone wanted or needed me to stay, they would pull me back in.

When they didn't, I wandered into the staff office to inform the PICU team that Nicky was dead.

"He was gone for a while," Dr. Williamson said before I had the chance to speak.

"How do you know?"

"I never took the EKG leads off," he explained. "I just turned off the monitors in the room but kept them on in here."

I nodded, realizing I probably should have thought of that.

"I don't stay in the room anymore," he continued. "It's just too fucking sad."

I wasn't in any position to judge because he'd been doing this work a lot longer than I had. And unlike me—whose job was to guide and comfort and, in some people's view, to get the DNR—his really was to fix kids. Maybe he felt like he'd failed Nicky somehow, even though he'd done everything possible to help. As I was learning, feeling like a failure only deepens your sense of grief.

But for reasons I had yet to identify—since that cocktail party conversation with Dave was still a few years off—I didn't feel a heart-piercing sadness like Nicky's family was experiencing. My reaction was more of a righteous rage at a world that was going on its merry way, complete with red and green ornaments hanging from the walls, indifferent to the death of a child. Soon another patient would be stretchered into the room where Nicky had taken his last breath. That had always seemed wrong to me, dating back to the first patient who died while I was doing my chaplaincy internship. I'd come to care for him deeply, and it felt like a violation when a stranger was wheeled into what I'd come to think of as Mr. Kral's room.

It's not like the hospital had a choice, of course, because it couldn't exactly memorialize every room where a person had died or else there wouldn't be any place left for sick patients. And from a human standpoint, you can't perpetually mourn every deceased patient. Normal people might go months or even years without losing someone they care about, let alone someone whose well-being they were responsible for. But physicians—especially those who work in high-mortality specialties like critical care or palliative care—lose a lot of patients, and the cumulative grief would be crushing.

The other feeling I experienced was an ache of absence as I put on my coat and headed home, where my own son and daughter (then ages two and four) were fixated on Santa's imminent arrival. My wife listened patiently as I shared my experience with Nicky, but I don't think she really understood. It was hard for me to put into words what he and his family had gone through, and even if I'd managed to, I don't think anyone really *wants* to understand. It's easier to believe that sick kids always get better and death comes only for those who've lived a full and fulfilling life.

Sipping hot cider and noshing on fresh-baked cookies, I tried to share in my family's Christmas Eve joy, but my mind kept returning to the very different holiday that Nicky's family was experiencing. I wondered whether they would attend Midnight Mass, either out of duty or strength of habit or simply to escape the emptiness of a house where Nicky would never again tear open the presents waiting for him under the tree. I wondered why, given even odds, Nicky had to inherit his mom's "bad X" and how missing one single enzyme—out of more than a thousand in every human cell—could cause such terrible disease. And why I had two children, both perfectly healthy, while Lorraine had lost her only one.

Once my kids were asleep and the presents laid out under the tree, I took a ceremonial bite out of a special chocolate chip cookie the kids had baked just for Santa, and as I laid the remaining fragment next to a half-drunk glass of milk on the fireside table, I thought of Christmases to come. I couldn't have known it then, but the stockings on our mantle would grow in number from four to six with the arrival of two more daughters. Our kids had many years left of believing that, if you were nice, each Christmas there would be a bevy of presents waiting for you under the tree. Which is really just another way of thinking that we are in control of our lives and that, as long as we stay off the naughty list, good things will come our way.

If I hadn't yet realized how untrue that was, I finally saw it that night. As I ascended the stairs, anticipating being awakened at dawn by squealing children, I thought of Lorraine, not just on that Christmas morning but on all the ones to follow. Nobody wants to make an agonizing decision on the eve of what is supposed to be a festive occasion, but in the process of caring for her son up to the very end of his life, sorrow and joy would now forever coincide on her calendar. Images of Nicky gleefully ripping open presents would commingle with those of him lying puffy and motionless in the PICU. As I fell into an exhausted sleep, I prayed that, over time, the final ones might give way to those where hope was still waiting under the tree.

Chapter 2

A very good life

— Hannah: Part two —

It wasn't surprising that I questioned whether I made any difference in Nicky's life; I tended to do that for even my favorite patients, dating back to Hannah from my medical student days. As I transitioned to new experiences and opportunities, I assumed they'd moved on with their lives, too. I doubted they'd even remember me.

Which is why I was shocked, nearly a year after Hannah's surgery, to get a phone call from a med school classmate, telling me about a six-year-old girl he'd seen earlier that day on his orthopedics rotation. Waiting for the surgeon to arrive, the girl had picked up the Fisher-Price phone she carried with her everywhere and started talking to "Dr. Bob." Her mother explained that this had been a daily ritual for Hannah since her surgery the previous summer.

"She's coming back next week," my classmate told me. "You could stop in and see her if you want."

I wasn't sure how to respond. It didn't feel like I'd done anything that special for Hannah, just spending a little extra time with her when the rest of my work was done. Not even out of some noble sense of duty but just because she was honest, funny, and enjoyed playing cool board games. At the time, she seemed to appreciate the attention but probably because there wasn't anything else to do when she had to remain prone all day long. I never dreamed, though, that the time we spent together had been that meaningful to her.

This wasn't the first time that someone had reached out to me, but I couldn't feel their touch. It was as if, over time, my emotional receptors had become calloused, like the sole of a foot—which as a baby begins soft and vulnerable—that hardens over time after repeatedly being scraped and pierced. As if an impenetrable barrier had formed between me and others, protective but ultimately isolating.

I can still remember, back in medical school, trying to assess a patient's emotional needs and respond appropriately, yet always feeling like it wasn't really me reaching out to them. It was almost as if I were watching someone with my name on his white coat provide assistance to a patient or family in need. In the end, I took consolation in having nobly discharged my duty, but I never had the sense of truly connecting with another human being.

That doesn't mean that I was oblivious to nonverbal cues or couldn't establish emotional connections. I'm blessed with lifelong friendships—as an introvert, those tend to be fewer in number for me and deeper in nature—and have what my kids describe as an adolescent sense of humor (which probably isn't intended as a compliment and, in truth, might be a tad generous). It just means that I'd often wait until I felt safe again—either alone or with my family or a very few close friends—to let myself truly feel. At that point, huge tears would flow and not just at profound moments. Sappy movies are more than enough to open the floodgates, despite my claim that an allergy attack caused my sniffles during the scene in *Cloudy with a Chance of Meatballs* where the gruff dad discovers the thought-translator that allows him to truly communicate with his son. (My kids are quick to point out that we saw that movie indoors during the winter.)

After thanking my classmate for letting me know about Hannah's appointment, I paused to wonder whether I might have actually made a difference in another person's life. Even scarier was the possibility that I had meant something to Hannah at some point but no longer did. How awful would it be if I finally dared to believe, only to show up at her appointment and have her struggle to remember who I was? Or ask what I was doing there?

The day of the appointment came and went. I never saw Hannah again.

— Clinical ethics —

After Nicky's death, palliative care consults started to trickle in to the PACT team—although rarely from the PICU, where I'd failed to get the DNR—and usually involved symptom management. That wasn't surprising since pediatricians have relatively little experience in treating severe pain, so I came to be viewed as the local expert in using morphine and even more powerful opioids.

Historically, kids' pain has been terribly undertreated, frequently justified by the erroneous belief that "they won't remember it anyway," which explains why, up until recently, newborn circumcisions were performed without any analgesia. People also suspected that kids weren't accurately reporting their level of suffering. That suspicion proved to be well-founded, except rather than over-reporting pain, it turns out that kids under-report because they don't want their doctors or parents to feel unhelpful. Plus, if admitting you're in pain means getting a needle jabbed in your arm or thigh—supposedly to make you feel better—would you fess up?

Most of my time was still spent on medical ethics, which seemed like work I was destined to do. From a young age, I'd been laser-focused on right and wrong with such a monochrome outlook that my best friend's mom once bought me a black-and-white vertical striped jersey for my birthday, having recognized that, while the rest of the kids liked to play games, I preferred to assess penalties for rules violations. Reminding teammates not to cut corners as they ran warm-up laps before practice, grumbling when some brilliant classmate got a better grade than I did without studying as hard—let's just say I wasn't in the running for most fun guy to hang out with. In theological terms, I resembled the older brother in the Parable of the Prodigal

Son: dutiful, hard-working, and likely to take offense if others received unearned rewards. It's worth noting that the older brother isn't the hero of that story.

The most vivid example of my hyperattuned sense of justice occurred when I was five. My parents thought it was time for me to overcome my aversion to water, so they hired the lifeguard at a nearby hotel to teach me how to swim. Sensing my trepidation prior to my first—and, as it turned out, only—lesson, they introduced the lifeguard to me as Uncle Dick. Not wanting to disappoint this never-before-seen relative, I started off by doing exactly as I was told: letting go of the edge of the pool, venturing beyond the shallow end, trusting that someone would be there to save me. It helped that my "uncle" promised if I swam the entire length of the pool, then I could take a breath on a scuba tank, which felt like the equivalent of the pot of gold at the end of the rainbow. After I'd bravely completed my assigned task, however, he told me I'd have to also swim *back* in order to earn that precious breath.

"But I already did what you said I had to do," I said.

"It's not far," he replied from the other end of the pool.

That may have been true, but the length of the pool was immaterial. It was the principle that mattered.

I got out of the water, dried myself off, and waited in silence for my parents to eventually return. Uncle or not, Dick was a liar, and complicity was not an option.

Given that starting point, the fact that I ended up studying philosophy in college and ethics in divinity school shouldn't come as a surprise, but the fact that I didn't really enjoy them might. However stimulating it was to sit around for hours discussing complex issues like euthanasia, all we seemed to accomplish was discovering that the issue was actually much more complex than we'd initially thought. We never seemed to arrive at an answer, and progress was measured in humility rather than certainty.

That might have been the end of the story—and I might never have realized there was such a thing as a clinical ethicist—were it not for a fortuitous drought. My newlywed wife, Pam, and I were living in

New York City and looking for someplace to start a family. Vermont seemed intriguing, so we decided to explore the state by taking a kayak trip down the Missisquoi River, near the Canadian border. Record low rainfall, however, put a crimp in our plans in the form of rock scrapes on the bottom of our tandem kayak. So, after pulling out and spending the night at a nearby bed and breakfast, the next morning, I read the *Burlington Free Press* for the first time. On the last page was an editorial on the use of feeding tubes in patients with advanced dementia, written by someone named Bob Orr (whom I'd never heard of) who worked as a clinical ethicist (a job I didn't know existed) at a local hospital called Fletcher Allen Health Care (which I'd also never heard of).

In the spirit of "nothing ventured, nothing gained," upon our return to Manhattan, I wrote Dr. Orr a letter of introduction, mentioning my seminary training in ethics and work as a physician. He responded with an invitation to visit him in Vermont, where we quickly recognized how much we had in common in terms of vocation as well as faith. He was moving toward retirement and liked the idea of three-day weekends, so he offered me the chance to be the Friday ethicist in order to see whether I had a knack for the work. I was able to supplement that with half-time jobs both as a primary care pediatrician and as a parish priest, and a year later, Pam (then seven months pregnant with our first child) and I moved from our Greenwich Village apartment into a church rectory in the "smallest city in America," population one thousand.

The hospital in Burlington was a far and welcome cry from the ivory towers in which I'd trained. Its humble origins date back to a frail but generous woman named Mary Fletcher who bankrolled the first hospital in the state—a rather modest brick building that is now physician offices—in 1879. As many hospitals do, it expanded in stages, with each new wing reflecting the needs of the time and the architecture of the period, including a newly erected expansive façade that most people referred to as "the airport" because it looked like a terminal (which is probably not the most desirable word to associate with a hospital). Not surprisingly, the architect who designed it had never worked on a hospital before because, up until that time, he'd been focused primarily on (you guessed it) airports.

In the early 1990s, what had once been Mary Fletcher Hospital merged with the Fanny Allen Hospital (named for Ethan's daughter) to create a new entity that an advertising firm was paid millions of dollars to produce an original name for, which I'm pretty sure I could have arrived at on my own, much more economically. A few years after I arrived, Fletcher Allen Health Care itself was renamed the University of Vermont Medical Center.

Over my first few years there, Dr. Orr mentored me as he scaled back further, eventually doing his best—though, thankfully, ultimately failing—to completely retire. Along the way, he became a surrogate grandfather to our growing brood who call him Grandbob, and his wife, Grandma Joyce. Whereas some ethicists are noted (or notorious) for avoiding patient contact—preferring to meet privately with medical professionals before dispensing confidential recommendations—or engaging in protracted ethical analysis complete with references to famous philosophers like Immanuel Kant, Dr. Orr took the "clinical" in his title as seriously as he did ethicist. He stressed the importance of meeting patients and families where they were, empathizing with their concerns, and gathering as much relevant information as possible.

Most of all, he taught me that ethical advice had to be practical. This wasn't some graduate school seminar where it was enough to acknowledge how complex or challenging a question was. That was obvious to the medical team or else they wouldn't have requested our help, and they would be unlikely to do so again if all we did was validate their uncertainty. They needed to emerge from the consult with greater clarity than they had before. That's why clinical ethics is sometimes described as the search for the least bad option, because if a good one existed, someone would have already found it.

— Linda —

I soon discovered that some ethics consult requests aren't ethical at all. Instead, they involve a failure of communication, a breakdown in relationship, or staff experiencing moral distress from being prevented from doing what they believe to be right. For all the philosophical arguments I'd studied, a lot of my work involved listening, mediating, and negotiating compromise. While those sorts of dilemmas might not technically fall under the purview of ethics, they're nevertheless profound.

And some actual ethics consults are so profound that they end up affecting the ethicist's life.

One of those involved an elderly woman whom I'll call Linda. She suffered from schizophrenia and what was then called "mental retardation"* and had been institutionalized in a psychiatric facility since she was twenty-two years old. She also had severe peripheral artery disease, which was causing such terrible pain in her lower leg that, not long after Nicky died, she was admitted to our hospital. Her doctors recommended amputation, which prompted an ethics consultation because she couldn't comprehend the medical situation, let alone render a decision based on her goals and values. So Dr. Orr—who was on call at the time—phoned the patient's daughter, Shirley, who provided informed consent.

In the days following the amputation, Linda became more and more withdrawn, which is understandable given that she was in an unfamiliar environment and didn't understand why the doctors had removed part of her leg. She was also refusing to eat, causing malnutrition that would make it impossible for the surgical wound to heal. The clinical team wanted to insert a nasogastric (NG) tube to infuse nutrition and hydration, so they called ethics again to obtain permission. It was Friday by that point, so this time they got me.

Dr. Orr had taught me that the first thing you do in an ethics consult is talk to the patient. I knew that Linda wasn't able to give informed consent, but that didn't mean she didn't have any rights or that she shouldn't be treated with respect. So I tried to get to know her by stopping by her hospital room, introducing myself, and asking generally how she was doing.

She was so agitated, though, that she wouldn't even meet my gaze. Practically cowering in the corner, she seemed very far from home—if

---

* This is the term used in the patient's records for what is properly referred to as "intellectual disability."

a psychiatric facility, even one you'd lived in for most of your life, could ever be considered home. In our hospital, she was shuttled between the psychiatric floor to the operating room and then back, since she was too mentally ill for the surgical unit and, at times, too medically unstable for the psychiatric floor.

After returning to my office, I called her daughter, expecting a rather straightforward discussion along the same lines as the previous one which had addressed amputation. It did begin that way, as I described what an NG tube was and why the doctors were recommending it. There was one major difference this time, though: whereas the amputation had been a last resort to treat intractable pain, an NG tube isn't a comfort measure. (Indeed, NG tubes are among the least comfortable interventions hospitalized patients undergo.) Rather, it was a life-prolonging measure, with the goal being wound healing so Linda could return to the familiar confines of the psychiatric facility, where, hopefully, she would start eating and drinking again.

Shirley hesitated, unsure of what to say. I assured her I wasn't asking what she thought was right; rather, I was asking what her mother would want, if she were able to make the decision for herself. That's never a simple question, because no matter how well we think we know someone, people still manage to surprise us. Even more so in this case, because Linda's profound mental illness meant that she had probably lost decisional capacity long ago.

"Maybe we could just start with you telling me a bit about your mom," I said, trying to reframe the question in more manageable terms. "Then, hopefully, we can figure out what's most important to her."

"I don't know if I can."

"I know it's hard."

"I don't think you realize just how hard," she said before launching into a story that was so remarkable that, were one to come across it in a work of fiction, it would surely be rejected for being patently unrealistic. Except it really happened.

Shirley proceeded to tell me that, when she was three years old, her father had her mother committed to a sanitarium, despite Linda's pleading screams not to take her away from their young daughter. He promised her it was only temporary and that they would return for her one day. Despite his reassurances, Linda was afraid he'd never come back and rightly so: with his first wife now institutionalized, Shirley's father soon remarried. Not only that, he convinced young Shirley that her stepmother was actually her real mother. It was as if Linda hadn't just been institutionalized; she'd been erased, not only from their home but also from her daughter's memory.

Years later, when Shirley was eleven, her stepmother was scheduled to have spinal surgery which required a prolonged hospitalization to recover. Upon arriving at the hospital, however, her stepmother was so appalled by the conditions that she refused the surgery and promptly returned home, only to catch her husband *in flagrante* with another woman.

She announced her intention to leave him, and Shirley begged to go with her. That isn't hard to understand, given her father's habit of abandoning members of his family. Shirley's stepmother didn't want her, though, so she broke the news that she wasn't actually Shirley's mother. Faced with the prospect of being left alone with her father, Shirley still pleaded with the woman she now knew to be her stepmother to take her away, which the stepmother did. Characteristically, her father never kept in touch with her.

The spinal surgery eventually happened at another hospital, and the recovery took even longer than expected. In the meantime, Shirley was handed off between various relatives, but when her stepmother was finally able to come home from the hospital, she didn't take Shirley back. In fact, she broke off all contact with her.

"I guess you might say I was thrice-orphaned," Shirley told me.

I'm pretty good with words, but that rendered me speechless.

Shirley was left to find her way in the world, which she did, ultimately marrying and starting her own family. Then one day, when she was twenty-five years old, Shirley received a postcard in the mail from someone named Linda, who shared Shirley's maiden name. Shirley responded mostly out of curiosity and included her phone number. Sometime later, she received a call from a nurse at a psychiatric facility.

"Your mother would like to speak with you," the nurse said.

Up to that point, Shirley hadn't known whether her real mother was alive or dead or why she'd dropped out of her life in the first place. But Linda had never given up. Held against her will, fighting through the haze of schizophrenia with voices in her head and medicine's most potent drugs coursing through her system, she never stopped trying to find her daughter. Even though it took twenty-two years—even if it had taken forever—she was going to find the little girl she never wanted to leave.

One phone conversation led to another and then to Shirley driving several hundred miles to the sanitarium to see her mother for the first time in over two decades. Though suffering from a profound illness, she was the one adult in Shirley's life who hadn't chosen to abandon her.

I wish I could say that Shirley sprang Linda from her captivity and they lived together as a family, but my patients' stories almost never end in "happily ever after." Linda was still battling severe schizophrenia, and Shirley had made a life for herself several hours away. She did keep in touch with her mother in the years that followed, though, trying to care for her as best she could and in ways that no one had ever cared for Shirley despite—or in the absence of—their best efforts. She also welcomed her mother into her life and those of her children to the degree that mental illness permitted, sharing photos and cards and stories and visiting as often as possible.

"I've had a very good life," Shirley said.

At first I thought I'd heard her wrong. Separated from her mother, lied to by her father, abandoned by him as well as the woman she was led to believe was actually her mother: it seemed a recipe for resentment and maladjustment without even taking into account the genetic risk of mental illness.

Yet, instead of dwelling on overwhelming injustice, she chose to focus on the positive. Despite the perpetual trauma of her own childhood, Shirley had built a nurturing marriage and was blessed with four healthy children. She may have lost twenty-two years with her mother, but eventually, they were reunited. Never had I met someone who started with so little and overcame so much. I'm not sure if she used the word "grace" or if it just kept popping into my head as I listened to her describe her present life.

When we came back around to the question of whether to proceed with the NG tube, she started to use more explicitly religious imagery. "Would that tube be considered ordinary care?"

From my theological training, I recognized that as a historically Roman Catholic distinction, whereby the faithful were required to accept ordinary treatment but were granted discretion whether to accept the *extra*ordinary variety. The problem with that construct is that medical interventions are inherently contextual: what's ordinary for one patient in a particular situation might well be extraordinary for another. Take intubation, for example. Mechanically ventilating a premature baby for a few days until they can breathe on their own—as they'll continue to do for hopefully the next eighty years—seems rather ordinary. Not so for intubating an elderly patient with metastatic cancer who'll never be able to breathe independently again.

That distinction has largely been replaced in Roman Catholic thought by the concept of proportionality of benefits to burdens, so I described the burdens associated with the NG tube, especially for a psychiatric patient who might not understand why there was a tube snaking through her nose down into her stomach. Linda would probably need to be restrained (if not also sedated) for the tube to be inserted, and she would remain so to prevent her from pulling it out. Since the psychiatric facility wasn't allowed to keep patients in restraints, she would essentially become a prisoner—literally lashed to the bed—at our hospital.

It felt like Shirley was about to authorize the NG tube, not because she thought that's what her mother would choose—since it was pretty much impossible to tell what Linda really wanted—but because she felt obligated to. At that moment, without much forethought, I found myself saying, "You don't have to."

"What do you mean?" she asked.

"It's okay not to put in the NG tube."

"From a medical perspective, you mean? But doesn't that mean she'll die?"

I was at a fork in the road, and each time before and since, I've taken the same turn: speaking as a physician. Very few patients I work with know that I'm also a priest, and then, only from other staff who happen to let it slip. One reason I never mention it is to prevent roles from getting confused because patients might not want to tell their priest some things that their doctor needs to know (like their sexual history). Being bi-vocational is also a touchy subject among fellow ethicists, some of whom don't think clergy belong in their ranks—and definitely shouldn't tout their ecclesiastical bona fides—because of perceived bias or "divided loyalties" (which isn't hard to understand if you've watched a dying patient be subjected to prolonged burdensome treatment while their family prayed for a miracle that never arrived).

But somehow I felt deeply connected to this person on the other end of the phone, whom I'd never met, whose life of being abandoned by her parents and shuttled from home to home initially appeared so very different from my own. At the time, I thought it was merely sympathy for someone who was treated far worse than she (or anyone) deserved. Only now, as I pen these words to describe that fateful conversation, am I finally able to recognize that the reason I broke my cardinal rule for the one and only time is that Shirley and I had both weathered a childhood full of lies as people who claimed to love us treated us in terrible ways. Even over a telephone line, that created a sacred bond.

So I confessed that I was also a priest, making sure to specify that it was of the Episcopal variety. My goal wasn't to offer spiritual counsel but to assure her that I understood the theological distinction she was drawing.

"That's pretty close," she said.

I still didn't tell her what she should do; I only told her what she didn't have to do. It wasn't as simple as ordinary or extraordinary because benefits had to be balanced against burdens, some of which could be extreme.

"I never thought the tube was right for her," she sighed with relief. "But what will happen if we don't?"

I explained that we'd continue to offer Linda food and drink, which she was free to accept or not. If she continued to refuse, over time, she would become dehydrated and less responsive. Eventually, she would slip into a coma and die.

"Nothing extraordinary," I said. "No tubes. No restraints."

"And she can go back . . ."

Shirley couldn't quite bring herself to say the word "home," and neither could I. Home had been taken away from Linda—and from Shirley—a long time ago.

"Yes," I replied. "She can go back to her psychiatric facility."

"Okay. That sounds like the best thing for Mom."

So that's what we did. Linda ended up drinking very little and eating even less, but she seemed comfortable now that her foot wasn't there to cause excruciating pain. With no NG tube, she didn't require restraints, and without restraints, she could go back to the psychiatric hospital. That's not usually something to be grateful for, judging from the facilities I've seen with their locked doors, padded rooms, and empty stares. But that had been all Linda had known for the majority of her life, and someone there had cared enough to help her find her daughter. When Shirley's children visited Grandma, that's where they went.

Even if Linda kept refusing to eat and drink, at least she would be surrounded by people who knew her as she died. A tiny part of me remained hopeful, though, that back in familiar surroundings and gradually coming to grips with the loss of her leg, she might drink a little something. Shirley might bring her a homemade pie or some cookies the kids had baked. Maybe that way, Linda would live a while longer, relieved of some of the suffering that she'd experienced for so long.

I never found out what actually happened to her, which isn't uncommon in my work. Over the course of a solitary day (Lorraine) or even just a phone conversation (Shirley), I might discuss some of the most important things in life with someone and then never see them again. That could be because the question I was asked—like about whether the patient is able to make their own decisions and what is in their best interest—had been answered. Or sometimes, like with Hannah, because I didn't dare to believe that I'd connected with another person, as if it were someone else (who happened to resemble me) who'd helped a patient or family through a difficult time in their life.

I wondered whether I would ever feel such a connection or if the calluses around my soul—which allowed me to function in a world full of pain—would always prevent it. With palliative care being more about empathizing and ethics more about theorizing, maybe ethics was where I belonged. My knowledge of the distinction between ordinary and extraordinary treatments certainly seemed to have helped Shirley, whereas all I'd managed to do for Lorraine was hang around longer than some other people, until she reached a point that she likely would have without me.

For all I knew, this new PACT team thing might not even clear the exceedingly low bar of being better than nothing. If so, maybe the most I could aspire to was doing ethics with a pastoral twist. Better to hang up my palliative care shingle now, saving a lot of wasted effort and sparing more disappointment down the road.

That's what was going through my mind when, a few days after Linda went back home, the PICU called, saying that Nicky's mother had stopped by to drop off some treats for the hospital staff. And she wanted to talk to me.

— Nicky: Part three —

In the months since Nicky died, I'd moved on the same way I had with Hannah. After incorporating the lessons I'd learned, like turning off the monitors in the room—for back then, my palliative care learning curve was near-vertical—I came to think of Nicky less and less as I focused on other patients. He would occasionally come to mind when I saw another kid with a mucopolysaccharidosis, but that condition is extremely rare. I didn't reach out to see how Lorraine was doing because she seemed well-supported and, as far as I could tell, her expressions of thanks had reflected politeness rather than true gratitude. I made sure, though, to add his name to the remembrance list for the annual memorial service that the children's hospital holds.

As I stepped into the elevator to head up to the PICU, I didn't know what to expect. Was there something that I should have done that I didn't—or didn't do that I should have—that she wanted to share with me, with the benefit of a few months of hindsight? Or had she just made a list of all the people involved in Nicky's care and wanted to make sure nobody was left out?

By the time I got to the PICU, Lorraine had already visited with most of the staff. After greeting her, I said what an honor it was to have taken care of her son. I also thanked her for the delicious cookies she'd baked. Then I asked her how she was doing.

As polite a question as that may seem, when you stop to think about it, it's a bizarre thing to ask someone who's lost their only child. How was she supposed to be doing? That inquiry also risks opening up uncomfortable avenues of conversation, ranging from blame to depression to regret. I couldn't help but think of a common saying among courtroom attorneys: "Don't ask a question unless you're ready to hear the answer." I wasn't sure I was ready to hear Lorraine's, especially as it might involve ways that my best efforts had come up short in her family's time of greatest need.

"Could I speak to you privately?" she replied.

It wasn't like I could say no—no matter how much I wanted to—so I suggested we go back to my office. On the way there, my mind went down the long list of things about palliative care that I needed to learn more about, ranging from complex symptom management to empathic communication. But were there areas that I didn't know I didn't know? Places where my ignorance might end up leading to suffering, like whatever Lorraine was about to shine a light on? If so, the PACT team might actually be *worse* than nothing.

Once we arrived at my office, Lorraine started talking about how she was coping with the loss of Nicky. She mentioned giving away some of his toys to kids who could still use them and how hard the last day of school had been because Nicky's aunts and uncles used to always celebrate when he'd completed another year. She spoke of fragmented sleep and often curling up in his bed because that was the closest she could get to him now.

"Is that normal?" she asked.

"Yes," I replied, grateful to finally get a question that I knew the answer to. I'd already relinquished the goal of fixing things, but I still dreamed of making things a tiny bit better.

It felt like the conversation was wrapping up. Grateful that I hadn't done something egregious on Nicky's last day—or that Lorraine was too polite to mention it if I had—I was about to stand up when she uttered words that barely computed with me. There was nothing wrong with the grammar or syntax, but I still struggled to process their meaning. So much so that I can barely remember my response, other than being fairly sure it was polite. I imagine I cut the conversation short after that, conjuring some excuse for needing to be somewhere else.

I didn't mention to anyone the words that Lorraine had said, even my wife. In fact, I couldn't even bring myself to write them down in my journal for several weeks. They just didn't seem to make sense based on how I viewed my place in the world. Even if they had, it all just seemed too much to hope for. Much more convenient to forget and move on as I had so many times before.

When I finally brought myself to face the words Lorraine had said, this is what I typed in my journal:

> *Nicky's mother told me I was her rock while her son was dying and that she didn't know how she would have made it if it weren't for me.*

I feel a little awkward pasting that journal excerpt into this book, as it might come across as self-promoting. But Lorraine's words weren't confirmatory for me; they were challenging—even perplexing. As if she were speaking a foreign language, leaving me to wonder if I'd understood her correctly.

Up to that point, I had simply been following a faint calling—like a still small voice, somewhere off in the distance—to at least try addressing an unmet need that resonated deeply in me for reasons I still didn't fully understand. But the operative word is *try* because I never thought I'd actually be able to pull it off. I'd been powerless to stop the suffering in my own life, so what made me think I could accomplish that for others? All I could do was keep trying my best until it became painfully obvious that wasn't good enough. Much more than a case of endearing self-effacement, this was imposter syndrome on steroids.

Such soul-searching was reminiscent of seminary days, when various ecclesiastical committees assessed the veracity of my calling and whatever pastoral skills I might have developed.

"I don't doubt how much I care about other people," I remember saying to my mentor in the ordination process, an older and far wiser priest, "but I'm just not sure if I can communicate that to them. The real question is will they feel cared for by me."

Even in a ministerial capacity, though, there were still concrete skills to fall back on. Just as the ethicist has valuable knowledge of the law and professional codes, also the priest can provide some benefit through articulate sermons and judicious parish administration. Indeed, during periods of self-doubt, I'd sometimes wonder if eloquence rather than spiritual presence had gotten me through the ordination process, as the final committee was so impressed by the way I described my shift away from my childhood fundamentalism to the progressive Episcopal church—"a necessary respite from the perpetual Lent of my youth"—that they might well have overlooked glaring pastoral deficiencies.

There are practical aspects to palliative care, too, like prescribing appropriate medications and enhancing care coordination. But Nicky hadn't needed any of those from me, and what helped his mother was something entirely different. Typing her words into my journal certainly didn't wipe away the self-doubt I'd been battling my entire life. They didn't even "validate" my career shift toward palliative care. All they did was tell me I had to keep trying until the day came when it would finally become clear I didn't have it in me to succeed at what felt like a sacred calling.

But at least that day wasn't today.

Chapter 3

Why is this so important to you?

So the palliative care shingle stayed out, and over time, the Pediatric Advanced Care Team came to be well-accepted within the hospital, with residents routinely consulting us for patients approaching the end of life, even in the PICU. (This makes sense because most deaths in children's hospitals occur in the ICU.)

Funding remained a barrier, though, since palliative care takes a lot of time, and our signature procedure is leading family meetings, which isn't nearly as handsomely reimbursed as even a brief surgical operation. The rest of the PACT team—nurses, a social worker, a child life specialist, and a chaplain—were essentially volunteers, stealing time from their official responsibilities to work together. (I often referred to them as "dedicated in spirit if not in time.") And I continued to divide my work between clinical ethics and palliative care, which, at first, didn't seem like such a terrible thing. Since some consults seemed to call for a blend of both, sometimes I wouldn't even ask which one the person was asking for. I'd just ask, "How can I help?"

It's the sort of open-ended question that I never dreamed would get me into trouble.

— Tony —

I did that with Tony, as I'll call him, an eight-year-old with bright red hair. Raised in a communal setting linked to a fundamentalist Christian sect, he'd led an uncomplicated life—save for his parents' divorce—of going to school, riding his bike to friends' houses, and playing baseball. Then he contracted Guillain-Barré Syndrome (GBS), a rare neurological disorder in which a patient's own immune system attacks their peripheral nerves. Numbness generally follows, as can paralysis. If the paralysis extends to the diaphragm—the muscle responsible for breathing—GBS becomes life-threatening.

Tony's mother, whom I'll call Gloria, had little use for modern medicine. Tony had never been immunized and had only seen a pediatrician twice—for ear infections as a baby. But when he became so weak that he couldn't walk, Gloria had no choice but to bring him to the local emergency room.

The first step in treating GBS is to give an antibody called gamma globulin to tamp down the immune attack. Until it has time to work, patients may require a ventilator to breathe for them. Gloria initially refused both interventions, saying that she preferred "natural healing processes." Recognizing that Tony was about to die from respiratory failure, the local ER doctor threatened to call the Department of Children and Families (DCF), at which point Gloria—who'd had previous encounters with DCF over her refusal of immunizations—begrudgingly gave permission.

Tony was then life-flighted to our PICU, where he progressed to complete paralysis. Gloria never left his bedside, reading to him and reassuring him how much she cared about him. She may have rejected the thing that pediatricians love the most—immunizations, which keep kids from getting sick in the first place—but she exceeded our devotion to the thing that comes in a close second. I'd never heard of someone as old as Tony getting breast milk, but with Gloria's infant daughter cared for by relatives back home, she expressed her milk to provide for Tony through his nasogastric tube (since paralyzed patients can't swallow food or drink).

As if being paralyzed wasn't scary enough, the breathing tube inserted down Tony's throat into his lungs was extremely uncomfortable. That's why we always give intubated patients strong medications for pain and anxiety. Gloria refused, though, out of concern that Tony might become addicted, instead focusing on homegrown herbal remedies, which, not surprisingly, proved ineffective. Meanwhile, Tony—still too weak to even wiggle his fingers—consistently scored a nine or ten on the nonverbal pain scale. The scale only goes up to ten.

The medical team listened to Gloria's concerns at great length, then provided verbal and written education regarding the beneficial role of medication and the almost nonexistent risk of addiction for time-limited illness. A hospital chaplain was consulted to address spiritual issues impacting care, but Gloria seemed to question the chaplain's religiosity for not recognizing what she saw as similarities between Tony's situation and Jesus' tribulations on the cross. She remained adamant that symptomatic medications not be used, and even though Tony's father disagreed, he wasn't willing to defy his ex-wife.

That's when the resident called me, asking for help. An ethics consult would clarify whether Gloria actually had the right to refuse pain medication for Tony, and—if not—palliative care could conveniently assist with symptom management. After hearing the story, I wondered whether my theological background might also come in handy, given Gloria's spiritual rationale for refusing recommended medications.

Pediatric ethics consultations are comparatively rare. (Indeed, one reason I was drawn to pediatric palliative care was that I rarely got to work with kids as an ethicist.) In contrast to hospitalized adults—who often have lost decisional capacity, so we have to figure out what the patient would have wanted and who they preferred to make medical decisions for them—most kids haven't developed decisional capacity in the first place. It doesn't make sense to explore what they would have decided if they could since they had never been able to.

The decision-maker is also clear in pediatrics—the parent(s)—and usually the treatment plan is too. For while it's reasonable to consider the burdens and benefits of potential treatment for an adult patient, in pediatrics, there's a strong presumption toward intensive treatment. I often say that when an eighty-year-old is diagnosed with cancer, you have a conversation; but when an eight-year-old gets cancer, you start chemotherapy. We're talking about kids, after all, who aren't supposed to die.

Parents are also granted wider latitude in making decisions for their children, even to the point of pursuing burdensome treatment that has a very low probability of benefit. Gloria, though, was exercising her parental discretion in the other direction: refusing treatment that would be extremely beneficial for Tony. That right is more limited as the Supreme Court famously said, "Parents may be free to make martyrs of themselves, but they're not free under the same circumstances to make martyrs of their children."

"We should just issue a 'no trespass' order for the mother," Dr. Williamson said when I checked in with him before introducing myself to the family. "That way she'd be barred from the hospital, and we could do what we need to do."

As a private institution, we did have the right to determine who was allowed on our property and who wasn't. But, as I explained to Dr. Williamson, the potential media blowback over evicting the mother of a critically ill child from his room—especially with Gloria free to share her side of the story while we were bound by patient confidentiality—would be significant. That wasn't the main reason I thought that kicking Gloria out was a bad idea, though. Unlike Dr. Williamson, I knew what it felt like to be helpless and alone. To have pain overwhelm you with nowhere and no one to turn to. Forced to choose between companionship in the midst of pain and abandonment with less physical suffering, as a kid, I always chose the first, and I wasn't convinced that Tony would choose the second.

Dr. Williamson had clearly been expecting me to support his "no trespass" plan, so I tried to put the frustrated look on his face—which I was making quite the habit of eliciting—out of my mind as I walked toward Tony's room. I had plenty of other things to work through—first and foremost, my feelings of anger toward Gloria, who I hadn't even met yet. The chart painted a vivid picture of the pain Tony was experiencing. What kind of parent, when their child is suffering, would actively prevent people from helping him?

But then I remembered how my mentor, Dr. Orr, had taught me to begin ethics consultations with a spirit of humble inquiry. No matter how egregious someone's behavior may appear—or even turn out to be—they probably have good intentions. Something was driving them to make harmful decisions, and if we could figure out what that was, we'd have a better chance of resolving the situation.

Gloria had straight red hair down to her waist and favored long, patterned skirts; her arms were usually folded in a defensive posture. She also wasn't much for small talk.

"Life is hard," she said after I'd identified myself as the ethics consultant, clearly not needing me to explain why I was there.

"It sure is," I replied. "And while we can't prevent suffering, we can at least reduce it in some cases. Like Tony's."

"Some people choose to suffer, like women in childbirth."

I nodded, thinking back to the two (and counting) unmedicated births my wife had. "And that was their choice, in order to be fully present during a sacred experience."

"But pain itself can be redeeming. Just look at Jesus."

Her argument was shifting rapidly, with suffering going from inevitable to voluntary and now to beneficial. In the process, she hadn't just cracked open the door to talking about religion; she'd flung it wide open. Normally when that happens, I'll say something personal and nonspecific, along the lines of, "I'm also a person of faith." That way, I don't claim to be of their religion or assert any ecclesiastical authority, while letting them know that I respect the role that faith plays in their life.

That's particularly important because of the chasm between physicians and patients when it comes to spirituality. Over 80 percent of Americans believe in God, and patients generally want physicians to be aware of their spiritual beliefs, which might explain the decisions they're making or the metaphysical challenges they're facing. Conversely, less than two-thirds of physicians believe in God, and we only inquire about spirituality about one-third of the time, often reducing religion to the pragmatic impact it can have on patient care, as in the well-known refusal of blood transfusions by Jehovah's Witnesses. During my pediatric residency, for instance, it was not uncommon to come across a patient intake form where the religion box simply read, "Accepts blood," as if that was the only relevance of faith to a child's care.

But even though Gloria had opened the religion door, I chose not to walk through it. The beliefs she was espousing bore no resemblance to my own. As I see things, suffering was never Jesus' goal, which is why, on the night before he died, he asked God to spare him from it. At the same time, he recognized that speaking truth to power would likely lead to the cross and that, by walking the path of sorrows, he could somehow save the people he loved. In other words, suffering isn't the worst thing that can happen, but you have to have a really good reason for enduring it. Jesus had one. Tony didn't.

Yet Tony continued to suffer and not just from the endotracheal tube. GBS essentially attacks the outer sheath of the nerves in the body, and when that layer begins to regenerate, it causes an exquisite, painful sensation that's referred to as neuropathic pain. Think of the tingling you feel when your foot falls asleep and then starts to wake up, only multiply that by about a hundred and have it happen to every part of your body.

I tried to steer the conversation back to Tony's comfort, but Gloria kept returning to the right of parents to do what they thought was best for their kids. All the while, the phrase, "make martyrs of their children," kept going through my mind.

"And the pain will eventually go away on its own," she added. "You said so yourself."

Technically, she was right, but the problem was with the word "eventually." For Tony, lying there unable to move or substantively communicate, a few hours—let alone days or even weeks until his nerves fully regenerated—probably felt like eternity.

Realizing that an appeal to Tony's present suffering wasn't going to yield much headway, I went on to describe the long-term implications of pain in childhood. Repetitive stimulation of pain receptors produces a "wind-up" phenomenon, causing subsequent painful stimuli to hurt even worse. Children who suffer pain are also at increased risk of anxiety and even post-traumatic stress disorder later in life. For each argument I made, Gloria had a counter-argument, generally based on anecdotes and bred of deep mistrust of Western medicine.

Months earlier, when Dr. Williamson had first consulted the PACT team to get the DNR for Nicky, I'd focused on listening to and empathizing with his mother. This time, though—now acting mostly as an ethicist rather than a palliative care consultant—I really did try to persuade Gloria to change her mind. She was clearly not acting in the best interests of her child, given how severely and unnecessarily Tony was suffering.

And once again, I failed, leaving the PICU team no choice but to follow the American Academy of Pediatrics recommendations on how to respond to possible medical neglect by formulating a written plan that delineated between optional treatments (which Gloria had the right to refuse) and the standard of care (which she didn't). In an attempt at compromise, the only opioids we included in the latter category were for pretreatment for physical therapy, which can be particularly excruciating in the context of nerve regeneration. By preserving Gloria's sense of control, we hoped she'd be amenable to treating Tony's underlying pain with non-opioids like gabapentin, which I recommended because it has no risk of addiction.

She refused even that, though, based on a report she'd found on the internet which associated gabapentin with suicide attempts. Never mind that gabapentin is actually used to treat depression and that studies have shown that it reduces the risk of suicide attempts in psychiatric patients. In one of our many follow-up conversations, I struggled to keep my voice even as I observed that Tony's risk of self-harm appeared to be quite low because he couldn't *move*.

In the end, after all the listening and educating and striving to establish some semblance of trust, Gloria remained steadfast. She also never left Tony's bedside because she suspected (rightly) that we might take that opportunity to provide Tony with symptomatic relief. That left us no choice but to make a report of medical neglect to DCF.

Not wanting that to take her by surprise—and thus annihilate whatever shred of trust might have been fostered—I took her aside to inform her of why I'd felt obligated to make the report. (While it was a team decision, I personally made the referral because it was better for her anger to be directed toward a consultant like me, rather than the PICU team who had primary responsibility for Tony's care.) I explained that this wasn't about permanently separating her from Tony or putting him in foster care since he would definitely return home with her once he was well enough to be discharged. This was about treating Tony's suffering now.

I was prepared for her to be enraged and never want to talk to me again. Instead, she took the news in stride, as if she'd been expecting it. With the DCF visit looming, she even gave us permission to start gabapentin for neuropathic pain, although she continued to tell Tony that the doctors "are just trying to make you a zombie" and warned him that the medication could "make you want to kill yourself."

Without much else to say—at least until DCF rendered a verdict—I thought our conversation was over. But then, Gloria moved a little too close to me and asked me a question that unnerves me to this day.

"Why is this so important to you?"

It was reminiscent of the question Dave had recently asked me at that cocktail party, but whereas he'd been trying to help me understand more about myself, Gloria seemed bewildered by the fact that some doctor who'd never even met her son before this hospitalization (and likely would never see him again after discharge) would fight so hard to treat something that she viewed as a temporary inconvenience. And it was only when I thought back to my response to Dave's question—"Because I don't want anyone else to hurt the way I did when I was a kid"—that I stumbled on the answer to Gloria's.

— My story —

On the surface, I wouldn't seem to have much in common with Tony—whereas he endured a prolonged and searingly painful hospitalization, I've been blessed with solid physical health—nor, for that matter, with Shirley, who was thrice-orphaned, while my parents were married and very much a part of my life for nearly fifty years.

Instead of rare diseases and impossible decisions, my life includes a smart and wonderful wife and four healthy kids who are awesome and imperfect and loved. As a straight, cisgender, white, upper-class male with multiple Ivy League degrees, I practically ooze privilege.

I was also abused like hell—literally—as a child.

It's hard to believe I actually typed those words because, at this moment, only a handful of people know that: my wife, my sister, and three of my closest friends. Nobody else. Not the rest of my family. Not my other friends. And certainly not the people I encounter on a daily basis who have no reason to suspect anything might have been terribly wrong in my childhood.

Evidently, I hide it really well, even from people close to me. Heck, my med school roommate ended up specializing in child sexual abuse yet never suspected he was sharing an apartment with a survivor. If you were to meet me, you'd think I had a storybook childhood—complete with traveling the world and hobnobbing with the rich and famous as long as I played the part of Exhibit A—followed by a steady and rapid upward trajectory in my personal and professional life.

I bought into that story for a long time, too, until I started to wonder why I had all of two memories from before I was ten years old. And why I've always hated the word *molest*—whose soft vowels sound almost poetic—when the harsh cadence of *abuse* rings honest and true. And why my body used to stiffen and my eyes clench shut when an adult male showed any kind of affection for me (even the not-over-the-line variety) as I prayed for it all to stop. And why, even as our fellow pediatric residents would usually remember to tell the children they saw in clinic that no one was allowed to touch them except their parents and their doctor, a close friend (who had survived abuse herself) and I were the only two who made damn sure every single kid knew that.

There had to be some reason for all of that, but I was too busy claiming to be perfectly happy to spend much time wondering what it was. Maybe it wasn't worth the effort because there was nothing I could do now to change it. My only choice was to cover up like a wounded boxer on the ropes, shielding my most vulnerable parts—in this case, my soul—while leaving the rest of me undefended. Trying desperately not to collapse, I prayed for the bell to finally ring.

The blows kept coming, though, and eventually, I stopped feeling, the calluses around my soul protecting me from further trauma. Losing the ability to deeply connect with other human beings was the price I gladly paid for blotting out the ungentle touches that came in the dark.

Along the way, I also stopped trusting that what I believed in the deepest part of myself might actually be true. For so many years, I'd been reassured that what felt manipulative was a purer form of love. Any confusion—let alone resentment—that I might dare to feel was actually a sign that something was wrong with *me*. I learned to reserve judgment until I saw what other people thought about something, instead of leaning on my clearly errant sense of right and wrong.

I was living in a Bizarro World where up was down and wrong was right. It was only many years later, when I shared with a friend a common example from my childhood—probably in a casual tone because I'd been told for so long that it was normal—and they, paling, demanded, "What did you just say happened to you?" that I started to recognize the Bizarro World for what it was.

It doesn't take Sigmund Freud to figure out why I gravitated toward the role of referee in pickup football games or became an ethicist once grown up. I wouldn't be the first person to spend their life searching for something sacred that had been stolen long ago. (In my case: past wrongs acknowledged and penalized, and future wrongs prevented.) But it would take many more years to dare to truly feel the horrors of my childhood, for initially all I could acknowledge was that it happened to someone who looked like me and bore my name.

Dissociation came naturally to me, having been forced to ignore and forget in order to survive as a child.

Maybe that's why I tend to be very patient with parents who at first can't accept their child's serious diagnosis. While some condemn denial as a crutch, I see it as a parent's self-protection in the same way that dissociation once was for me. Eventually, they'll come to see the truth, just as I did. And in the meantime, I remind myself of the old pastoral care adage: "Even if denial is a crutch, you better not take it away before you give that person something else to lean on, or they'll fall down."

In addition to soul calluses and deep-seated self-doubt, the third thing that inescapable trauma cultivated within me was a profound sense of helplessness. Too young and small to fight back, I long ago relinquished any expectation of being able to truly impact the world around me. All I could do was my meager best in the face of what always felt like an inevitable outcome. I would take on some very challenging endeavors, like simultaneously attending medical school and divinity school, becoming a certified instructor for the National Outdoor Leadership School, and sailing to Antarctica to raise awareness about pollution in the region. Noble in intention, to be sure, but always with the expectation that the time would come when it finally became obvious that I hadn't made a difference—to a single person, let alone the world—because I'd never been able to before.

My purpose here is not to go into gory detail about my story because others have shared similar narratives with greater power and eloquence. I'm not concerned with the details of when, where, how, or especially who, for the thieves of my childhood have long ceased to threaten anyone. This book is not about revenge or blame; there's too much pain and suffering in the world already without adding any more.

It's also not a plea for pity because—as I've learned from the parents of the kids I treat—"Why me?" is a nonsense question. It comes perilously close to wishing one's own bad fortune on another, as if one were asking, "Why couldn't this have happened to somebody else instead?" The real question is, "Why anyone?" because in anything that remotely resembled a kind and just world, no kid would be abused or get sick or especially die. The injustice isn't that something terrible happened to me but that it happened at all.

And if it was going to happen to someone, why would I think I'm sufficiently special to be exempted from consideration? Viewed in that light, I should cast aside any sense of special privilege or protection and ask a more honest question: "Why *not* me?" At least that way I wouldn't have to feel guilty, too, for having done something—which I can't even pinpoint, although Lord knows I've tried—that caused the pain I endured.

If only all this pain was random, then I could let myself believe—in a statistically invalid though intuitively comforting way—that my suffering spared someone else a similar fate.

Until Dave's question at that cocktail party, I'd never made the connection between my past and my present. Up to that point, I'd attributed my choice of pediatric palliative care to a thoughtful search for a way to blend my medical and pastoral lives, as well as high familial expectations. After making his mark on the business world, my father turned to philanthropy, founding a tiny charity in his corporation's spare office that eventually became the largest private healthcare charity in the world, credited with saving literally millions of lives. Realizing I'd never come close to that number, I relinquished the aspiration of saving any lives by focusing on reducing suffering in a line of work that most people don't even know exists, and a line of work that others generally flee from as quickly as they can.

I learned that the hard way. When I first got involved in pediatric palliative care, I was so excited about the possibility of helping children at the moment of their greatest need that I wanted to share that enthusiasm with anyone who inquired.

"So what do you do?" somebody would ask me at a cocktail party.

"I practice pediatric palliative care."

"Pallia-what?"

"Palliative care," I'd say slowly. "It means caring for children with serious or terminal illness."

My erstwhile conversation partner would stare at me blankly, as if I were speaking some foreign yet faintly demonic language, before retreating to the bar for the rest of the night. No matter how freely the booze flowed, though, there was never enough to drown out what I'd just said.

The same holds true for my fellow physicians. My med school classmates who went into pediatrics often did so precisely because children don't tend to get serious illnesses. The few who ended up in palliative care almost exclusively treated adults, and when I mention I treat kids, they'll often say, "Oh, I could never do that." And they take care of dying people every day.

Dave—and later Gloria—helped me see why I was really drawn to pediatric palliative care: because I didn't just recognize how awful it is to suffer as a child. I could feel it in my bones, having experienced that pain firsthand. In kids like Tony, I saw myself: not understanding why this awful thing is happening or when it will end or why other people aren't doing anything to stop it. Even though I seriously doubted that I could truly make a difference, given the stakes, I knew I had to try.

Plus, I seemed ideally suited to the work. While the suffering of kids like Nicky and Tony discouraged most pediatricians from doing palliative care—or cut short the careers of those who did, as sorrow accumulated over time—the calluses surrounding my soul blunted the pain. What drove others to choose a different specialty (or belly up to the bar) was bearable for me precisely because the nerve endings in my soul had died long ago in a last, desperate act of self-preservation. Now my greatest weakness would also be my strongest protection.

Yet—as I realized over time and through provocative questions from the likes of Dave and, yes, even Gloria—sheltered deep within me were the vestiges of innocence and hope. However distant my memories of those noble traits might have been, there was nevertheless an utter certainty of how precious and irreplaceable they were. If I could do even one small thing to shelter them in others, then not only would another child be better off, but it just might cast a faint, redeeming light on the horrific events that had brought me to this place.

— Tony: Part two —

That Gloria's inability to understand why I would want to spare her son needless pain played a role in my self-discovery was ironic at best and perverse at worst. Needless to say, I didn't share my epiphany with her; I had discoveries of my own to process while we waited for DCF to investigate. In the meantime, a nurse overheard Gloria expressing confidence.

"As long as they can't prove a greater than fifty-fifty chance of death," Gloria said to someone on the phone, drawing on her previous experiences with DCF, "I should be okay."

She turned out to be right. The PICU team was forced to admit that Tony, by that point, was no longer at risk of dying and that Gloria had been a consistent presence at his bedside. In his report, the DCF worker also noted that Gloria had consented to life-saving treatments like intubation in the outside ER, seemingly overlooking the fact that she did so only after the staff there threatened to report her to DCF.

After being informed of DCF's decision not to substantiate the accusation of neglect, Gloria took me aside and said, almost nonchalantly, "I probably should report you to the American Medical Association, but that would violate my moral beliefs."

I didn't inquire about what moral beliefs those might be since, clearly, they weren't violated by allowing her son to endure unrelenting pain. Meanwhile, Dr. Williamson seethed.

"I don't just want freedom of religion," he said. "I want freedom *from* religion."

It was a curious statement to make, given that we'd worked together long enough for him to know about my other job. But if he was talking about the sort of religion that viewed suffering as inherently redemptive and ignored the pain of an innocent child, I'd tend to agree with him.

Medication negotiations with Gloria continued, although, without the threat of DCF intervention, she had even less incentive to accept our recommendations. Meanwhile, Tony toiled daily at physical therapy, enduring intense pain that we were powerless to treat, and eventually regaining the ability to eat, sit up, and stand on his own. Tony walking out of the hospital under his own power was one of the more inspiring sights I'd ever seen, a testament to his inner strength and perseverance.

I thought of Tony often after that, but I didn't attempt to check on how he was doing. That was less because I was scared (as I'd been with Hannah) and more because I doubted that Gloria would even take my call.

A couple of years later, though, his dad phoned me out of the blue.

"Tony's pretty much back to where he was before all that stuff happened," he said, although I still worry about the long-term impact of what Tony endured. "I really appreciate all you did for him."

I appreciated that he didn't say, "Tried to do for him." I'd wanted to do so much more for Tony, but the gabapentin—and the opioids before physical therapy—had hopefully lessened his suffering to some degree. Which made me think of something the parent of another patient once said to me.

"I finally figured out what you do for a living," Khanti had mused, years after his son, Kaiden, was born with an incredibly rare genetic condition that, from early studies, sounded awful: developmental delay, prone to violent outbursts, limited life expectancy. But then we did a little more digging, and it turns out that some kids with the condition go to school, most seem very happy, and the mood swings might not be worse than most other teenagers. So he and his fiancée, Kerri, chose to remain optimistic, which proved to be prophetic. Kaiden is now in eleventh grade and has yet to encounter an obstacle he can't overcome. Along the way, he acquired two younger brothers—whose names also start with K—and also proved to be a very dapper ring-bearer at his parents' wedding at which I had the honor of officiating.

"Do tell," I said, momentarily tuning out the music at the folk festival that Khanti and I were attending with our kids.

"You take a really shitty situation," he continued, "and make it less shitty."

So much for lowering the bar of success; it was now practically lying on the ground. But however far short of the standard of care Tony's symptom management had been, I dare to hope his medical team did something more profound for him: we acknowledged his pain and called it out as wrong.

I, too, know what it feels like to be powerless as a child to protect yourself, even though my paralysis had been emotional while Tony's was neurologic. I so, so wish that someone would have made those nighttime visits to my bedroom stop. But even if no one was brave or powerful enough to do that, it still would have meant so much to me for someone—anyone—to have *seen* me. It felt like the world was going on its merry way, indifferent to the suffering I was experiencing, leading me to wonder if maybe I wasn't worth noticing, let alone fighting for.

Tony's medical team ultimately failed to provide him with what he deserved, but it wasn't for lack of effort or dedication. We tried everything we could to ease his suffering, and I hope he remembers how hard we fought for him. But one thing I know for sure, from the many times we asked him how he was doing and pledged to do everything within our power to ease his suffering, is that he felt seen, which is—speaking as someone who never felt that way—sacred.

I think having survived childhood abuse myself helped me care for Tony by not shying away from the pain he was experiencing and also recognizing that, for all her tragic flaws, his mother was his emotional lifeline during an unspeakably difficult time in his life. That's why, instead of barring her from the hospital, I spent so much time presenting her with empirical evidence about medication safety and listening to her rant about the supposedly redemptive nature of Tony's suffering.

But being a survivor also inspired rage at a person who should have been protecting her child, which prevented me from doing what might really have helped Tony. Now, with years of hindsight, I can see that I should have focused less on convincing Gloria that she was wrong and more on identifying what she needed. I learned that lesson from a remarkable book called *Nonviolent Communication*, whose primary counsel in a conflictual situation is to observe the feelings it provokes, without judgment (which is no small task for an ethicist). The next step is to identify the needs—both yours and the other person's—that prompt those feelings so you can each make requests for how all those needs can be met.

I hated that book when I first read it. It seemed to be saying that we should give people like Gloria a free pass, despite her seeming disregard for her son's suffering. But I eventually came to recognize that judgment undermines meaningful dialogue, and even seemingly heartless actions arise out of unmet needs, which call for compassion rather than condemnation. It was convenient to write off Gloria's views of God and suffering as distorted and destructive, but deep down, she had needs just like Tony and I. She needed to see herself as a devoted mother and, maybe, to assert her authority in the formally educated, empirically based, male-dominated world of medicine.

Without her realizing it, Gloria's question—"Why is this so important to you?"—was very much in line with nonviolent communication. However unintentional, it was her way of asking me what needs I had in relation to Tony, which I'd revealed to Dave at that cocktail party: "To not have anyone else hurt the way I did." I still wonder what would have happened if I'd reflected the question back to her.

"Gloria," I could have asked, if only I'd been wiser, "why is this so important to *you*?"

If I had, maybe she would have said something about feeling helpless to protect her son. Maybe she felt guilty about past decisions she'd made. Easy as it was to judge Gloria, she was not an evil person, in the same way—I can now say, after a whole lot of therapy—that the person who abused me was not. She had profound, soul-level needs that likely were never recognized and that ultimately manifested themselves in harm against others, a cycle which, without deep reflection, is bound to repeat itself. As Richard Rohr says, "Pain that is not transformed is transmitted."

I wish I could go back in time to whatever they lacked in their lives—whatever formative events created those needs or prevented them from subsequently being met—and change history. I wish I could do it to spare them pain; as human beings, they didn't deserve to endure what they did. But, mostly, I want to spare people like Tony and I, who would eventually suffer at their hands, and to stop a cycle of pain from which no good ever comes.

Chapter 4

When hello means goodbye

The birth of one's child is usually among the most joyous moments of a person's life, while the loss of a child is incomprehensibly painful. When those two events happen in rapid succession—or even simultaneously—it's little wonder that parents aren't really sure how to feel. They're feeling everything imaginable, all at the same time, which is why palliative care for newborns is especially hard.

— Lily —

As devout evangelical Christians, Daniel and Miriam, as I'll call them, were thrilled that God had blessed them with a pregnancy only a few months after their wedding. Like all first-time parents, they eagerly awaited the first ultrasound to get a glimpse of their child and learn the gender. They never expected the grainy images to reveal that their daughter Lily's brain was missing a band of nerve fibers that joins the two hemispheres, and there was a hole in the muscular wall that separated the two sides of her heart. Taken in isolation, neither of these were overly serious: the brain abnormality doesn't necessarily cause any symptoms—indeed, a lot of folks are probably missing that part of their brain and just don't realize it because they've never had a CT scan or MRI—and the heart defect isn't very complicated to repair. But it's rare for someone to have both of these conditions unless they're caused by a syndrome, and most syndromes that cause things like that are serious.

I know that, not only from my medical training but also from personal experience. Midway through my wife Pam's second pregnancy, a fetal ultrasound detected bilateral polydactyly, otherwise known as six fingers on each hand. (The extra finger is usually just a nubbin that falls off on its own soon after birth.) The benign version is autosomal dominant—so if either parent has it, the baby has a fifty-fifty chance of having it, too, which makes it one of the most common genetic defects.

The only problem was that neither Pam nor I had six fingers when we were born. So, barring a case of misattributed paternity, there were only two other possibilities. One was that our son, Noah, actually did have the benign and common gene, either inheriting a version from my wife or me that we didn't exhibit or developing a spontaneous mutation. The other possibility was that this was part of a larger syndrome, like trisomy 13.

Normally, a person has twenty-three pairs of chromosomes, but a trisomy occurs when a patient has an extra copy of one. Trisomy 21, for example, is the medical term for three copies of chromosome 21, and is more commonly known as Down syndrome. Trisomy 13 is sometimes called Patau syndrome, but most people just call it T13. And it's bad.

Many affected fetuses die in utero and, of those born alive, half die within the first week of life. It's so serious, in fact, that the Neonatal Resuscitation Protocol at the time included it in the handful of conditions—along with absence of the brain and being born prior to viability—where non-resuscitation in the delivery room was appropriate. In other words, even if the parents requested intensive treatment for their newborn, a pediatrician was on firm ethical ground to refuse.

My nonmedical wife and I reacted very differently to this possibility. While Pam had an intuitive sense that everything would be okay, part of my job is to prepare for the worst case scenario. It didn't help that I was a doctor and thus very superstitious. That may sound strange when you consider how many years physicians spend in school and how focused we are on empirical evidence. But that doesn't stop us from dreading full-moon nights because we just know an ER shift will be more chaotic than during other points in the lunar cycle. Our superstitions run so deep that we even do studies to test them, ultimately finding no effect of a full moon (or, since we were already looking, Friday the thirteenth or a particular sign of the zodiac, either). And yet, despite such incontrovertible evidence, those superstitions persist, as we know from even more studies.

Another of our deeply held beliefs is that bad things happen to good people, partly because the cruelest cases are impossible to forget. Not that anyone deserves to get a life-threatening illness, but it's easier to make sense of cancer in an eighty-year-old lifelong smoker than an eight-year-old kid whose worst habit was forgetting to make his bed. Even decades later, we still remember the supremely loving and supportive families who did absolutely nothing to deserve the cruel hand fate dealt them.

To all appearances, my wife and I belong to the "good people" group: we donate to charity, always send flowers to our moms on Mother's Day, and our rap sheet is an index card listing a couple of speeding tickets. That's why, when we learned as newlyweds that we were pregnant, I was even more worried than the average first-time dad. Our goodness seemed to place us in a high-risk group; so in order to protect our daughter, I decided to get mean.

First came the terse emails without benefit of salutation or concluding well-wishes. Then I tried to scale back on the pleases and thank yous, although they still slipped out occasionally, habit being so strong. I even lost my temper once or twice, if raising your voice a fraction of a decibel counts.

Yet instead of provoking rage or indignation in the person I was talking to, more often they responded with amusement and curiosity.

"What's up with you today?" they'd ask, when I was hoping for an "Am not!" or an "Oh really?" or, if I dared to dream, a "How could you?"

Try as I might, I couldn't pull it off. That's because I am, by my own admission, a pathologically nice person. That may seem an odd way of describing what in almost every other context is a laudable trait, but "pathologically" isn't some kind of über-superlative, even stronger than "extremely." It's a recognition that sometimes being nice isn't helpful. Sometimes you need to stand up for yourself and express the feelings that arise from your unmet need for things like direct and honest communication. As you'll see in the pages to come, I didn't do that nearly enough.

I'd given up my doomed misanthropic quest by the time we got pregnant the second time with Noah, whose ultrasound findings left me feeling helpless. There's no therapy for trisomies, so the only decision my wife and I faced was whether to do an amniocentesis to know for sure whether he had one. There's an old saying in medicine, though: don't do a test unless it's going to change management. Pam and I knew that even if Noah did have T13, we weren't going to terminate the pregnancy, so the only reason to do an amnio was to emotionally prepare for what lay ahead. But the amnio came with a small risk of inducing a miscarriage. Causing the death of a healthy fetus was an even worse scenario than him being born with T13, so we waited: me intensely worried and my intuition-driven wife much less so.

Late one winter night, Noah entered the world. He's the only one of our four kids I examined in the delivery room, as I try really hard to just be Dad. But I needed to know, and only when I saw his healthy chest and limbs—and heard his heart beating strong and clear and murmurless—did I finally breathe easy. That extra nubbin on each hand was a sign that he was special, not that he was dying.

Brain and heart defects are a whole lot more serious than sixth fingers, though, so Miriam and Daniel went ahead with an amniocentesis, which confirmed their worst fear: Lily did have T13. They wouldn't have the fifteen years that Lorraine had with her child, but they could still hope that Lily would survive delivery so they could welcome her into the world and hold her in their arms.

People respond in very different ways to situations like that. Some hold out a tender hope that the doctors are wrong, although, under a microscope, three copies of chromosome 13 look very different than two. Some crumple under the weight of grief, either in the direction of their partner so that neither fall or in the opposite direction so that both do. And some pray for a miracle.

That last group of parents often possess—or have hurriedly acquired—what might be called a "transactional faith," according to which God repays devotion by honoring a prayerful request. In the case of pediatric palliative care, that request is worthy and noble, as different from a big house or a fancy car as you can get. A miraculous healing might seem less like granting a wish than making amends for a past wrong.

Some parents don't merely pray for a miracle; they expect one. There's no possible way God could permit a righteous person to lose a child, the argument goes, seemingly ignoring the biblical example of a blameless and upright man who lost all ten of his children, as well as his animals, crops, and his health. Admittedly, God later replenished the supply of each, which might have squared things for Job but didn't do squat for his original ten children, who were still dead.

This creates an all-or-nothing scenario: the parent either leaves the hospital with child and faith intact or bereft of both. I'll never forget one mother who was utterly convinced that God not only could heal her son of cancer but had told her through prayer that he would do precisely that. She fully expected to take a healthy son home from the hospital, rejoicing with fellow parishioners for his miraculous healing. When he eventually died, her faith did, too, so closely were they intertwined.

Daniel and Miriam definitely prayed for a miracle, but their faith wasn't contingent on one happening. They derived reassurance from a deep belief in God's sovereignty, relieving them of responsibility for things outside their control. They took great comfort in imagining Lily with God in heaven someday, liberated from the extra chromosome and every other burden, waiting—in a direct reversal of the natural order—for them to join *her* someday. Eternity is infinitely longer than anyone's life on Earth, so no matter how intense the pain might be now, they still had things to look forward to as a family.

That didn't stop them from crying. Sometimes the injustice got to be too much, like at the birthing classes they took when it seemed unkind to taint the other couples' joy by sharing that Lily was different. They derived comfort from Jesus' example, especially when he wept at the grave of Lazarus, despite knowing that his friend would soon come to life again. They understood that to mean that sorrow is compatible with deep faith and that it's normal to be overwhelmed when we're separated from someone we love, if only temporarily. But even granting eternal salvation to look forward to, Daniel and Miriam would nevertheless have to wait decades to see their daughter again.

They prepared for Lily's delivery with a degree of courage and openness I'd never seen before, sharing her diagnosis with those closest to them, including their church community. I'm not sure if any child has ever been the recipient of more prayers or if any couple has had more food delivered to their door. Their pastor stood ready to baptize Lily the moment she entered the world, no matter what time of day or night.

Meanwhile, Miriam, who wore her brown hair in a bob and favored blouses buttoned all the way to the top, set about knitting a onesie for her daughter. Many expectant parents do that so that their baby will have something handmade to wear home from the hospital or be baptized in. It was unlikely, though, that Lily would ever leave the hospital, and her baptism would be an emergent procedure given the uncertainty about how many minutes—or even seconds—she might live. The onesie Miriam was knitting would be for Lily's burial so that something of her parents could continue to hold her even after she died.

Daniel, a carpenter, not only had the best posture I've ever seen—he practically sat at attention—he was also among the kindest people I've ever met. Were he to have modeled my quest for meanness, he would surely have failed even more spectacularly than I did. Instead, he devoted his energies to crafting a coffin for Lily. Since then, building your own coffin has become a trending spiritual exercise, offering an opportunity to reflect on—and come to peace with—one's mortality. But parents rarely do that for their children, mostly because, if the world were a kinder and fairer place, parents wouldn't have to attend their child's funeral, let alone provide the supplies for it.

Daniel was different: he lovingly crafted the vessel that would hold his daughter's lifeless body, choosing the design, cutting and sanding the wood. If I end up half as brave as Daniel one day, I'll have reason to be proud.

#

One of my responsibilities was helping Daniel and Miriam create a birth plan for Lily. Most of it was pretty straightforward, given the certainty about her diagnosis: maximize time with family, avoid painful procedures. If Lily was born alive—which was very important to the family, in large part because baptism is (in theological parlance) a "sacrament for the living"—the delivery room team would quickly suction out any fluid from her mouth and nose, dry her off, wrap her in a warm blanket, and give her to her parents, where she'd remain until she died. The family pastor was on standby, and we'd have medicines drawn up for pain or shortness of breath, but I doubted she would live long enough to need them.

That was the plan until subsequent ultrasounds revealed that, like many fetuses with T13, Lily was developing hydrocephalus. Colloquially referred to as "water on the brain," it's caused by a blockage in the outflow of cerebrospinal fluid, causing the head to grow very large. So large, in fact, that the obstetricians were worried that it might get stuck in the birth canal, prolonging labor and increasing the chances that Lily would die during delivery. So Daniel and Miriam asked that I include a caesarian section in the birth plan if that seemed like the only way Lily would be born alive.

There was just one problem: Miriam's obstetrician didn't want to do a C-section.

"It's not worth the increase in maternal morbidity," he told me when I inquired.

He didn't need to explain. Cutting into the uterus isn't a trivial thing. There's a small risk of complications that could necessitate a hysterectomy, and if a woman has a trial of labor in a future pregnancy—which many hospitals don't even allow—there's a risk of uterine rupture along the previous C-section incision. For a young woman like Miriam who wanted more children, that was a big deal.

But so was Lily being born alive, at least to her parents.

I spent a lot of time trying to convince her obstetrician to consider a C-section if it didn't seem like Lily could survive a vaginal birth. I noted that one of out of every forty births in the United States is via C-section by maternal request, for reasons that include a pregnant patient's planned vacation about to start. If wanting to minimize the amount of parental leave you take is a good enough reason for a C-section, how can wanting to hold your living baby not be?

In the end, Lily took the decision out of our hands by deciding to come early, which isn't something that pediatricians are generally in favor of. (Prematurity of even a few weeks substantially increases the risk of respiratory, neurologic, and infectious complications.) But Lily and her family were always the exceptions to the rule, and a smaller head is easier to squeeze through the birth canal.

Lily was born vaginally and immediately gave a vigorous cry. For a split second, it felt like any other delivery—the same joy, the same hopes—until the family pastor rushed to the warming table to baptize her. Dried, suctioned, and breathing a little unevenly, Lily was brought to her parents. I stepped back to the edge of the room, struck by the concentric circles of love that surrounded this little girl: her parents holding her, behind them her grandparents, broadening out to include friends and members of their church.

For the first time, I wondered if eternity might not only describe time but also depth and devotion. If so, eternal love filled that delivery room.

In my first consult, with Nicky, I'd felt guilty for not doing more. This time, I was merely thankful that Lily was surrounded by love and receiving everything we had to give, even if it wasn't as much as she needed. The hour her parents had with her was far less than they'd prayed for, but they still cherished every second.

"Holding her," they would later say, "we felt like the luckiest unlucky parents in the world."

#

There's a debate in medicine about attending patient funerals. Some argue against it for reasons ranging from fairness—"If you go to the funeral for one patient, you should go to them all"—to self-care, since palliative care docs, especially, would end up going to a lot of funerals. Others believe that physicians should companion patients to the very end, including providing comfort to families in their grief.

The practical reality is that physicians usually don't attend their patients' funerals and for a very human reason: the last place a doctor wants to go is somewhere where everyone might blame you for the fact that they're heartbroken, not recognizing that you might be, too. That might be why palliative care docs are more likely to attend patient funerals than other specialties. Nobody ever looks to us for a cure, even though we never stop hoping for one.

I don't go to the funeral of every one of my patients who die, but I did go to Lily's. It took place in the small country church that Daniel and Miriam attended. The pastor gave an honest and encouraging sermon, simultaneously recognizing the congregation's present grief as well as their eternal hope. After the service, he led us out of the church and around back to the parish cemetery. That's where I first saw the coffin that Daniel had crafted.

Sanded so smooth that it glinted in the fading afternoon sun, with lovingly carved adornments that reminded me of medieval churches I'd visited in Europe, the coffin was far beyond anything I could have dreamed of creating. But the size was what hit me hardest. I knew on some level that it wouldn't be "normal size" since Lily was a baby (and a premature baby at that). I guess I was prepared for something slightly smaller, which would still have let people believe—if they needed to—that inside was just a person of short stature, who might well have led a rich and full-length life.

A three-foot-long box permitted no such delusion.

While Daniel and Miriam watched through tear-filled eyes as Lily's tiny, beautiful coffin was lowered into the ground, I suspected they were looking ahead to another blurry moment in the distant future, when they eventually arrived in heaven, too. No matter what might have happened in the intervening decades, the first thing they'd do was look for Lily. They wouldn't have to search long because she'd be waiting for them. In many ways, that's what she would have been doing all the years in between: eagerly anticipating being together again, as a family, the way it should have been all along and now would be forever.

It was a comforting vision, and to soothe my soul, I let myself rest in it as well. That's not often the case because I don't presume to know what happens after people die. Such an admission may be surprising coming from a priest, but I've long since given up the binary of eternal bliss in heaven or punishment in hell, determined entirely and forever by what someone did (or didn't) do or believe during earthly life. My best guess is that a loving God will honor the people we've become, which may mean seeking communion with God or could also mean a different path. Not one of torment in the flames of hell but rather a life without the divine, like the one that C. S. Lewis describes in *The Great Divorce*: a gray town where it rains continuously and people follow routines without purpose. The people there are free to leave, but the almost painful vividness of heaven—where, at first, the bright sunlight hurts their eyes, and blades of grass pierce their spectral feet—leads most of them to return to what is familiar and unthreatening.

In that moment, though, I let Daniel and Miriam's faith carry me, too, deriving comfort from the belief that eternal bliss would far outweigh earthly struggles. At the same time, I hoped that Lily's presence here on earth, however brief, would never truly be forgotten. For while heavenly visions are comforting to people of faith, the image of a pain-free life where God takes care of everything, to my mind, pales beside the courage and devotion that Daniel and Miriam showed to their daughter in an often cruel world.

— Thomas, Amelia, and Ethan —

Daniel and Miriam had months to consider what was best for Lily, ultimately focusing on her comfort and those precious few moments together as a family. Some parents, though, barely have time to think, as terrible decisions are thrust upon them without warning. I saw that firsthand some years later, on a Friday night after a long week of work.

I'd just gotten home, and judging from the loud giggling and sound of slamming doors, my three little kids were upstairs, hopefully only destroying things that were replaceable. My wife had uncorked a bottle of wine and was tending to savory stews simmering on the stove. Surrounded on all sides by people I loved, I almost forgot that, beyond the steamed-up windows, the ground was frozen, and not everyone in the world was safe inside.

Then my pager went off, revealing the number of the labor and delivery floor.

"A patient just rolled in," the obstetrics resident said when I called her back. "She's ruptured at twenty-two weeks."

Those last five words were enough for me to form a mental picture: "ruptured" referred to the pregnant patient's amniotic membranes, commonly known as the water breaking. And it had happened really early: a full-term pregnancy is forty weeks; less than thirty-seven weeks is premature; less than twenty-eight is extremely premature. There wasn't even a name for twenty-two weeks.

"How solid are the dates?" I asked, searching for some shred of hope.

Because fetuses grow at different rates, the later the ultrasound, the more uncertain the stage of pregnancy. Second-trimester ultrasounds can be off by ten days or even more, meaning this baby could be twenty-three weeks or even twenty-four. That was a huge deal because the cusp of viability—the point before which babies can't survive—had moved up over the years, from twenty-eight weeks a few decades ago to twenty-three as of that night. Despite all the wonders of medical technology, there are some things only time can accomplish.

"First trimester ultrasound," the resident responded somberly, referring to the gold standard for dating a pregnancy. "And she's in labor."

"Any chance of stopping it?"

There are lots of medicines that can slow labor down, which could buy us another day or two. That might not seem like much, but forty-eight hours of intravenous steroids for the mother can significantly accelerate a premature baby's lung development.

"I wish," the resident muttered. "It won't be long now."

Then, almost as an afterthought, she added, "Oh, and she's carrying triplets."

"You're kidding," I said in not my most sensitive moment. This was beginning to sound like someone's bad idea of a practical joke.

"Do I sound like I'm kidding?"

It was the first time I'd heard her voice break.

"How can I help?" I asked.

In my mind, I'd already identified several questions the resident might be asking. Some were straightforward—"No, there's no obligation to resuscitate a baby born that premature"—and could be communicated over the phone. The others were much harder and needed to be addressed in person: explaining to the parents why resuscitation wouldn't work and what we'd do to keep their babies comfortable.

"The parents want everything," the resident said.

We all want everything for our kids, I thought. Somewhere upstairs, I could hear one of my daughters singing, "Let It Go" from *Frozen* for the eight millionth time.

"I'm happy to talk to—" I began.

"And the neonatologist thinks they're going to need your help making decisions."

"What decisions?"

The hardest thing about some cases are the impossible choices parents are forced to make, but this one was agonizing because there weren't any options to choose from.

"About how far to keep going," she said.

I struggled to believe what I was hearing. "We're going to resuscitate?"

"Let me put it this way," the resident said. "I'm standing in the operating room, looking at three neonatal teams prep their warming tables."

#

It was a twenty-minute drive to the hospital, but before leaving, I hurried upstairs to see for myself that my kids were okay. They were fine, of course, and patiently tolerated the interruption to their karaoke rendition of the *Frozen* soundtrack. They'd gotten used to me hugging them long and tight for no apparent reason, unaware of how my work is a perpetual reminder of how powerless I am to protect the people I love. Many nights, after all the lights were out, I'd make rounds of my children's rooms, standing in the doorway and just listening to them breathe.

When I arrived on the labor and delivery floor, there were three people in the patient's room: a dark-haired woman in her thirties, lying in the bed, who, from the size of her abdomen, looked much farther along than twenty-two weeks; a man about the same age in a red flannel shirt, sitting beside her and holding her hand; and an older woman who would be a grandmother very soon—and a bereaved one for the rest of her life—weeping in the corner.

I started off by trying to build rapport with Tom and Mary, as I'll call them, by empathizing with the impossible situation they found themselves in and building rapport by asking them a little bit about themselves, like where they lived and worked. Their replies were factual and polite—no other children, stable jobs—up until I inquired about the babies' names. Mary and Tom looked at each other and paused before responding, leading me to wonder if they'd even decided yet. When they'd woken up that morning, they'd thought they had months left to choose.

Or maybe no one else had asked. We all knew these babies weren't going to survive, so getting to know them better would just make it hurt more later.

After a moment, Mary recited the names so precisely that there could be no mistake: "Thomas. Amelia. Ethan."

When she didn't say anything more, it felt like she was waiting for the reassurance that no one else had given her and that I couldn't, either.

"What have the doctors told you," I asked, "about the situation?"

At that point, Mary started crying, too, so Tom spoke for both of them. Everything he said was accurate: the gestational age, the ruptured membranes, the unstoppable labor.

"But I just wonder," he said, "if there could be some mistake."

"You mean about the dates?"

After he nodded, I talked about the early ultrasound and the estimated fetal weights, each well under one pound.

"I wish we were wrong," I said as he nodded again, slower this time. "And I imagine my colleagues have talked about the probabilities."

There's an online database used to determine the percentage likelihood of survival based on gestational age. The only problem is that it only goes down to twenty-three weeks, but I was pretty sure what the number would be for twenty-two-week triplets: zero.

"I've been doing some research on the web," Tom said, "and I found reports of babies this young making it."

I suspected that any twenty-two-weekers who survived were singletons who'd gotten a full course of steroids, but I was a father, too. I owed it to him to be certain, if only to spare him and his wife the doubt that might come later.

"Let me check on that for you," I said.

#

The labor and delivery conference room was standing-room-only with three times the usual number of doctors and nurses. After confirming with the obstetrician that the resident's report was accurate, I sought out the senior neonatologist.

"No way," he said, when I asked if the kids had any chance of survival. "And we've all told the parents that."

"But you're still going to try?"

"They're fully informed," the neonatologist said with a hint of resignation, "and it's what they want."

I looked at the other people in the room; they knew the numbers as well as I did. They all had somber looks on their faces, realizing what we were about to do and just as surely what the result was going to be. None of us, though, could bear to say no to parents who'd done nothing to deserve this terrible situation, which explained why we were all gathered there while the family grieved alone.

At that point, an ethicist's work would have been done. The parents understood the treatment options and their likely outcomes, and the clinicians were aware of their professional obligations. There's no ethical dilemma when parents accept a treatment that the medical staff is willing to provide, no matter how poor the likely outcome may be.

But the team hadn't specifically asked for an ethics consult. They'd called me, and I'd asked, "How can I help?" With Tom and Mary desperately clinging to hope and a roomful of dedicated medical professionals standing by to enter into an unwinnable battle, there had to be more that I could do. I thought back to all the palliative care books I'd read with their lists of what to say and what not to. Once again, I was struck by how different the pediatric version is than the adult. The basic components may be the same—goal-setting, psychosocial support, and symptom management—and every death a cause for sadness, but at least in adult palliative care, you can try to extract a sense of meaning. Approaches like "life review" and dignity therapy can help adults appreciate all the things they've accomplished and hopefully come to peace with the approaching end.

That's not relevant, though, in pediatric palliative care, where patients are cheated out of so many foundational experiences—graduation, marriage, parenthood, professional opportunity—that there's precious little life to review. When patients may never even make it out of the delivery room, you need to sit with the injustice for a much longer time, rather than trying to move past it to establish a treatment plan.

So I returned to Mary's room, more because I'd promised I would than because I knew what to do or say. The creases around Tom's eyes had deepened, almost as if he'd aged in the past few minutes in a desperate attempt to accelerate time so that his children would be old enough to survive.

"So you're sure there's no chance they'll make it," he said as I sat down in what had been Mary's mother's chair before she couldn't take it anymore and had to step out. "Not even one of them."

"I'm so sorry, Tom."

He stared straight ahead, as if he could peer through me and into the operating room across the hall. As if he could see what the future held, and he wasn't about to turn away.

"But if we don't try . . ." Mary began.

"We'll keep them comfortable," I said, using another phrase the textbooks recommend, which after a few years of practicing palliative care was starting to come naturally. "I can promise you that."

She kept going as if I hadn't said anything. "They won't have any chance at all."

All parents have to let their children go someday, but it should be decades down the road after we've taught them all we know. And we should be the ones to leave, not them. I couldn't explain why my three kids were safe at home and, hopefully, had many years ahead of them while Tom and Mary's only had a little while left.

"That's right," I said, realizing I'd probably say the same thing as Mary if the roles were reversed.

The three of us sat in a heavy silence. Tom and Mary already knew the numbers conveniently collected in an online database, and they'd heard all our empathic statements. They needed something else.

"I would give anything to change things," I said, leaning forward with my elbows on my knees, "but no matter what we do, your babies are going to die. And if we stick with the current plan, as soon as they're born, they're going to have tubes put in their throats and IVs placed in their belly buttons, and then they're going to be whisked off to the NICU. They might survive for a few hours or even days but not longer than that."

I'm pretty sure Tom and Mary were crying, and I know I was. Up to that point, I'd just described the situation a little more boldly than I had before, like by using the "D-word." They'd heard it all before, though. The feeling in the room hadn't changed.

In that moment, I was struck by how, for all our emphasis on "reframing"—shifting from negative descriptions of what we think should be withheld (like CPR) to positive descriptions of what we hope to provide (like comfort and dignity)—words often remain so generic as to be meaningless, especially when compared to the tangible reality of three tiny babies about to be born.

That's when I uttered words that didn't come from any textbook. I'd never said them before. I hadn't even thought of them, truth be told. It was almost like someone was cuing me from offstage, prompting me with words that were not my own.

"If we try to resuscitate your babies," I said, "they're going to die in an incubator in the NICU. But if we focus on comfort, you'll be able to hold them for their entire lives."

I don't remember what we said after that, but it wasn't much. It probably involved some combination of silence and nodding and a promise from Tom and Mary to consider everything we'd talked about.

What I do remember is that the room felt different. It was as if that one phrase—"Hold them for their entire lives"—had turned around the terrible question Tom and Mary were wrestling with, allowing them to see it in a whole new light. It tapped into a primal urge to protect your children at whatever cost, through any sacrifice. Their children were yet to be born, but Tom and Mary were already parents, and no matter what they decided and no matter how long their babies lived, the only certain thing was that they loved their children and would do anything to keep them safe.

Tom and Mary had always known there was something to be gained by resuscitating: the slimmest chance at life for their babies and reassurance for themselves that they never gave up. But now they saw that there was something to lose, too.

Out in the hallway, I passed the three neonatal teams as they strode purposefully toward the OR, where the resuscitation tables were prepared. Soon Mary, whose contractions were getting stronger and closer together, would be wheeled in.

It would take time, though, to deliver three babies, even more to insert breathing tubes and umbilical catheters and transfer the triplets to the NICU. Once we started down the path of intensive treatment, it didn't make sense to consider changing course until we had relevant data like blood tests and X-rays, the results of which wouldn't come back until morning.

At that moment, I had an overwhelming need to see my own three kids, who suddenly seemed incredibly fragile. I knew that I could return immediately to the hospital if called, but before leaving, I—in a hopeful and surely pointless action—clipped comfort care order sheets to the front of the three waiting charts, waiting to be signed if the parents changed their minds.

Everybody was asleep by the time I got home. I nuked the bowl of stew my wife had left in the fridge without bothering to stir it halfway through, which meant it was scalding on top but cold in the middle. Even though I wasn't particularly hungry, I still ate it all, not wanting to hurt her feelings. I knew she'd ask me when I slipped under the covers how things had gone at the hospital and that I'd answer in generalities. No names, few details. Less out of concern for confidentiality than because she didn't need to be reminded of all the things that can go wrong in the world.

I was just turning off the kitchen lights when my pager went off again.

"Change of plan," said the same resident who'd paged me before. "The parents say they just want comfort care."

Normally I would have commented on her use of "just," which seemed to suggest that comfort care was easy or somehow deficient. (I often say that palliative care can be just as intensive as ICU care, just with a goal of comfort rather than prolonging life.) But not that night, not after all she and the team had gone through. I simply took a deep breath and thanked her for letting me know.

Before going to bed, I made my usual rounds, only this time, instead of standing at the threshold, I stepped inside each room and kissed each of my three kids on their forehead. They didn't stir, and I doubted they'd remember in the morning. But I still treasure the memory of holding them safe and close when not every loving parent has that chance.

Tom and Mary's babies were born around the time I closed the last bedroom door. They were dried and warmed and cuddled. There were no catheters or tubes or chest compressions. They lived for twenty-three, thirty-one, and forty-two minutes, respectively, a precious instant on what should have been a long journey. I never asked which of those times belonged to Thomas, Amelia, and Ethan because it didn't really matter. I only knew that their mom and dad held each of them for their entire lives.

Chapter 5

When the "right" answer isn't

Some of the stories in this book might seem so unbelievable that if you came across them in a novel, you probably wouldn't keep reading.

"That could never happen!" you'd think.

Benjamin's is another such story, except you need to understand the ethical and cultural context to appreciate just how remarkable it was. Despite his never having said a word—and my not even meeting his family—he made a huge impact on my life by calling into question things I'd always taken for granted. And by helping me see how I hadn't just added a dash of palliative care to my ethics work, I was beginning to leave one behind for the other.

— Benjamin —

Still sore from my disagreeing with him about the no trespass order for Tony's mom—and not wanting any palliative care to creep into an ethics consultation—Dr. Williamson made it crystal clear what he was calling me for this time.

"I have a straightforward ethics question for you," he said, prompting me to wonder if there even was such a thing. "I realize it's only hypothetical at this point, but I want to be ready."

I appreciated his proactive approach because most ethical conflicts could have been conversations if our department had been involved earlier. The right answer to the question of when to call an ethics consult—or a palliative care consult, for that matter—is short and sweet: the earlier, the better.

Dr. Williamson explained that a family had been involved in a head-on motor vehicle collision on the New York State Thruway, just across Lake Champlain from Vermont. The father had been driving while the mother was nursing their infant son, whom I'll call Benjamin, in the passenger seat. She had died on the scene from her injuries, while Benjamin had suffered severe head trauma and was airlifted to our hospital.

As I listened to the story, I was acutely aware of the parallels to my own life. Earlier that year, my wife had given birth to our fourth child, Charlotte, and on long road trips, she would sometimes breastfeed Charley (as we called her) in the backseat of the minivan. To be clear, Pam is even more of a stickler for car seats than I am—which is saying something, seeing as I'm a pediatrician—but she also happens to be a yoga teacher, which explains how she managed to breastfeed while Charley remained strapped in.

Dr. Williamson was concerned that, even with maximal treatment, the brain damage was so severe that Benjamin would likely be declared dead by neurological criteria (colloquially known as "brain death").

"I just want everyone around here," he said in conclusion, "to be clear that 'dead is dead,' okay?"

I didn't need to ask what he was referring to. Families often confuse brain death with coma or vegetative state, from which patients can sometimes recover. It's not hard to understand why. Brain-dead patients don't look much different than the living patients in the ICU: the EKG monitor traces the electrical activity of their hearts, and their chests rise and fall with each breath from the ventilator. We do so much, in fact, for critically ill patients—breathing for them, dialyzing their blood when the kidneys can't filter out enough toxins, even circulating blood through their body when their hearts no longer can—that, sometimes, it's hard to tell whether a patient is dead or alive.

But they have to be one or the other. With all due respect to Miracle Max from *The Princess Bride*—who claimed that "mostly dead is still alive," a colloquial sentiment that offers many families hope—there is no middle ground. Just like you can't be sort of pregnant, you also can't be sort of dead.

There are two ways of determining death: heart/lung and brain. You'd think heart/lung death would be straightforward because a patient who isn't breathing and whose heart isn't beating is what most people picture when they envision someone who's dead. But even that patient may not be dead, at least not yet. For death to be declared, failure of the heart and lungs has to be irreversible. A patient in cardiac arrest who is successfully resuscitated was never dead in the first place, or else the "R" in CPR would have to stand for "resurrection."

Death by neurological criteria is even trickier to determine. The concept had been batted about for a while—previously going by other names like "irreversible coma"—until 1968, when a committee at Harvard coined the term "brain death." In 1981, the Uniform Determination of Death Act (UDDA) established the standard definition: irreversible cessation of function of the entire brain, including the brain stem.

A clear understanding of brain death serves two important purposes. One is clarifying professional obligations toward a patient whose entire brain has permanently stopped functioning. Up until that point, goals of treatment might include prolonging life, minimizing suffering, and respecting patient autonomy. But once a patient is declared dead, medicine's obligations shift to treating the body with honor and reverence, and there's no longer any ethical obligation to provide mechanical support, even if the family requests it. That's what Dr. Williamson wanted the ethicist—the institutional expert on brain death, who taught courses on it and had written scholarly articles about it—to make sure the staff understood.

The other reason for the UDDA is that transplant waiting lists are very long. One of the fundamental ethical precepts of organ donation is the dead donor rule, which says that you're not allowed to retrieve vital organs (i.e., those necessary for survival) from living patients or else you'd be killing them. Once a patient is declared dead, though, you can retrieve the heart, liver, pancreas, and pairs of lungs and kidneys. All the better if the dead patient's heart is still beating, thus keeping those organs perfused with blood up until the moment they're removed.

But even if a patient has been declared "brain dead," there's no ethical obligation to immediately discontinue mechanical support. If the family consents to organ donation, for example, the ventilator is routinely continued to give the transplant team time to arrive. Even when organ donation isn't an option, most doctors will keep going for a little while if family members are on their way to say goodbye, so they can see the patient while he still appears to be alive.

Understandably, families have a harder time accepting declaration of death by neurological rather than heart/lung criteria, and a few state laws actually treat them differently. The most famous is New Jersey, which doesn't allow physicians to declare a patient brain dead if "such a declaration would violate the personal religious beliefs of the individual." This is largely in recognition of the fact that Orthodox Jews—who make up an active voting bloc in that state—generally believe that, as long as the heart and lungs are functioning, a patient is still alive.

The other well-known state happens to be New York, whose law is broader than New Jersey's—encompassing moral as well as religious objections—but also less demanding. While New Jersey law could preclude a declaration of death by neurological criteria, New York's law merely requires hospitals to make "reasonable accommodation of the individual's religious or moral objections to use of the brain death standard." (While the car accident took place in New York, once Benjamin was life-flighted across the state line, Vermont law took precedence.)

But beyond ethics and the law, there was a baby lying in an oversized bed in the PICU, his face badly bruised and head severely swollen. An adult patient in that condition would have required surgical removal of part of the skull to relieve pressure on the brain, but Benjamin's head was free to expand thanks to skull plates that had yet to fuse. The ventilator breathed for him, as multiple drips propped up his blood pressure and infused nutrition and hydration into his veins.

Gazing at him through the open doorway, I couldn't get over how drastically his life had changed in the blink of an eye. The day before had probably been like every other in his young life: nursed by his mother whenever he showed signs of hunger, all of his other needs—which seemed so modest in comparison to those he had now—met by his loving family, a long and healthy life in front of him. Up until the crash and the extraction and the intubation and the life-flight left him clinging to life.

No family was present, so I turned to his chart for more information. That's when things got really complex. It turned out that the family were Orthodox Jews, making any declaration of brain death more complicated, if not legally then at least ethically. Not only that, the father was a rabbi and wasn't at the hospital because he'd taken his wife's body back to Israel to sit shiva. His last exhortation before departing was: "Do everything you can for my son."

"Damn sad," Dr. Williamson said, when I stopped by his office.

"And Dad won't be back for a week?"

He nodded. "The kid'll probably be declared brain dead way before that."

I tried to imagine how Benjamin's father would react to that news. Just because we weren't in New Jersey or New York didn't mean that he'd accept that his son was—contrary to all appearances—actually dead. Understandably, physicians get concerned that parents might never accept the diagnosis. It's one thing to compassionately grant a few extra hours for a loved one to visit, but it's quite another to have no end in sight. And given the prohibition of the family's religious tradition on accepting that Benjamin was actually dead, it felt like his father's absence might be our one chance to let him go without provoking additional conflict.

The ethics department expects written recommendations to be entered into the chart within twenty-four hours of the consult being requested or whenever all relevant data is obtained. Unable to reach Benjamin's father, I had all the information I was going to get and, of all the ethical questions I get asked, this actually was one of the more straightforward. Over the years, I'd given countless lectures featuring a slide that read: "There is no ethical or legal obligation to continue mechanical ventilation of a patient declared dead by neurological criteria."

But something held me back from writing those words in Benjamin's chart. I kept hoping his father would call to check in and I'd have the chance to talk to him. Or maybe Benjamin would make a miraculous recovery, rendering the entire question moot.

There was no word from his father, though, and Benjamin's condition didn't improve. I spent utterly unproductive time standing on the precipice of his hospital room, trying to convince myself that he'd moved an arm or leg or even just one finger. Yet he remained perfectly still, save for the rise and fall of his chest, in such perfect rhythm that it clearly wasn't part of the natural world but rather the result of the hulking machine at his bedside.

When my office phone rang the next day, I instantly knew who was calling.

"I don't see an ethics note in the chart," Dr. Williamson said, without bothering with a "How are you?" or even just a "Hello."

"How's Benjamin doing?"

"The same. We're just holding off on the brain death exam until we're on solid ground proceeding."

He didn't need to spell it out for me: Don't do a test unless it's going to change management. And for Benjamin, that test was a formal brain death examination, which included temporarily stopping the ventilator and monitoring his response to falling oxygen and rising carbon dioxide levels. If he made no attempt whatsoever to breathe, brain death would be confirmed. The change in management would be removing his breathing tube, leading to a lack of oxygen that would cause his heart to stop. Then there wouldn't be any more debate about whether he was dead.

"His dad will be back in a few days, right?" I asked.

"So he said, but anything could happen."

"You're not considering waiting for him?"

It was more of a statement than a question, but I would have been fine if Dr. Williamson had disagreed.

"He's not going to get the kid's brain working again," Dr. Williamson muttered.

It would have been so easy to just say, "Okay, go ahead." There was plenty of ethical precedent to fall back on, and it wasn't as if Dr. Williamson technically needed my approval since he was the attending physician, and I was just a consultant. It would look bad, though, if "ethics wasn't on board," especially if this ever got ugly, either in the newspapers or in the courts.

Instead, I said, "Are you in your office? I'd love to talk in person."

One reason for the in-person conversation was that whereas medical school teaches you that "dead is dead"—regardless of which criteria are applied—but the bioethics community isn't quite that certain. Some critics question whether brain-dead patients are actually dead since the legal definition requires that the entire brain no longer be functioning. But even patients who have been declared dead by neurological criteria maintain some hormonal function, which is stimulated by the pituitary gland and the hypothalamus, both parts of the brain. So how can a brain-dead teenage girl enter puberty?

Others take the polar opposite position, arguing that the entire brain doesn't need to stop functioning for a patient to be declared dead. If you think about it, everybody's brain stem is pretty much the same: it takes care of autonomic (i.e., unconscious or unintended) functions like blinking when something touches the surface of your eye or gagging when something tickles the back of your throat. What makes a person unique is the cerebral hemispheres, where memory and emotion reside. So if both hemispheres are beyond repair, why claim a patient is alive solely on the basis of a tiny bit of thoughtlessly functioning neural tissue in their brain stem?

Such a higher brain criteria for brain death would certainly increase the number of organs available for transplant, but it's a slippery slope. Pretty soon, we could be deeming patients with profound dementia—so severe they can't recognize their family or eat or even form words—not just severely ill but dead. It's worth noting that, in addition to sometimes retrieving their organs, there's one other thing we do to people after they die: we bury them. Patients whose brain stems are still working could conceivably breathe on their own, and are we really ready to bury people who are still breathing because we're pretty darn sure they're actually dead, contrary to all appearances? If so, we might need to bring back so-called "safety coffins," eighteenth-century devices with ventilation pipes and signaling devices for emergency use in case of premature burial.

"I'm not sure what we should do," I said once I reached Dr. Williamson's office, although academic debates didn't feel like the only reason.

"It seems pretty obvious to me," he replied.

I nodded. Over the last four decades—out of concern for thousands of patients waiting for an organ transplant and wanting to spare families the terrible decision of whether to remove a loved one with no brain function from a ventilator—brain death had become almost a litmus test of medical orthodoxy.

"We don't ventilate cadavers here," Dr. Williamson said through gritted teeth.

It was a pithy argument; I had to give him that. But I couldn't bring myself to apply the word "cadaver" to the bruised baby whose heart still beat and chest rose and fell, even if machines were doing all the work. I wasn't sure whether he was alive or dead. I just knew that while his father was half a world away, grieving his wife, praying for his son, it felt wrong to stop those machines.

Felt wrong. Definitely not the language of an ethicist guided by principles and rational argument.

"Couldn't we just wait a little while longer?" I asked.

"For what, exactly?"

"For the dad to come back," I said softly.

"So he can just tell us to never stop?"

I wanted to argue with Dr. Williamson, but I had no idea what Benjamin's dad would say. I'd never even talked to him.

"So I'm supposed to just keep the vent going," Dr. Williamson said sarcastically, "for him and every patient like him."

He had a point. Justice is one of the four core principles of bioethics, demanding that we "treat like patients alike." So if we'd withdrawn the ventilator from other brain-dead patients in the past, we should do the same for Benjamin.

But at that moment, precedent—so revered by ethicists—didn't seem that important anymore, at least compared to a little boy lying motionless in an oversized bed. Sure, the fact that his father's faith was often associated with the rejection of brain death increased the possibility of an impasse, but shouldn't we at least give him a chance to listen to what we had to say and reach his own conclusion? Not to do so would be to assume that he fit our preconception of what an Orthodox rabbi would do or believe, which doesn't always turn out to be true. I knew that from personal experience: when I applied to medical school, one of my interviewers—noting my master's degree in theology—asked me if I planned to use medicine as an "evangelistic tool." His question was as offensive as it was misinformed since pretty much the only thing the Episcopal church I attended had in common with evangelicalism was the letter "E" at the start of their names.

Even if we were treating Benjamin differently from previous patients who'd had their ventilators disconnected, that didn't necessarily mean we were doing something wrong. Maybe the circumstances in this case were unique such that the precedent didn't apply to Benjamin. Or maybe those other patients should have gotten different treatment, like the kind we were considering now.

And the patients who would follow him? Even forgetting the New York complication, realistically speaking, how many babies of Orthodox Jewish rabbis were going to show up at our PICU, teetering on the cusp of brain death? But should one arrive at our hospital, we would deal with them with integrity and reflection, drawing on the lessons we'd learned from Benjamin's care to do even better—although perhaps not the same thing—next time.

This was yet another example of how, in the years since I'd started the PACT team, my approach to the hardest problems had shifted.

Whereas once I'd analyzed them through an ethical lens by focusing on rights, precedent, and fairness, I was increasingly aware of the importance of feelings and relationships in making heartbreaking decisions. Usually those approaches are complementary—adding heart to head, if you will—but with Benjamin, they were pulling me in different directions.

Dr. Williamson had made it crystal clear that he wanted an ethics consult, but my black-and-white striped referee jersey no longer seemed to fit. I found myself unable to quiet the more palliative voice inside me—which recognized that sometimes the supposedly right answer doesn't feel right at all—or to give him what he was looking for.

#

Over the next few days, and with rising levels of indignation, Dr. Williamson made a lot of excellent arguments in favor of proceeding with brain death testing, like the moral distress of the staff, especially the nurses. While doctors flitted in and out of various hospital rooms over the course of the day, ICU nurses usually took care of only one patient. For twelve hours at a time, they had no escape from the tragedy of a baby whose lungs and heart were propped up by machines and who might actually be dead if only we had checked.

If Benjamin really was dead, so many things that had once been obvious no longer would be. For instance, we turn unconscious patients every two hours in order to prevent bedsores because bedsores can cause infection which may lead to death. Dead patients aren't at risk of dying, though, because they've already died. Even basic comfort measures like giving morphine before painful procedures no longer make sense because dead patients can't feel pain.

I understood Dr. Williamson's position, even if comments like, "We don't ventilate cadavers here," could have been phrased differently. I was trying to be compassionate to Benjamin's father, but sometimes you "must be cruel, only to be kind," as Hamlet observed. However awful it would be for him to return to find that his son had died, perhaps it would be worse to be asked for permission to let Benjamin go, in violation of every paternal instinct and possibly religious obligation. Maybe, on some level, he'd be grateful that the doctors had done what they thought was best, sparing him a decision that I could scarcely comprehend, let alone make.

But I just couldn't bear the thought of him returning from mourning his wife to find some other patient in the room where he expected to find his son. I was a father, too, and I could at least try to imagine how I'd feel if Pam died and the doctors were worried that Charley might, too. Returning from Pam's memorial, I'd race to the ICU to check on Charley, and if she wasn't there, I'd probably assume I'd gotten the room number wrong and check the ones on either side. Not finding her there, either, I would become desperate, beseeching everyone nearby to tell me where she could be. Only when I ran out of places to look would it truly begin to sink in that my baby was gone and that the doctors had let her go while I was away.

Lorraine was able to rest her forehead on her son Nicky's, surrounded by family and friends as the ventilator went silent. Daniel and Miriam were blessed to welcome Lily into the world for those few precious minutes. Tom and Mary got to hold their triplets for their entire lives. But if we removed Benjamin's breathing tube, his father would never get the chance to hold his child as the ventilator provided one last breath.

I can't be absolutely sure—because I've never been in that position myself—but I think I would have wanted to see Charley again. I would have wanted to hold her hand and tell her I loved her, no matter that the doctors said there was no way she could hear me. Even if they were right about her being brain dead, my child still would seem alive to me, and we'd have had those final, precious moments together.

That was the moment I realized that my perspective hadn't just transitioned from that of an ethicist to that of a palliative care doc; I was responding as a father. A fellow cleric with a child the same age, this rabbi whose name I don't recall—if I ever knew it in the first place—seemed like kindred. Even though he was on the other side of the world, his pain felt immediate and raw. I'd companioned many parents who were about to lose their child, but this man was on the verge of losing his entire family.

Many people think pediatrics is only about kids. And, yes, patients should definitely be our primary concern with the parents expected to act in their child's best interest. But at some point, the focus begins to shift slightly. There are times when a child is beyond suffering—brain death being the ultimate example—and the well-being of the family becomes a more significant consideration. They're the ones who will have to live on, after all, with the memories and the grief.

If Benjamin really was brain dead, he'd never again feel pain. But his father still could.

#

The pressure to make a decision grew with each passing day as Dr. Williamson's feelings for me transitioned from anger to betrayal, as if he suspected (rightly) that I'd shifted my allegiance from the physicians (who acknowledged brain death and its impact on our legal obligations) to the family. Both were worthy perspectives, and without the other as counterbalance, each could lead to harmful extremes: either a return to the paternalism of the past—when physicians made decisions based solely on what they thought was right—or forcing children to endure disproportionately burdensome treatments based on the parents' unrealistic expectations. It wasn't uncommon for physicians to come down in slightly different places when trying to find the proper balance, but the chasm between Dr. Williamson and me seemed vast.

Then, just as he was getting ready to proceed with brain death testing even without having ethics "on board," something remarkable happened: Benjamin's eyelid seemed to flutter. At first I didn't dare get my hopes up. Sometimes you see what you want to see, and I'd been fooled before.

Not long after, though, the monitors detected the tiniest hint of spontaneous respiratory effort. So small that it was invisible to the naked eye, so I couldn't have imagined it. He was alive in there.

Suddenly, nobody was talking about a brain death exam anymore.

Some patients get a little better after a head injury, which isn't always a blessing. To still be incredibly limited—but now be able to appreciate yourself just how limited—is not a fate everyone prefers. Some have even called a state of profound impairment "worse than death."

Benjamin didn't stop at mild improvement, though. Over the next few days, he regained movement of his entire body and relied on the ventilator less and less, until he didn't even need it anymore. Sometimes it helps to be a baby whose skull plates are free to stretch and flex only to fall back into perfect alignment when the brain shrinks back to where it started.

My greatest fear had been that his father would return to find a stranger in what used to be Benjamin's room, and the most I'd dared hope for was that Benjamin would still be there, only apparently alive. But he left that tender hope in the dust by being awake and alert, sucking on a bottle, and staring curiously at the now-silent hulking machines when his father, fresh off the plane from Israel, walked into his room. With no ethical dilemma left to resolve—or anything to palliate—I didn't even introduce myself to him. There was no point in even mentioning the tense debate over what would have happened if Benjamin had progressed to brain death, because he never did.

That was a purely academic question anyway because, let's be clear, it's not like I saved his life. If we had gone ahead and done a formal brain death examination, it would just have shown that he was still alive—which subsequently became obvious—and we would never have considered removing the ventilator.

In an ICU where kids like Nicky die despite the highest quality care, and many survivors face limited life expectancy or significant disability, a kid like Benjamin—who looked like he was going to die (or might already have) but ultimately makes a full recovery—is cause for celebration. So there was quite a party when his father proudly carried him out of the PICU, flanked on either side by rows of cheering nurses and doctors, and into the winter sunshine.

Yet for all the joy and relief that day, this wasn't a happily ever after ending to their story. Benjamin had lost a mother, after all, and his father had lost a wife. But Benjamin did have a long life still ahead of him, which is happier than many endings in palliative care.

I thought Benjamin's discharge would be the end of the story, but Dr. Williamson wasn't about to risk a repeat of the brain-death-exam-that-never-was. So he invited—although given his seniority, attendance might not have been entirely optional—the directors of all the other ICUs in the hospital to a debriefing. The only other person on the guest list was me.

It might simply have been the only space available, but the imposing conference room—with a twenty-foot mahogany table and portraits of past chiefs of surgery hanging on the walls—felt intimidating. Forgoing any open-ended questions about individuals' opinions, Dr. Williamson dived right in and summarized our professional obligations in succinct terms.

"Dead is dead. We don't ventilate cadavers in this hospital. Once brain death is confirmed, the ventilator is disconnected. No ifs, ands, or buts. And no waiting around."

Not bothering to explain what (or who) shouldn't be waited around for, he scanned the room, hoping for clear affirmation but willing to take silence as agreement. Outnumbered and still bruised by his judgment in Benjamin's case, I kept mum. A few seconds passed without anyone responding, and it felt as if this might be the shortest meeting in human history. As if everything that needed to be said already had been.

But then the head of the Medical ICU said, "Well, unless there's family on the way. They might need some time."

Dr. Williamson paused as if considering whether to argue or make a modest concession. He opted for the latter. "How long are you talking about?"

"A few hours," the MICU director said.

"Like four?"

The MICU director was nodding when the Surgical ICU director said, "It could be longer if they have to travel a long way."

"Just how much longer?" Dr. Williamson demanded.

The SICU director shrugged. "I don't know. Twelve hours? Maybe as much as twenty-four, I suppose, in special circumstances."

Dr. Williamson's voice rose a couple of decibels. "Special circumstances?"

He seemed ready to go at it when the Trauma ICU director, the elder statesman of the group, muttered so softly it was like he was afraid someone else might overhear, "I'm not sure I really believe in brain death."

Mic drop.

"It didn't even exist back when I was in medical school," the TICU director explained apologetically as Dr. Williamson gaped at him. This amounted to medical heresy; heck, even the rogue ethicist acknowledged that brain death was real. I'd merely advocated that we not remove the ventilator the precise moment it was declared.

I really tried not to smile. After all, it wasn't like anybody had said I was right to advocate for continued support for Benjamin. The other ICU directors had merely confirmed that questions aren't always as straightforward as we wish they were and that the answers aren't as obvious as they once seemed to be.

I never found out whether they thought Benjamin's case qualified as "special circumstances" because Dr. Williamson abruptly adjourned the meeting, which had fallen far short of what he'd hoped to achieve.

I left the imposing conference room with renewed appreciation for how dedicated physicians can profoundly disagree. Even though we were all looking at the same important issues—a child's tenuous life, a parent's excruciating decision making, the moral distress of staff—we balanced them differently and reached distinct conclusions. I hoped that, as tempers cooled, we would all look back on our discussion with a sense of humility, hopefully having learned from one another and remaining open to new perspectives.

Unfortunately, if there's one thing that every palliative care physician knows all too well, we don't always get what we hope for.

CHAPTER 6

The finite miracle of modern medicine

— Grace —

Hunched over and with thinning hair from years of chemotherapy, Grace reminded me of a wizened elder, only without the wrinkles. She was fifteen years old when I met her, already well into her journey with cancer. Neuroblastoma, to be specific, which, in a word, sucks. That may not be the most eloquent description, but it's accurate. For all the amazing success stories about childhood cancer—some forms of which have gone from uniformly fatal to eminently curable in recent decades—neuroblastoma is still incredibly hard to treat and can cause intense pain, especially when it metastasizes to bones. It's so bad, in fact, that at various points it's topped the charts of "My Most Hated Disease."

Many patients with neuroblastoma don't live long enough to even have what you might call a "journey," but with the help of her dedicated pediatric oncology team, Grace soldiered on. When one kind of chemotherapy stopped working, they always managed to find another that did. There was a lot of pain along the way, though, requiring extended hospital stays and even stronger opioids than morphine, like Dilaudid.*

Hospital days can be long and boring, often with the only reprieve coming from silly and creative activities devised by child life specialists. After checking on Grace's pain and modifying her regimen appropriately, she and I might pass the time by watching Buddy Valastro create a four-hundred-pound cake in the shape of Wrigley Field on *The Cake Boss* or by playing cards. Rest assured that she didn't go easy on me, her normally pallid complexion—thanks to the persistent anemia—lighting up when she won.

I probably would have gotten in trouble if my boss found out I was spending work time on such non-billable activities, but I never viewed them as a waste of time. The way I figure it, if all palliative care does is have tough conversations and break bad news, and I were a patient and saw the palliative team walking toward me, I'd run/scurry/wheel myself—even crawl if necessary—in the opposite direction. Anything to avoid having to go through *that* again.

Some palliative care folks would call playing cards and watching TV "filling the rapport bucket," a strategy that allows you to cash in good will when heavy discussions are necessary. That's always felt a little transactional to me, though, as if we only give patients what they need now so they'll do what we want later. The reason I spent time with Grace (as I had long before with Hannah) wasn't to fill some work-related bucket but because I genuinely enjoyed her company.

Despite her frequent hospital stays, Grace remained a valued member of her high school class, especially on stage. I was fortunate to see some of her plays, sometimes dragging med students or residents with me long after they should have been allowed to call it a day. Speaking as someone who participated in drama long ago and then only under extreme peer pressure, I figured she'd be nervous performing in front of so many people. Toss in missed rehearsals for

---

* By convention, generic drug names (like morphine) aren't capitalized, while brand names (like Dilaudid, the most commonly used version of hydromorphone) are.

unexpected hospitalizations and side effects of medications; I'd have scarcely been functional if I were her.

Yet she seemed at home on stage with a quick wit and a sly sense of humor. Often cast as younger characters—prolonged chemotherapy forces downward revisions of projected height—Grace had a presence. It was as if all the trials and tribulations that came before were worth it precisely because of that one moment when she had a chance to put her stamp on a part, daring to forget, if only for a few precious seconds, that she was a cancer patient and that her kind of cancer was just as stubborn as she was.

"So what do we try next?" she asked one afternoon in the clinic after her oncologist had told her what she already knew: the current therapy was no longer working. By that point, the metastases in her spine had become so painful that she was forced to use a wheelchair.

"I'm sorry, Grace," he replied, the pain audible in his voice. He was known throughout the hospital for always wearing a baseball cap except when he had to break bad news.

"There's got to be something more," she said, which was understandable since, up to that point, there had always been something more. Diagnosed in elementary school and given only a few years to live, somehow she'd made it to the end of her junior year of high school.

He brushed back the hair on his bare head. "I'm afraid we've tried it all."

That's why the trip to Europe was so important. Her whole class was going, the first opportunity many of those kids would have to see another part of the world, but this would be Grace's only chance. Her teachers were ready to do whatever it took—wheel her around, even taking extra staff to help—as long as the doctors cleared her.

Recognizing how high the stakes were, we explored every possible option: sending opioids with her on the plane (which isn't simple given the high doses she required), identifying hospitals in the cities the class would be visiting in case she got worse, formulating an evacuation plan if everything went to hell. In our hearts, we were desperate to help Grace get there, but our heads ultimately prevailed. If her wheelchair rolling over the smallest bump sent shock waves up her spine, the cobblestoned streets of medieval villages would be excruciating. No matter how hard it would be to tell Grace that the trip wouldn't be possible, allowing her to go would lead to even more pain.

In palliative care, we're taught to "fire a warning shot" before giving bad news so the patient has an inkling that something big and bad is coming. This time, though, the warning shot seemed to go straight through Grace's heart. She'd been holding on for this trip, the kind of dramatic last hurrah that would have been so Grace. And now we were taking that away, too.

I wasn't surprised when her pain immediately spiked. There's a concept in palliative care called "total pain," which refers to the fact that your heart, soul, mind, and circumstances have a role in suffering, not just your body. I sometimes give a glib example: if the sun's shining and you just aced a test and the person you like feels the same way about you, you probably won't even notice if you stub your toe. But if it's cold and rainy and you flunked that test and your significant other just dumped you, a stubbed toe will hurt like hell.

Grace had plenty of physical reasons to feel pain—infinitely more than a stubbed toe—and now she had a big soulful one, too. The problem is that it's hard to tease out how much of a patient's suffering comes from each source because when you ask someone to rate their pain on a scale of zero to ten, you only get one number. That day, Grace would probably have rated her pain a twenty if that had been an option.

Instead of going home from the oncology clinic, she went straight to the pediatric floor in a full-blown pain crisis. Standard practice is to use oral pain meds as long as a patient is able to swallow and isn't vomiting. There are two big reasons for that. The first is that oral meds take effect a little more gradually, causing less of a "high" that can contribute, if not to addiction, to prolonged courses of pain meds in order to recreate that high. The other is that most patients don't leave the hospital with an IV, so the quicker their pain can be controlled with oral meds, the sooner they can go home. That was my reasoning for ordering oral Dilaudid.

"But I'm in a lot of pain!" she said to me, tears welling up.

"And we're going to help you with that," I replied.

"You always said that I know my body best."

She was right. We'd talked a lot over cards, including me paraphrasing one of the famous sayings in palliative care: "Pain is whatever the experiencing person says it is, existing whenever the experiencing person says it does."

"And you do," I said.

"So why won't you give me what I need?"

"I think starting with oral meds is the best plan."

"But they'll take longer!"

"They'll start working soon. I promise."

Everything in me just wanted to give her what she was asking for since she was getting precious little of what she dreamed of—and deserved—in life. I'd done that before, truth be told, at other times when things weren't going well and her pain took over. Sometimes it felt like writing, "1 mg IV Dilaudid now," in the chart was another way of saying, "I care about you," in the only language that Grace could understand at that moment.

This time felt different, though, because it wasn't just a bump in the road; it was the end of the journey. Intravenous Dilaudid would just knock her out—which is probably what she was asking for—and when she woke up, the pain would still be there.

She stared at me, and I wish I could forget the look of abandonment in her eyes. "Why won't you help me?"

"Because Dilaudid can't cure a broken heart."

In my memory, the conversation stopped there. There may have been a couple more back-and-forths, some further attempt on her part at negotiation and compromise. Whenever the conversation did finally end, it wasn't because she'd recognized the truth of what I'd said. She'd just realized that I was also as stubborn as she was, and it was time to wait for the oral medications to take effect. Then, ever so briefly, she wouldn't have to think about shattered dreams.

— Pediatric hospice waiver —

By that point, I'd been practicing palliative care for a few years, and I'd seen the many hurdles that patients like Grace and their families were forced to overcome: complex symptom management, inscrutable bureaucracies, nowhere to turn for help. A big reason was that hospice—which is an incredible blessing to patients approaching the end of life—is designed for adults, not kids. Originally implemented in 1982, the Medicare Hospice Benefit funds exquisite interdisciplinary care if you have less than six months left to live, as long as you agree to forgo life-prolonging treatment. That might make sense for an elderly patient who is clearly dying, but it leaves parents of seriously ill children with a terrible choice: either get amazing hospice care at home or try a last-ditch treatment that might just save your child's life. You couldn't have both.

The Affordable Care Act (a.k.a. Obamacare) saved parents from that terrible choice by allowing children within the last six months of life to enroll in hospice while still pursuing life-prolonging—or even potentially curative—treatment. But that still didn't address the needs of seriously ill kids who either weren't in the last six months of life or might be but their doctors didn't recognize it. That occurs pretty often with doctors frequently overestimating how long patients have left to live, which is a big reason that most hospice patients die within three weeks of enrolling.

To address that deficiency, some states had passed waivers that allow them to provide an intermediate level of hospice services to kids who might not be imminently dying but still weren't expected to live into adulthood. Obtaining legislative approval for such a waiver isn't fast or easy. For example, it took California—whose advocates were highly organized and well-funded—nearly a decade, during which pilot projects were initiated, evaluated, and modified. But in a small state that has one-sixtieth the population of California, one person can make a huge difference. In Vermont's case, that person was State Representative Bill Frank, who, one day, after I'd testified about advance directives before his subcommittee, asked me what the legislature could do to help sick kids.

"Funny you should ask," I replied before explaining to him the Catch-22 that families found themselves in.

"Let me see what I can do," Bill said.

Evidently, he could do a lot, because only a few weeks later, I was testifying at the state house.

"Less than one percent of hospice patients are kids," I explained to the joint house and senate committee, specially convened to discuss the subject. "As a result, most hospices aren't comfortable taking care of kids, especially babies. But a Medicaid waiver would allow hospice workers to get more training in pediatrics so that when kids approach the end of their life, they'll get the care they need. And deserve."

"Do you think there's any way to balance the books?" one of the senators asked.

His tone was hopeful because, after all, who doesn't want to help sick kids? And the question was logical since adult hospice actually saves money by preventing costly hospital admissions. But there's a limit to how much money can be spent on hospice care for adults since only patients in the last six months of life qualify. If the pediatric waiver passed, a child could conceivably receive modified services for years.

The obvious answer to his question would be: "Yes I do, Senator." As a physician, I was expected to provide clinical perspective, not financial analysis. Heck, I was free to think anything I wanted. The legislators would have a much easier time justifying a new budget outlay to their colleagues if there was at least the possibility of budget neutrality.

"I'm not sure," I replied, wondering if I should add "honest" to my list of pathological qualities, right next to niceness.

The senator nodded somberly. I'd answered the question he'd posed, though not the one we should have been asking.

"But what does it say about us," I said slowly, my voice trembling as images flooded back to me of kids whose stories couldn't be told by statistics, like Nicky—whose mother had to fight every battle by herself—and all the others who didn't have anyone to fight for them, "and the importance we place on the lives of children facing serious illness if we'll only do something if it doesn't cost us a cent?"

As far as extemporaneous remarks go, that was a pretty good one. But my five minutes of fame were up, and it was time to let the real stars of the show take over: bereaved parents I'd invited to the hearing, some who'd lost a child in infancy, others in adolescence. For some, their grief was a fresh wound; for the rest, it was a deep and familiar ache.

One by one, they told variations of the same story: doctors and nurses and other staff who did a wonderful job caring for their child, often despite a system that wasn't made to take care of kids. They offered palpable examples of uncoordinated care, unavailable resources, uncontrolled symptoms, and undeserved frustration compounding their sorrow. Finally given a chance to make a difference for other families enduring the same experience, they didn't hold back.

When it was her turn to speak, one mother gently placed a framed senior photo of her deceased son on the witness table. Tom had died before I started practicing palliative care, so I didn't know whether his smile was a brave one in the face of a foreshortened future or an innocent one where the most pressing question was who to ask to prom. All I knew was that she handled that photo with the reverence of a holy relic.

As her voice rose in intensity, describing the final painful days of Tom's life, it felt like he was right there beside her, an innocent man at the mercy of the court with her as his defense attorney. Near the end of her testimony, she rose, cradling the sacred photo in her arms, and came around the table that separated her from the people in power. Then she "walked" her son down the row of legislators, making absolutely sure they didn't just hear a story or jot down a statistic but saw the smiling face of a young man who deserved more out of death.

The chairperson of the joint session—an experienced and tough-skinned legislator—leaned back and sighed. Initially, I feared the worst, attributing her wounded expression to her having to tell a group of bereaved parents that there just wasn't enough money in the already deficit budget to fund the waiver. But then I noticed the tears in her eyes, which is something—having on several occasions watched her calmly mediate heated testimony in her cramped committee room—I'd never imagined.

"Just tell us what you want," she said with an air of resignation.

Within two weeks, both the house and senate had added amendments to their respective healthcare bills, allotting $170,000 of Medicaid funds—on a per capita basis, equivalent to over ten million "California dollars"—for a pediatric hospice waiver. By the end of the year, our tiny state had its very own Medicaid-funded pediatric palliative care program, which over the past decade has supported hundreds of seriously ill children and their families through the hardest of times.

— Grace: Part two —

Meanwhile, Grace's cancer, now untreated, continued to spread, and with her high school class having returned from Europe, there didn't seem to be much left for her to hope for. It may seem odd to talk about hope in the context of terminal illness—especially when death is imminent—but everybody needs to hope for something. Dying can be painful and tragic, but without hope, it's even worse.

Pediatric palliative care folks talk a lot about hope because not only is it a hallowed concept, it also frames the decisions people make. Rather than asking patients—or their parents—what treatments they want or don't want, we often start with what they hope for, and we don't stop with the first thing they mention. That one's obvious: cure leading to a long and happy life. If that were a given, though, palliative care probably wouldn't be involved. And sometimes it's impossible.

So then we ask, "What else do you hope for?" It might take them a second, but they usually come up with something. We listen and explore and then ask what *else* they hope for. And we keep going like that until they run out, which may take a while. One study found that parents are able to identify an average of seven distinct hopes, not all of which are consistent with the others. Parents often start off with cure and prolonging life and seeing their child get married and have a family of their own, but they also mention comfort at the end of life and holding their child as they take their last breath. Unless we identify all those hopes, we won't know what to work toward when the ones at the top of the list can't be achieved.

Grace was plenty able to speak for herself, so we moved down her list of hopes. Cure wasn't possible, and time was limited. The Europe trip was out. Even starting her senior year—just a couple of months away—seemed unlikely. Only one thing was left on her list: Broadway.

She'd always dreamed of starring on the big stage, and just seeing the marquees for herself would be awfully cool. Easier dreamed of than done, though, given the logistical problems with getting her there. A six-hour car ride from Vermont to Manhattan would be excruciating for someone with spinal metastases. But Grace wasn't going to get any better, and if we didn't go now, it would never happen.

Enter Beth, a nursing student who took care of Grace on one of her clinical rotations. Beth lived on a farm on the New York side of Lake Champlain, complete with a grass landing strip. Each morning, while her neighbors who worked in Vermont took a ferry or drove north to the closest bridge, Beth would hop in her single-engine plane and zip over the lake to Burlington Airport, where her "jalopy" was waiting for the two-mile drive to the hospital. Even though she lived in a different state, her commute was shorter than mine.

Having heard about the Broadway dream—and clearly more creative than I—Beth managed to score not just wheelchair-accessible tickets to *Wicked* (Grace's favorite show) but a visit to the set of the *Cake Boss* just across the river in New Jersey, courtesy of Buddy Valastro himself, who, somehow, Beth had managed to get in touch with.

"But how are we even going to get her there?" I asked, still landlocked in my thinking.

"That's actually the easy part," she replied.

Evidently, when you're a pilot, a lot of your friends are pilots, too. Two worked together—Don, who had prostate cancer, and Chaz, whose wife was a palliative care nurse—and, upon hearing Grace's story, asked their boss if they could borrow the company plane for a special weekend trip to New York City. Which is how I came to be parked in front of a private hangar at Burlington Airport on a

Saturday morning. Beth was already there, along with Nicole, one of Grace's favorite nurses from the pediatric floor. (Since Beth was still in school, she wasn't permitted to administer meds without supervision.) A few minutes later, Grace and her mother, Linell, pulled up, and I wheeled Grace—whose smile lit up her blanched face—across the tarmac to the corporate jet of PC Construction.

The flight crew treated us like we were bigwigs, literally rolling out the red carpet leading up the jetway and serving delicious snacks en route. When we touched down at Teeterboro Airport, a huge black SUV was waiting for us courtesy of the Make-A-Wish Foundation (which also covered the theater tickets and hotel rooms). As I'll say several more times in this book, palliative care is a "team sport," as that unforgettable trip illustrates.

But even the short ride to *Cake Boss* headquarters set off spasms of pain in Grace's back, requiring additional pain meds, which, in turn, made her sleepy. Before getting out of the SUV, I gave her a small dose of Ritalin, which is used to counteract the sedation caused by opioids. It was a tightrope that we would walk—with comfort on one side and alertness on the other—for the rest of the weekend.

Inside, the cast was about to start shooting an episode, but Buddy called time-out to welcome Grace and introduce her to everybody on the set, most of whom he was related to in some way. He was just like on TV: warm, focused, and apt to repeat how wonderful things were and how much he loved everyone around him (as long as they didn't mess up any of his cakes). The other characters from the show were there, too—like Mauro and Lil Frankie—as were a cadre of wives and cousins who I had trouble keeping straight since they all had bleached-blond hair, wore stilettos, and appeared to have iPhones sutured to their palms.

When filming eventually resumed, it was obvious how much Grace loved watching the real-life banter and exchanges between the various characters on the show. She even got the chance to pie one of Buddy's relatives, even though the guy had to know what was coming when Buddy's kid told him that the pie Grace was holding on her lap smelled funny, so he should lean over and sniff it for himself.

I could tell she was getting tired, but every time I asked her how she was doing, she claimed to be fine. She'd waited too long for this moment to have it end early.

Finally, when it was obvious that she was really fading and not wanting to endanger the plans for the evening, we convinced her to go. Before we left, Buddy took us all back to his office where he gave her bagfuls of *Cake Boss* bling, along with his business card, which had his personal email address on it.

"You need *anything* from me," he said, "you just call. We can talk on the phone or Skype or whatever."

Some folks say stuff like that out of politeness, but I had absolutely no doubt that he meant every word.

The SUV then whisked us into Manhattan where we checked into the hotel so Grace could get some rest before the evening performance. After a light snack—going out to dinner would have used up precious energy—I gave her another half-dose of Ritalin and wheeled her down the sidewalk to the Gershwin Theater. From there, I wished her well as she and her mom, along with Beth and Nicole, melted into the crowd, searching for their seats. Make-A-Wish had generously bought four tickets, and it made sense for me to stay behind since I'd recently seen the show with my oldest daughter as a special eighth birthday present.

Never a huge *Wizard of Oz* fan—those flying monkeys scare me nearly as much today as they did when I was a kid—I'd been surprised by how much I loved *Wicked*. Yet for all the wonderful songs Catie and I heard that night, the thing that meant the most to me was her reaction. Early in Act II, it was becoming clear that the green witch, Elphaba, had simply been labeled as wicked by the despotic Wizard because she was fighting discrimination. I can still remember Catie turning to me and saying, "Does that mean that just because someone says you're bad doesn't actually mean you're bad?"

Leave it to a musical to help her grasp what I'd been trying to teach her her whole life.

And I remember crying—just as I would when I later saw the show with her younger sister and then her youngest sister—as Elphaba and the über-blond "good witch," Glinda, sang their final duet:

*I've heard it said
That people come into our lives for a reason
Bringing something we must learn*

*And we are led
To those who help us most to grow
If we let them
And we help them in return.*

Those lyrics—which I knew by heart by the time Grace saw *Wicked*, thanks to the well-worn soundtrack CD back at my house—filtered through my head as I waited outside the backstage door of the Gershwin. The show had ended a while ago, but the cast insisted on giving Grace a private tour so she could see the inner workings of a real Broadway musical. When she finally emerged, she was positively aglow. As I wheeled her down the sidewalk toward the hotel, she proudly showed me dozens of photos on her phone with cast members—like Glinda in her curly blond wig and a practically fluorescent Elphaba—kneeling beside her wheelchair so they were all on the same level, smiling ear to ear.

When you added up all that she'd done over the last twelve hours, Grace's back should have been killing her. But this was the opposite of the day she'd learned that the Europe trip was off. Back then, a broken heart had amplified the pain, but now her spirit was soaring high above whatever nerve signals might have been traveling up her spine.

As she chattered on and on about what an amazing night it had been, I was reminded of that cocktail party in Boston. Even before Dave's persistent questioning about why I went into palliative care brought on my epiphany, I'd been struck by how I'd finally found "my people." That night in New York, it felt like Grace was surrounded by hers.

By the time we reached the hotel, exhaustion had set in. Nicole checked on her regularly over the course of the night, giving additional Dilaudid as needed for pain and letting Grace sleep in as long as she liked. By the time she woke up, I had fresh-from-the-oven New York bagels waiting for everyone.

With the jet not scheduled to take us back to Vermont until late afternoon, we filled the morning with classic Manhattan activities like a carriage ride through Central Park. Since we didn't have access to the SUV anymore, we needed to take taxis to get around. Fortunately, quite a few New York cabs have lifts, so Grace didn't even have to get out of her wheelchair. For the few that didn't, I gingerly picked her up and gently set her down in the backseat. More than once, I wondered if my major contribution on that trip wasn't as a physician managing symptoms—since we had all of two oral medications with us, which Nicole was plenty capable of administering—but as "the muscle," transferring Grace from place to place.

After the carriage ride, I wheeled her over to FAO Schwartz, just off Central Park. Normally, she would have been entranced by the unique and amazing toys, but by that point, it was obvious that we couldn't walk the pain/sedation tightrope anymore. Grace had given her all, and it didn't feel right to give her more Ritalin when what she really needed was rest.

So, while Linell and Beth and Nicole window-shopped along Fifth Avenue, I sat on the floor in a quiet corner of FAO Schwartz next to Grace, whose head tilted to the side to rest on her shoulder. She'd rouse every once in a while, usually just long enough to glance over at me and then, reassured she wasn't alone, fall back asleep in her wheelchair. Occasionally, she'd mumble something about how great *Wicked* had been or reminisce about the clip-clop of the horse's hooves on the carriage ride. Then we'd chat for a minute or two before she drifted off again.

We didn't talk about any of the big stuff, like the fact that she was dying. That was partly because she was so drowsy and partly because we didn't need to. We'd covered those topics before, and while she might still have had things left that she needed to say, it would have felt wrong to talk about them then. It was clear to all of us (including Grace) that there was only one reason that the Cake Boss freed up an afternoon for her and the construction company loaned her the plane, but just because end-stage neuroblastoma had brought us all there didn't mean we wanted to spend extra time talking about it. We were in the most famous toy store in the world, for God's sake, surrounded by life-size teddy bears and exorbitantly priced gadgets that you didn't know existed until you realized you couldn't live without them. If there was any place on earth that Grace should have been allowed to just be a kid again, we were sitting in it.

As she dozed, I thought about how much she'd taught me. My self-doubt still lingered, the kind that had kept me from metaphorically picking up the Fisher-Price phone when Hannah came back for her check-up and led me to focus on practical things I could provide, like prescribing medication for symptoms. But on that terrible day in clinic when Grace learned that she'd never see Europe, I'd done something more personal than practical, and somehow, she hadn't hated me for not giving her what she asked for.

In New York City, my main job was to carry her to where she dreamed of going, which more creative folks than I had made possible. And you don't need a medical degree to sit next to a dying patient in drowsy silence on the floor of FAO Schwartz. You just need to be willing to open your heart, even though you know it's going to get broken real soon.

It was a quick hop back to Burlington, but Grace still needed extra Dilaudid to get through the flight. After landing, when I carried her down the steps from the plane, she groaned louder than she had before. Even though the tarmac was smoother than Manhattan sidewalks, I pushed her extra slowly toward Linell's waiting car.

Over the past couple of days, Grace and I had improvised all sorts of transfers: from the plane to the wheelchair and between the wheelchair and SUV, the horse-drawn carriage, and a bunch of taxis. This was the family car, though, so I could just ask her how she usually got in. I'll never forget her response.

"Usually you carry me," she said.

My soul calluses had always protected me from overwhelming emotion, at least temporarily. I used to be able to hold it together until the work was done and I got back home, and only then would I let myself break down. But evidently, those soul calluses weren't quite as thick as they once had been, judging from the tears that tumbled down my cheeks as I set Grace's cancer-light body down in the passenger seat.

#

I drove straight home to hug my kids. They were still young enough to erupt in jubilation upon Dad's return from an overnight trip, and it didn't take much for them to convince me to take them out to a local arcade with a stop for creemees on the way back. We grilled burgers for dinner and roasted s'mores on the lakeshore, wrapped in towels after a dip in Lake Champlain. That time of year in Vermont's high latitudes, the sun sets late and far to the north, as if it's reluctant to leave people on earth who deserve a little extra warmth after a long winter.

When I tucked each of them in that night, I didn't skip a single bedtime ritual, which, among the kids, ranged from songs to book stories to tales from my childhood and even to backrubs that never seemed to last long enough for them. The older ones asked about Grace because I'd told them about her high school drama productions that I'd attended, and they knew why I'd gone to New York. I didn't feel like that violated patient confidentiality because there wasn't any identifying data—they only knew her first name—and certainly no privileged health information, which they wouldn't have understood anyway. In a way, not sharing what Grace had come to mean to me would have felt wrong because she'd long since gone beyond just being a patient I cared for. Her story was one of such immense bravery that it deserved to be told, then to my kids, and now here.

The next morning, as I started off on a long drive to attend a distant family graduation, I had no idea that Grace was on her way to the hospital. After a fitful night in her own bed, she'd woken up vomiting and in a terrible pain crisis. Everyone in the ER knew the drill: put in an IV and start patient-controlled analgesia, which would allow her to push a button and receive an immediate dose of Dilaudid. That had always managed to get her pain under control quickly, and over the next few days, the nausea would ease, and she could be transitioned back to oral medications and then home. It had become so routine that there was no reason to consult palliative care.

That's why the resident didn't page me until later that afternoon and then mostly out of courtesy because of how much I'd been involved in Grace's care. I listened patiently as he described her condition and treatment plan, which was a carbon copy of so many previous admissions. Except, somehow, this time felt different.

"I think this could be it," I said to the resident on the phone, without needing to explain what *it* referred to. "Please take good care of her."

When I'm worried about patients, I pretty much always go in to the hospital to see them, no matter the time of day or night. But by then, I was far from Burlington, and it felt like Grace and I had said all we needed to say. She was being well cared for, and—as she liked to remind me that I'd told her many times—she knew her body best.

Looking around the room at family and old friends gathered for the graduation, I also had the sense that Grace wouldn't want me to leave. From how she described the drama community at her high school—and seeing her response to the people she met in New York—it was clear she knew how important it was to be surrounded by your people.

That night, after a festive dinner, I was on the verge of falling asleep when my pager went off again. It felt like my very own warning shot, granting me a few precious seconds to rub my eyes before dialing the number which brought news that, on some level, I already knew. Grace had died comfortably, the resident said, surrounded by her family and the devoted staff whom she'd come to love as much as they loved her, barely twenty-four hours after the corporate jet had touched down at Burlington Airport.

#

I think Grace knew how much she meant to me, from all the card games we played and episodes of the *Cake Boss* we watched, even before the New York City trip. But I'm not sure if she realized how much she taught me. My life has always been dictated by shoulds. Children should be quiet and obedient. Good should be rewarded while bad is punished, whether by the referee in the striped jersey or the ethics consultant.

But the word that kept going through my mind a week later at her memorial service, as I listened to Grace's teachers, field hockey coaches, play directors, and oncology team speak about what a remarkable person she was, was *shouldn't*. First and foremost, Grace shouldn't have gotten cancer, but given the kind she had, she also shouldn't have survived as long as she did. She shouldn't have had the chance to meet the Cake Boss and hang out with the cast of *Wicked*. (Speaking statistically here rather than morally because, seriously, who gets to do stuff like that?) When so many patients with cancer seem to fade away, gradually losing their appetite and energy and even their ability to engage with the world, she shouldn't have still been living out her dreams the day before she died. And the high school gym shouldn't have been standing room only for the memorial service of someone who missed as much class as she did.

Grace had long ago stopped caring about what should or shouldn't happen; she was too busy living what the poet Mary Oliver refers to as her "one wild and precious life." To someone like me, raised to fulfill other people's expectations as Exhibit A, that was a revelation. A glimpse of freedom and possibility, which invited me to relinquish the litany of shoulds that had long dominated my life.

Which is exactly what I did with Grace. Always before, I'd followed the palliative care textbooks' instructions while relying on my soul calluses to shelter me from overwhelming grief. But those textbooks don't tell you how to transfer a patient from wheelchair to taxi, and they definitely don't teach you how to sit quietly beside a dying kid in a toy store. I was forced to figure that out on my own, which is an incredible challenge for someone drowning in self-doubt, who learned long ago to watch what others did and emulate that because whatever came from deep inside me must be unreliable and unworthy.

I'm not sure everything I did was right. A more compassionate doctor might have ordered the IV Dilaudid if that was the only way Grace could know that we cared about her. And accompanying her on the New York City grand finale—if only as the muscle helping her get where she needed to go—could strike some as a boundary violation, treating one patient as more special than the rest.

Thankfully, Grace didn't need me to be right all the time. She forgave me for not giving her what she was sure she needed (like on the day she learned the Europe trip was off) as long as she knew I truly cared. And as long as I was willing to try again tomorrow, which I definitely was.

That was a level of, well, *grace* that I'd never experienced before. Certainly not in my Exhibit A childhood, nor in the evangelical beliefs I once harbored, where God's pardon for what I then called "sin"—and now view as a kid growing up and making some mistakes along the way—felt begrudging and in limited supply.

The cocktail party conversation with Dave might have answered the question of *why* I practice pediatric palliative care, but those card games and heartbreaking talks and silent moments with Grace in the corner of a world-famous toy store started to answer the equally important question of *how*. Not by parroting stock answers from the textbooks but by daring to trust that my heart was worth following. It wasn't infallible, to be sure, judging from the many boneheaded comments and errant predictions I would go on to make (many of which are detailed in the following pages). But it was in the right place, which—thanks to Grace—I dared to believe would be enough for my patients.

As tears filled my eyes, blurring the poster-sized photo on the gym's makeshift stage of smiling Grace, and I thought of card games and the Cake Boss and Broadway and setting her down in the passenger seat that one last time, I could practically hear Elphaba and Glinda singing the final lines of their concluding duet:

> *Because I knew you*
> *I have been changed for good.*

Thanks to remarkable patients like Grace, the calluses that had formed in response to repetitive trauma were beginning to soften and heal. I had a sense that would make me a more present and caring doctor, but I did not yet recognize the emotional toll it would take. When those floodgates open, I would soon learn, you can't close them again.

CHAPTER 7

Never, never giving you up

— Hope —

Baby Hope was born premature but not extremely so. She needed a little help breathing and a bit more to prop up her blood pressure. Her kidneys were doing just enough to avoid dialysis, and her liver function tests were only slightly abnormal. Any one of those problems, by itself, is easily treatable. But when they all happen together, the patient usually has some kind of syndrome.

Which is why the NICU team did lots of extra tests, all of which came back negative. The doctors still suspected that Hope had something, but without a definitive diagnosis, it was impossible to tell how to treat her or what the future held. All we knew for sure was that Hope wasn't getting better. So the most optimistic thing we could say was that, on some days, she was stable.

Usually, that's a good thing for a patient to be, but not in the NICU. Healthy newborns make steady progress: gaining weight, weaning off respiratory support, tolerating larger volumes of feedings, and learning how to swallow on their own. Hope was struggling with all of these.

That was understandably hard on her parents, who'd waited a long time for a baby. Spencer—a wilderness adventure-seeker who remained unfazed in situations that would have rocked anyone else's world—took new developments in stride as he pressed the team to keep searching for a diagnosis. Kate, though, latched onto any reason to hope (even a modest normalization in lab values), only to have subsequent results reveal the improvement to be ephemeral. That's why particular words, whether intended or not, held such value.*

"When you take her home—" the nurse practitioner said one morning on rounds, before describing what would need to happen for that to occur.

Not if. *When.*

Looking back with years of hindsight, Kate—whose porcelain skin is practically translucent, as if you can see what she's feeling inside—isn't sure she actually believed that. At the time, though, she clung to the word "home," describing it as the fuel that kept her going. She and Spencer weren't demanding the perfect baby, just one who could enjoy life and feel the love around her, part of which was being home together as a family.

But before we could even conceive of getting Hope there, many questions needed to be answered, including whether she was able to see since she barely responded to light. Eye exams are commonplace in the NICU, where many of the babies are at risk for a serious condition called "retinopathy of prematurity." Hope was so fragile, though, that even a normally safe procedure tipped her over the edge. She never woke up from the sedation necessary for the exam.

By that point, I'd had many lengthy conversations with Kate and Spencer. We'd talked about their hopes and fears and their intense regret that Hope's entire life had been spent as a patient. The NICU, where she'd been immediately whisked from the delivery room, was the only home she'd ever known. While other babies her age were napping in their crib in the nursery their parents had lovingly prepared for them or being pushed in a stroller through the park, Hope had been desperately clinging to life, one in a line of incubators in

---

* Honoring the family's request for privacy, the names used for Kate, Spencer, and their surviving children are pseudonyms.

the alien world of the NICU, beside dozens of other babies doing the same.

Kate and Spencer now accepted that the burdens of ongoing treatment were greater than the benefits, but they were still hoping for even a brief period of time together as a family, away from the machines and all the other patients. So they opted for comfort care, trading in blood draws, x-rays, and antibiotics for a focus on treating pain and providing emotional support to the family.

If Hope had been more stable, we could have tried to get her home. But unsure how long—or even if—she'd survive without respiratory support, we tried to create a sense of normality in the NICU. We moved her into one of the private side rooms usually reserved for breastfeeding moms, which meant Kate and Spencer, at long last, had their daughter all to themselves. They could finally see her lovely face, liberated from the nasal prongs that had forced air into her lungs and the feeding tube snaking through her nose. Bending the visitation restrictions—which usually bar siblings and grandparents from the NICU because even the common cold can be dangerous to neonates—allowed some of the other people who'd long loved Hope to finally meet her in person.

When Hope died peacefully in Kate's arms a few hours later, I thought my work was pretty much done. I'd supported Spencer and Kate through the decision-making process—offering perspective and clarification along the way as well as recommendations based on the values they'd expressed—and navigated the transition to comfort care, signing the limitation of treatment orders (like Do Not Attempt Resuscitation) and safeguarding the family's privacy. In the process, we'd cried together more than once as the conversation turned to what a beautiful baby Hope was and how much joy she'd brought to her family over the course of a few short weeks.

But as I had with Nicky, I waited to see if the family needed anything else. I wasn't sure what that might be since some parents—after their child dies—are so overwhelmed with grief that they can't wait to escape the hospital. Others, though, can't bear to say goodbye. Stroking their child's face, gently brushing the tip of her nose: those are the things that meant so much when she was alive, and even if this was a different situation—a different world, now—they would never have that opportunity again. Leaving their child behind with no plan to return would be yet another finality, which is why some other hospitals have a cuddle cot that keeps babies cool after they die, delaying the physical changes that happen after death so parents can stay as long as possible.

I wasn't surprised that Spencer and Kate couldn't bear to be separated from Hope. I figured that would mean a few more hours of me waiting in the NICU, but Kate had a different idea.

"We want to take her home," she said, having never let go of that dream. "She deserves to feel the sun on her face and see the room we made for her."

It was a totally understandable request and also one that I'd never encountered before. It seemed like it should be simple to grant, though. Weighing only three pounds, Hope wouldn't require a stretcher to get to the hospital exit or a hearse to transport her home. Her parents could just pick her up and carry her out. Most people would assume that the baby in their arms was merely sleeping.

Unfortunately, in a world of rules and regulations, things are seldom simple.

"That's not normally done," the administrator of the hospital morgue explained when I called him.

"And this isn't a normal situation," I replied, wondering if such a thing even existed in pediatric palliative care.

The administrator patiently explained that only licensed funeral home directors were allowed to transport a dead body unless you had a burial-transit permit.

"So where do we get that permit?" I asked.

"I'm not even sure if we have any around here."

The way I figured it, if the morgue didn't have them, nobody else in the hospital would. Calling the State Department of Health would take time, the one thing we didn't have since Hope's body would soon start to decompose. But I couldn't believe that, after managing to fly Grace all the way to New York City to hang out with the Cake Boss and the cast of *Wicked*, we couldn't find a way to transport Hope a few miles down the road.

Kate and Spencer briefly considered just risking it without the required paperwork since they lived so close to the hospital. Part of my job, though, is to prepare for the worst, which, in this case, would be them getting pulled over for rolling through a stop sign or having an expired registration. It wasn't difficult to imagine the police officer asking about that baby with no car seat who didn't seem to be moving. Sure, a call to the hospital would eventually sort everything out, but Kate and Spencer had been through too much already.

So I called the morgue back and, since asking politely hadn't gotten us anywhere, resorted to begging. I described Spencer and Kate's heart-wrenching journey and how much it would mean to them to have even a few minutes at home with their only child. As far as stakes go, these definitely seemed high enough to justify a little emotional manipulation.

The administrator begrudgingly agreed to dig through the file cabinets lining the walls of the morgue, sounding nothing close to optimistic. He did, however, promise to call back if he found anything, leaving us to wonder if bending the law would be our only option. A few minutes later, though, the NICU extension rang with good news: he'd unearthed a long-forgotten stash of permits.

Without even being asked, a medical student sprinted down to the morgue to retrieve one, and not long after, with a signed and completed permit in hand, Kate sneaked Hope out of the hospital under her winter coat, comparing the feeling to smuggling contraband. They emerged into a crisp, sunny day where the wind was sharp and silent. Spencer brought the car around for them, and on the way home, he came to a full stop at every stop sign as well as one Thai restaurant, because you still have to eat.

After arriving home, they dressed Hope in a lovely outfit that Kate's sister had bought for her. Then they lay down beside her in the same bed where Kate's mother had passed away, not long before Hope was born. They whispered to her and kissed her forehead, taking roughly a million photos that are now spliced together in a video that begins with Hope being born and which they watch every year on her birthday.

It wasn't the homecoming they'd dreamed of for Hope—where she would have been cured of her illnesses and had a long life to look forward to—but it was a homecoming nevertheless. And for her parents, it was sacred.

#

Doctors sometimes ask nonsense questions. Like, "How are you doing?" to a parent who lost a child. Or, "Let us know when you're ready?" after parents make the indescribably hard decision to withdraw life-sustaining treatment.

No parent is ever ready. Regardless of how exhausted they are or how crushed their spirit, the bottom line is that this is the last time they'll see the gentle curling of their child's toes or feel a tiny hand close around their finger. Doctors might classify palmar grasp as a "primitive reflex"—all spinal cord and no emotion—but parents know that any touch is better than being apart from your child, which is one way to describe the rest of your life.

That's why, in palliative care, we try to take the responsibility for when upon ourselves. We explore what needs to happen before treatment is withdrawn—loved ones getting a chance to say goodbye, perhaps a religious ritual like baptism—and then suggest a time after all that has happened. The parents are free to say no, of course, but if they agree, hopefully they won't feel like they chose the moment of their child's death.

There's usually less to worry about after the child dies, especially if that occurs in the hospital. Even the most grieving parent eventually gets exhausted and returns home, at which point we transfer the child to the morgue. In this case, though, Spencer and Kate were already home, and I knew they'd never be ready to let Hope go. I also knew we couldn't afford to wait too long, given the time we'd spent searching for the transport permit and the lack of a cuddle cot. Their image of peaceful time together as a family didn't include rigor mortis (which becomes complete within six to eight hours). It wouldn't be the first time that an attempt to give parents a semblance of control in an out-of-control world ended up making things worse.

That's when an incredibly generous, previously uninvolved person stepped in, which is not uncommon in pediatric palliative care. Maybe it's because there aren't too many things in life that tug on your heartstrings more than a child clinging to life or parents who have just lost their baby. (Just think of Representative Bill Frank who brought his colleagues together to hear the stories of bereaved parents, prompting the legislators to forget about balanced budgets and allocate the funds for a hospice Medicaid waiver.) When I'm in a metaphysical mood, I sometimes wonder if that's the universe's way of apologizing, offering a morsel of kindness to kids who got a far worse fate than they deserved.

In this case, it was the director of a local funeral home that, I knew from past experience, provided free cremation for any baby who died. I was betting that someone who thought to offer something like that might be willing to go the extra mile for a grieving family. So, before Spencer and Kate left the hospital, I'd called him and asked for an unusual favor.

"Can you go to a house in exactly four hours to pick up a body?"

"Surely can," Tom replied after I'd explained the situation.

He rang the doorbell precisely on time. Seeing the Moses basket—woven from cotton rope and usually used for babies to nap in—in his hand, Spencer and Kate didn't need to ask why he was there. As they walked back to the bedroom where Hope lay still, they experienced a new onslaught of grief, confronted by the moment they'd so long feared, when they had to say goodbye to Hope. I'd like to think that having even a little time at home as a family tempered that sadness a tiny bit.

When they returned to the front door, bearing her body, Tom already had tears in his eyes.

"Never seen a human being this small," he whispered, as he gently laid Hope in the Moses basket, which had never seemed too big for anyone before.

Tom's compassion toward Spencer and Kate didn't end there. They didn't want Hope to be cremated, but—unlike with Lily—there was no handcrafted casket waiting for her. Arriving back at the funeral home, Tom perused the model coffins (miniaturized versions designed to give potential customers a sense of the real thing) on display in the front window. They offered a wide variety of styles and wood types, but he quickly realized that aesthetics wasn't the issue. The problem was size: a standard coffin would engulf tiny Hope. It would be like she was lost in another vast, strange world.

Then it dawned on him that a model coffin would actually fit Hope perfectly. He didn't offer to sell one to Kate and Spencer, though; he just gave them the nicest one he had, free of charge.

Tom's generosity might not have been enough to even the score on a metaphysical level, but it was just one more example of an incredibly generous, previously uninvolved person going out of his way to help a family in need. And thanks to him—as well as Spencer and Kate's determination, with a dash of emotional manipulation—Hope finally made it to where she should have been all along: home.

#

The NICU is a world unto itself, where the neonatologists are understandably protective of their unique and vulnerable patients. This is why it's frequently also the last place in a children's hospital to embrace palliative care. Getting consulted on patients like Hope was, therefore, a sign of how far the PACT team had come since that first consult with Nicky. Much had been accomplished with minimal funding, including passing the hospice Medicaid waiver and holding the first pediatric palliative care summit in northern New England.

Those successes also created some challenges. The director of the larger adult palliative care program at the hospital, whom I'll call Dr. Danvers, didn't like the PACT team functioning independently. She felt that there was an economy of scale that could be achieved by incorporating pediatrics into her team. And Lord knows I would have appreciated a night off once in a while after being on call essentially 24/7/365 for the past several years.

There's a flip side to economies of scale, though. On one level, it makes sense to join forces in order to address the palliative care needs of all patients, but the number of adults who need palliative care dwarfs that of children. I worried that a combined program—which understandably focused resources on its largest group of patients—would leave children out in the cold, their needs either unaddressed or left to primarily adult clinicians who struggled to talk to kids and their parents in a way that honored their uniqueness.

Control wasn't the only source of tension with Dr. Danvers. She had done things the right way by taking a year off to complete a formal fellowship where she was constantly supervised and mentored by senior physicians. I had grandfathered in to palliative care. That meant I was learning on the job and committing a bunch of rookie mistakes along the way, such as initially overemphasizing practical assistance (like managing symptoms and formulating treatment plans) while underestimating the importance of empathic communication. If the novelist Rita Mae Brown was right in observing that "good judgment comes from experience, and experience comes from bad judgment," then let's just say I was accumulating a lot of experience.

My not having done a fellowship wasn't the only reason Dr. Danvers questioned my commitment to palliative care. She frequently reminded others that I still split time with clinical ethics, bristling at the broader recognition I'd achieved through publishing articles and delivering presentations. Why would someone who merely dabbled in palliative care (her description) be invited to serve on national committees, while people who'd dedicated their lives to the field (like herself) didn't have the opportunity to do so since they were so busy taking care of patients?

The irony wasn't lost on me after spending most of my life emulating the dutiful elder brother in the famous parable, throwing the proverbial penalty flag whenever someone reaped undeserved rewards. But now I was playing the role of the Prodigal Son, at least in Dr. Danvers's eyes. Finally being on the receiving end of judgment was a novel and decidedly unpleasant feeling.

Intimately familiar with righteous indignation, I endeavored to explain to Dr. Danvers that I'd forgone a palliative care fellowship, not because I was engaged in dissolute living like the Prodigal Son but because Vermont was the only home my kids had ever known. (The closest fellowship program was in Boston, which would have meant either uprooting my family or spending a year away from them.) I also noted that devoting only a portion of my working hours to palliative care was more a reflection of the sparse rural population—which, thankfully, didn't have enough seriously ill kids to require a full-time palliative care pediatrician—than a lack of dedication.

That explanation didn't mollify Dr. Danvers, though, and professional disagreement gradually deteriorated to personal animus. Things got so bad that when we passed each other in the hallway—which was not a rare event, given that our offices were about thirty feet apart—she would literally plow right into me. I know that's hard to believe, given that a big part of palliative care is navigating powerful emotions and relational complexity, and from what I could tell, she was quite skilled at doing that with patients. But when things hit close to home, sometimes professional skills don't translate into the personal arena.

I tried everything I could think of to improve our working relationship, from seeking counsel from trusted advisors to reading every book on workplace conflict that I could find, like *Crucial Conversations* and *Difficult Conversations*. (If there'd been one called *Difficult Crucial Conversations*, I would definitely have read that, too.) I put their advice into practice by assuming good intentions, offering to help in ways I wasn't expected to, even writing notes of encouragement. Basically, I tried to "nice" my way through conflict, reasoning that if I responded to her with kindness, there was no way she could keep treating me that way.

As noted in the last chapter, doctors are terrible at prognostication. We tend to significantly overestimate things like how long our patients have left to live or (in my case) the prospect of improvement in my relationship with Dr. Danvers. My pathological niceness—which might appear noble but really was just a form of conflict-avoidance—only served to fuel resentment as well as hallway collisions. If it's true that "what you permit, you promote," then I helped promote behaviors that would come to take a much greater toll.

— Rider —

I'm glad Tamara and Joe gave me permission to share details of their son's story because I wouldn't have been able to come up with a cooler (or more appropriate) name for him than Rider. His parents ran a motorcycle dealership, and it wasn't hard to imagine Tamara taking off her helmet and shaking out her long, curly hair. Or—given Joe's sense of honor and commitment—to imagine Rider, one day, as the sort of person who'd stand up for what's right even if it was hard or dangerous.

To Tamara and Joe, he was the cutest, smartest, most awesome kid in the world. (Okay, so maybe he was tied with his five-year-old sister, Jada.) To me, though, Rider had started off average, which I say with the greatest admiration. The residents of Lake Wobegon might take pride in all of their kids being above average, but measures of success are skewed in palliative care. Compared to the alternative, average is practically a dream come true. It means that the child is as healthy as most children are, and all children should be.

But then, at four months of age, he started missing motor milestones, which is a fancy way of saying he wasn't doing what other kids his age were able to do. That's concerning because the bar for success rises quickly in the first year of life with a kid expected to consistently acquire new skills. At first, his doctor was reassuring because some kids just go at their own pace. But then Rider started *losing* milestones: his muscles grew weak, his cry faint, and his breathing labored.

He was admitted to the Pediatric ICU for respiratory support, where a thorough work-up revealed Spinal Muscular Atrophy (SMA). The disease is caused by a defective SMN1 gene, which can no longer produce a vital protein called SMN (standing for "survival of motor neuron"). Fortunately, the neighboring SMN2 gene can sometimes pick up the slack. The math is simple: the more copies of the SMN2 gene you have, the more SMN protein you make, the longer you live, and the higher your type of SMA. Type 4's—the highest you can go—don't even develop symptoms until their thirties.

Rider had Type 1.

Certain diseases, like cancer, have a variable trajectory. Some patients are cured; others go into long remission. Not SMA 1, where patients get progressively weaker to the point where they can no longer eat, drink, or breathe on their own. By the time I met Rider, the only part of his body he could move was his face, which is why the PICU nurses nicknamed him Mr. Smiles. They still talk about his dancing eyebrows.

Revolutionary treatments have subsequently been discovered which can delay the progression of SMA, prompting a host of ethical questions due to their exorbitant cost and the burden of frequent intraspinal injections. Tamara and Joe would have loved the opportunity to wrestle with those questions, but the only one they had to face back then was how much life support to use when even more of Rider's muscles eventually stopped working.

Some parents seek to prolong their child's life as long as possible, while others think a life without eating, drinking, speaking, and playing isn't much of a life at all. Many come down somewhere in the middle, perhaps accepting a surgical feeding tube to provide nutrition when a child can no longer swallow but drawing the line at a breathing machine that would require a tracheostomy.

Rider's parents asked thoughtful questions about how much care he would require and the burdens he would endure, like frequent hospitalizations and the risk of bedsores and infections. Heartfelt conversations followed, some with the doctors but mostly with the nurses who Tamara describes as "more family than friends." Especially Amy, the nurse case manager who was originally enlisted to procure parking vouchers for the family but ended up hanging around for more personal reasons.

What seems obvious to Amy isn't always so to others. Blessed with a passion for her work and an irreverent sense of humor, she routinely goes above and beyond the call of duty and seems perplexed why anyone would praise her for doing so. It seems to run in the family, as her parents (by that point in their fifties) had recently adopted a baby who had suffered severe brain damage from having been abused. Amy had watched her parents make the same decisions for her brother that Joe and Tamara were facing with Rider, which helped establish a strong connection.

"Plus," Amy recalls, "when you see Rider, you just have to keep seeing him. He just lit up the room."

Eventually, Joe and Tamara decided that Rider would never have the quality of life they wanted for him. But how do you let your child go when his mind—his smile, his *light*—were still there? Listening to them grapple with what was best for their son, Amy shared from her clinical experience that there can be beauty in death, which was hard for Joe and Tamara to comprehend. All they knew was that Rider seemed like a little boy trapped inside a failing body, and the thing they wanted most was for him to be free. But before that, they wanted him to be baptized.

Which is where I came in.

#

When folks who don't go to church need something liturgical—like when they get married or lose someone close to them—they have two options: let their fingers do the walking through the Yellow Pages to find a church that might resonate with them or rack their brains for someone they know from another context who fits the bill. Which explains how I ended up presiding at the funeral of a local French restaurateur who had no use for God but who'd once mentioned to his wife that he actually liked me *despite* my being a priest. And also how I came to "marry the babysitter," which is how our then-five-year-old daughter, Lucy, described me officiating at the wedding of our favorite babysitter and her fiancé. That's why I sometimes refer to myself as a priest for people who don't know any other priests.

Rarely did that happen in a hospital context because I strive to keep my medical and pastoral lives separate. In over a decade at the hospital, I'd only broken out my collar twice. Both experiences had been incredibly meaningful.

— Harry, Carrie, and Trey —

The first involved a twenty-one-year-old man* who needed a palliative care consult because he was dying of cancer. Over several conversations, Harry (as I'll call him) described all the things he longed to do in life, like marry his sweetheart—whom I'll call Carrie because, in real life, their names rhymed, too—and get a job and raise a family. At an age when most people are savoring their newfound freedom by staying out late on the weekends and sleeping in the next morning, it was almost as if Harry was trying to fast forward through life, to see and do as much as he could before time ran out. He'd even banked his sperm so that Carrie would have the option of having their children one day. But with his disease progressing quickly, it was becoming clear that the fairytale wedding they'd planned would never come true.

"Are you really a minister?" he asked me out of the blue one day, as Carrie sat beside his hospital bed, holding his hand.

Evidently, some of the staff had been talking out of school.

I thought I detected a tone of surprise in his voice, which wasn't uncommon. Lots of people, upon learning my secret, exclaim, "I never would have dreamed you were a priest!" I hope that reflects a narrow conception of what a priest is and not a negative assessment of my character.

"Guilty as charged," I said, trying to keep it light. I wasn't sure where Harry was going with this.

"So you can marry people?"

"I can," I said, beginning to understand. "The only requirement is that at least one of the couple has been baptized."

Neither he nor Carrie had been, though. But just as I was about to bend that rule—please don't mention that to my bishop—Harry asked, "How about we do them together? The baptism and marriage, I mean."

---

* Instead of graduating to the internal medicine service, many young adults opt to stay with the pediatric team they'd come to rely on, often over many years. Pediatricians have a reputation for being a little warmer and fuzzier than adult providers, cutting patients more slack than they can expect on general medical units.

I shrugged. Just because I'd never done a liturgical two-fer like that didn't mean there was a rule against it.

But Carrie, who had been sitting quietly beside his bed, didn't want to stop there. "What about me?"

Make it a three-fer.

Everything moved fast after that because there was no telling how much time Harry had left. The staff on the oncology floor transformed the solarium into a wedding chapel with balloons and flowers galore. A glossy photo still hangs on my office wall of my thumb—dripping with holy water—resting on Harry's forehead. He's leaning forward in his wheelchair with a slightly crinkled expression on his face, whether of pain or utter concentration, I'm not sure. Behind him, Carrie looks on, waiting her turn. She's slightly out of focus, but you can still see her wide eyes searing the images into her brain so as not to forget a single detail of his baptism or hers that followed and definitely not the wedding that rounded out an unforgettable day.

The other time involved a baby named Trey, who had the worst chest x-ray his NICU doctors had ever seen, leading them to doubt he'd ever be able to breathe on his own. They weren't even sure a ventilator could keep him alive, which is why they urged his parents—when he wasn't even a week old—to baptize him while they still had the chance. Beth and Randy felt like that would be a sign of giving up, though, so they kept advocating for him as he battled bravely, permanently tethered to a ventilator, eventually growing too big for the NICU and transferring to the PICU.

Five months later, in the middle of the night, when they weren't there, his heart finally stopped. The PICU doctors managed to bring him back, but it had become clear to everyone that he would never leave the hospital, and unless something changed, he would die with a resident frantically thumping his chest. His parents couldn't bear to see him continue to suffer, so they consented to compassionate extubation.

First, though, they wanted him to be baptized alongside his twin sister, Stella, who had healthy lungs. Unlike before, they didn't feel pressured into it. They simply figured that twins who'd spent nine months side by side in the womb should experience this sacred moment together. So they asked Trey's nurse if she knew any local priests.

"Actually," the nurse replied, "I happen to work with one."

The following day—the next-to-last of Trey's life—the PICU team set up an elaborate cascade of monitors, allowing grandparents and godparents to tune in via Skype from far-off locations. Beth and Randy were there in person, of course, and Trey's crib—which, as he became more mobile and curious, had sometimes seemed like a prison, with bars preventing him from exploring the world—felt more like a playpen now that his big sister (by two minutes) was in there with him. For a moment, as I picked him up and dripped water on his forehead, it was possible to overlook the tracheostomy tube in his throat and the whoosh of the ventilator keeping him alive and just think of him as an adorable and inquisitive little boy, unsure why he was the center of attention but in no way objecting to it if that's what it took for Stella and him to be back together again.

— Rider: Part two —

Tamara and Joe also had very personal reasons for wanting Rider baptized. They recognized that his life was coming to an end, and they felt this would complete his journey. Not in the form of some prerequisite for heaven because they weren't even sure that there was an afterlife. But just in case, they wanted to have that base covered.

"And I'd like to be baptized, too," Tamara said, making me wonder if two-fers were a thing, and I'd just missed that lecture in seminary. She explained that she was raised Methodist, and her parents had left it up to her about whether to be baptized. It hadn't seemed like the right time when she was a teenager, but things felt different now.

So, the next morning, I showed up at the hospital with a clerical collar rather than a stethoscope around my neck. I'd worked there long enough that most colleagues knew about my other profession, but it was the first time most had seen me in uniform. Which, in my experience, often evokes a vague sense of guilt in people, as if they're thinking back on whatever they might have done wrong, wondering if somehow I'd found out about it. Hopefully my co-workers knew me well enough to look past the collar and not worry about judgment.

Joe and Tamara arrived a few minutes later along with Jada, who made a strong first impression.

"How come Rider gets to be baptized," she asked indignantly, "and I don't?"

I knew from personal experience that just-turned-six-year-olds hate feeling left out of anything, but this was the first time I'd seen it applied to a liturgical rite of initiation. Of course I said yes.

Having some tall guy dressed all in black sprinkle holy water on your head can be a little intimidating for grown-ups, let alone six-year-olds. So I started off with a little show-and-tell, using the handmade stole that my wife had given me on our wedding day, embroidered with cloth cutouts of children and grown-ups holding hands.

"When Jesus himself was baptized," I explained to Jada, "a voice from heaven said, 'This is my child, whom I love, and with whom I am well pleased.' And that's exactly what God is saying to you today and to your mom and your little brother."

She blushed because what six-year-old—or, while we're at it, forty-six-year-old, as I was at the time—doesn't love hearing that?

The Rite of Baptism in the *Book of Common Prayer* starts off by quizzing the parents about whether they truly renounce Satan, the evil powers of this world, and all sinful desires, which puts a rather negative spin on what's supposed to be a joyous event. Which is why—and please don't tell my bishop about this, either—I often adapt services to the context. Rider's parents weren't Episcopalian, so they weren't expecting the traditional form or language. They just wanted what every parent wants: to celebrate their child with the people closest to them and hear some reassurance that, no matter what the future holds, God has a hand in it.

So I just skipped to the end and asked if they put their "whole trust in God's grace and love." Jada looked up at Tamara, and they nodded in unison. Then Tamara and Joe replied, "Yes," on behalf of Rider, although they didn't really need to. It was obvious to everyone that they'd been trusting in grace and love every day of Rider's short life, especially in the decisions they'd recently made.

Then we went down the line, starting with Rider and moving on to Jada and finally to Tamara. After dipping my thumb in a half-full Styrofoam cup, I made the sign of the cross three times on each of their foreheads and then sealed them with oil as "Christ's own, forever." Tamara describes the experience of the three of them being baptized all together as "a connection of the soul."

The baptism was truly a team effort. An administrator bent the visitation rules for Jada, nurses—some of whom weren't even working that day—took photographs, and a social worker brought in refreshments. Only Dr. Williamson didn't look pleased. A physician in a collar didn't mesh well with his hope for "freedom from religion," but since the baptism was Rider's parents' idea, there wasn't much he could do to intervene.

Later that night, the eve of Rider's extubation, Amy made a special trip to the hospital. The days of arranging parking vouchers were long past; she was there to cry with Tamara and Joe and say goodbye to Rider. Before leaving, she leaned over his bed and softly sang "Godspeed" by the Chicks, just like she did every night when she tucked in her two young sons.

> *God bless Mommy and matchbox cars*
> *God bless Dad and thanks for the stars*
> *God hears "amen" wherever we are*
> *And I love you*
>
> *Godspeed little man*
> *Sweet dreams little man*
> *Oh, my love will fly to you each night on angel's wings*
> *Godspeed*
> *Godspeed*

Listening to that song, Tamara finally understood what Amy had said weeks earlier about death being beautiful. Not as something to be passively accepted, of course, and certainly not to be sought. But when the question ceases to be if your child is going to die and becomes *how* he's going to die, there are a lot of options. Lonely and in pain is one, which is why there's such a thing as palliative care. And beautiful is another with the outpouring of love and support that Rider and his family received.

The breathing tube was removed the next morning, and Rider died in the same room where he'd been baptized. Joe and Tamara stayed with him for, coincidentally, the same amount of time that Spencer and Kate spent at home with Hope: four hours. In addition to the usual memory-making activities—saving a lock of hair, making molds of his hands—they did other things to specifically remember that moment. Like holding him in their arms in front of a mirror to burn that image in their minds forever. Even now, over a decade later, Joe says he can feel "the weight of Rider, the feel of his body up against mine."

They still sense his presence every day in unexpected ways. Like in the light above their sink at home, which they freely admit is on the ugly side. So much so that they never even tried to turn it on, occasionally wondering if it might have burnt out long ago. But after Rider died, it started to light up on its own, especially when they talked about their kids. Only it wouldn't just glow faintly in the darkness; it would blink and get brighter than it had any right to. They've taken to calling it the "Rider light," and they never once considered changing the bulb.

— Three degrees of separation —

It's probably obvious why Lily and the triplets share a chapter in this book—for they all died within an hour of birth—but not so for Hope and Rider, who died years apart and of very different conditions, one in the NICU and the other in the PICU. But if there are six degrees of separation in the world, there are probably only three in Vermont, a small and wonderful place where people's paths cross frequently, especially those going through similar experiences.

After what Spencer and Kate had gone through with Hope, no one could have blamed them for never wanting to see the inside of a hospital—especially the NICU—ever again. But they wanted to help others enduring difficult times, so Kate volunteered to hold hospitalized babies whose parents weren't able to stay with them. That was how she came to know the parents of the twins I baptized years before Rider: she was the only person to hold Trey in both the NICU and, later, when he was transferred to the PICU.

Spencer and Kate also longed to have another child. Since she was thirty-eight years old when Hope died, they opted to pursue in vitro fertilization, which is a long, expensive, and uncertain road. In the sort of confluence of beginnings and endings that isn't uncommon in pediatric palliative care, Kate's fertility doctor called with the joyous news that her pregnancy test was positive the day after Trey died, at the precise moment when his parents had stopped by to say goodbye to Kate and Spencer on their final drive home from the hospital. Nine months later, baby Ava was born, who now sometimes has playdates with Trey's sister, Stella.

Kate and Spencer weren't done growing their family or helping other people. It took quite a bit of time and effort to get pregnant again at age forty-two, also through IVF but this time with donor eggs. Feeling blessed to have defied the odds, they wanted to donate their leftover embryos to some other family hoping for a child.

The offer initially caught their fertility specialist off guard. "But now that you mention it," he said, after taking a moment to consider their offer, "I do know a couple who recently lost a child."

That couple, as you might have guessed, was Joe and Tamara, who had struggled with infertility for years. (Both Jada and Rider had been adopted.) After Rider died, they also tried IVF, which didn't work. They explored adopting another child, only to have that fall through. Running out of options, it felt like the universe was telling them to stop trying. Then their former fertility specialist—who also happened to be Kate's—played matchmaker.

The two couples met, instantly liked each other, and hatched what seemed like a perfect plan: Spencer and Kate would give the embryo they no longer needed to Joe and Tamara, who yearned to have another child. There was just one problem: Tamara wasn't sure she could carry the baby. The doctors had never been able to determine precisely why she and Joe couldn't get pregnant, whether naturally or through IVF.

It felt like trying to get Hope home and back: a sacred dream that needed outside help to achieve. That's where Amy, the nurse case manager whose official work with Tamara and Joe had finished long ago, came in.

After Rider died, she'd stayed in close touch with Tamara and Joe. They soon realized that Amy's oldest son was almost exactly a year younger than Jada, so the two families had begun celebrating their birthdays together. That year, bowling was involved.

"Why don't you let me carry the baby for you?" Amy said casually, a few weeks later, after leaving a hanging ten pin at Spare Time Lanes.

Tamara initially brushed off the suggestion, but Amy is nothing if not persistent. She explained that she and her husband, Dave, were content with the two kids they had.

"I actually *like* being pregnant," she went on to say. "And my uterus just happens to be available."

Joe and Tamara don't usually ask for help, but now they were going to need a lot of it. So they gratefully took Amy up on her offer.

There was one connection left to be made, though. Tamara was great friends with Amy, but Kate understandably wanted to meet the person who might end up carrying the embryo she was donating. So the three families got together with their assorted kids in a local park, and it didn't take long for Kate to discover that her best friend from high school was Amy's cousin, and Amy's aunt had been her bus driver in junior high. Three degrees of separation indeed.

With the grand plan in place, from that point on, Amy and Dave and Tamara and Joe did practically everything together: a Chicks concert where they remembered Rider's last night on earth, two weeks later the embryo transfer—right around the time Kate gave birth to her son, Wilder—and two months after that, the first ultrasound.

Amy's approaching due date prompted "family photos" with her and Dave and their two sons (then six and eight) and Joe and Tamara and Jada. Keeping three kids smiling through a professional photo session isn't easy, and when it was finally over, Amy muttered that she could really use a drink.

"Then you should have one," Tamara said.

Thirty-eight weeks pregnant with Tamara's baby, Amy gave her a questioning look.

"What's done is done," Tamara said. "It's not going to do any harm now."

So they found a nearby pub, where the first three adults ordered beers. Then it was visibly pregnant Amy's turn.

"Could I have some white wine?" she asked.

The responsible waitress turned to Amy's husband, Dave, who was sitting next to her, and said, "I guess you know what to get her when she delivers your baby."

"Not *my* baby," Dave replied.

Amy pointed across the table at Joe. "It's his baby."

Joe just shook his head. "It isn't my baby, either."

While the quartet at the table tried unsuccessfully to not bust out laughing, the waitress muttered, "I'll just get you some water."

Less than two weeks later, Amy went into labor. When she started pushing, Dave held one of her legs and Joe the other. Tamara rubbed her back and whispered encouragement until Amy practically had to order her to move down-bed in order to catch her son. It just so happened that, at the moment little Boden entered the world, the random playlist had landed on another Chicks song:

> *They didn't have you where I come from*
> *Never knew the best was yet to come*
> *Life began when I saw your face*
> *And I hear your laugh like a serenade*

Boden immediately went skin-to-skin with Tamara, and for nearly two hours, the couples remained together, cherishing that sacred moment of welcome. When Amy was discharged from the hospital the next day, she didn't bring a baby home, which was just fine with her two sons, who'd already had plenty of upheaval in their lives. Amy's adopted brother—their three-year-old uncle—had died the previous year.

"The boys knew both loss and love," Amy says, "and what love can bring."

Hospital policy guarantees employees eight weeks of maternity leave and conveniently doesn't require that you actually need to be taking care of a baby. Amy took every day she was entitled to, dividing her time between binge-watching Netflix and pumping breast milk. Evidently, she's very good at both because she watched a slew of movies and, between maternity leave and the first eight months back at work, produced enough milk for the first thirteen months of Boden's life.

The families still get together a lot, and how could they not after all they went through? Amy refers to Boden as her "belly buddy" because, in her words, "'Uterus buddy' sounds weird. Let's be honest."

Boden, for his part, keeps it simple. "I love Amy. She grew me."

And Tamara says what I've been thinking from the moment I heard about their grand plan: "I look at Boden sometimes, and I think, *I just can't believe this.*"

Which, in turn, reminds me of Mark Twain's famous words: "Truth is stranger than fiction, but it is because fiction is obliged to stick to possibilities. Truth isn't."

Occasionally, Kate and Spencer join in with their kids. Wilder may be nine months older than Boden, but they still look like twins, which, genetically, they are, explaining why Amy likes to call them "cellmates." They also look a whole lot like Spencer, who of the six adults involved is the only one they share any DNA with. But every one of those adults had a starring role in this amazing story, and whenever I think of them all together, my conception of family undergoes a major expansion.

I'm so grateful, after all they went through, that Kate and Spencer have Ava and Wilder, and Joe and Tamara (and Jada) have Boden. Those kids will have the chance to write their own stories one day, which is why this chapter focuses on Hope and Rider. Factually speaking, their deaths made Boden's life possible, or else Joe and Tamara wouldn't have been looking for an embryo to adopt, and even if they had, Kate and Spencer might not have had any left over to donate.

But while it's healthy to draw meaning out of tragedy—and to remain optimistic in the face of unspeakable sorrow—it's also important to reject any sense of a divine and wondrous plan behind all these events. There was no noble purpose in Hope and Rider departing way too early. They didn't die so that Boden could live; they lived in order to be loved. To make Spencer and Kate parents. To give Joe and Tamara a son and Jada a little brother.

If you met those families today—each with two happy, healthy kids in tow—you might reasonably assume that they're like so many other families who got what they'd always dreamed of. You'd have no way of knowing that both couples have a third child, who in many ways made those dreams come true. Hope and Rider deserve to be remembered for that and so much more, and it's them I think of now whenever I listen to the Chicks. I imagine Amy singing to "Mr. Smiles," just as she did the night before he died. Only this time, it's the song that was playing when his baby brother was born, carrying the love of so many along with a promise:

> *You can close your eyes when you're miles away*
> *And hear my voice like a serenade*
>
> *How long do you wanna be loved*
> *Is forever enough, is forever enough*
> *'Cause I'm never, never giving you up.*

CHAPTER 8

Return of sensation

— Sabbatical —

Billing less for hours of intense discussions than a surgeon can for a few minutes in the O.R., palliative care doesn't generate much income. Neither does pediatrics, in large part because Medicaid (the government program that covers children without private insurance, or at least some of them) pays only a fraction of what Medicare (which covers the elderly) does. That makes pediatric palliative care a double money-loser and explains why my hospital would never have gone out and hired someone to do pediatric palliative care.

Luckily for them (I'd like to think), someone already working there wanted to start a pediatric palliative care program. So much so, in fact, that I made it one of two conditions for accepting the promotion to director of clinical ethics after Dr. Orr retired. That had seemed to the administration like such a win-win—having a current employee request to do extra work—that they'd also agreed to the second condition: a sabbatical.

Sabbaticals are common in most of academia, traditionally occurring every seven years, but they're rare in academic medicine because physicians pay for their salaries by seeing patients. Since sabbaticals are so unusual, physicians often don't think to ask about them in contract negotiations, often prioritizing a higher salary or additional staff support. More precious to me, though, was time, as I was acutely aware that my kids were growing up, and some opportunities would never come around again.

It wasn't like I was looking to sip piña coladas on a beach somewhere. Working on a textbook as a visiting fellow at the University of Cambridge seemed like a pretty respectable way to spend six months. And while I never expected Dr. Danvers to throw me a going-away party, I did harbor some hope that absence might help the heart grow a tiny bit fonder, if only because it didn't seem possible to go in the other direction.

First, though, my family and I had to get to England, and packing up four kids (ages two, five, seven, and ten) in the dead of winter for half a year away in a foreign country is no small feat. As Pam and I worked through the final logistical details, I couldn't help but think back to the eve of another momentous journey. Twenty-five years earlier, having just graduated from my small midwestern college, I'd been preparing to fly to England to study theology at Oxford. I'd been equal parts excited and intimidated, having never lived abroad and wondering if I would be up to the academic expectations.

That turned out to be one of the best years of my life, in no small part due to the friends I made while there, especially my four housemates whom I remained close to. One of them shared my love of sailing, and over the years, Jon and I (along with assorted other friends) had chartered sloops for a week in far-flung places like Greece and Thailand. He was a wonderfully complex person: becoming pleasantly flushed after a couple of drinks but easily able to handle a great many more, and as comfortable grilling world statesmen over human rights violations as he was resting his head on a friend's shoulder, grinning in contented embarrassment as we told stories about him.

When I let him know about my upcoming sabbatical, he immediately hatched a plan to have a summer reunion of all the housemates—even the ones who lived in Australia and Canada—at his cottage on the coast of Scotland just before my family and I returned to the States. That seemed like the only time I'd see him, since he was a BBC correspondent currently posted to Egypt.

The eve of my family's departure for England also happened to be New Year's Eve, which we celebrated with the last of our leftovers supplemented by Chinese takeout. As Pam and I were doing the dishes, I noticed that a voicemail had come in earlier in the day. It turned out to be from Jon's wife, Maire, whom I knew from having officiated at their wedding in Ireland some years before. I assumed she and Jon were wishing us well on our grand adventure.

It turned out that Jon was sick. On the voicemail, Maire explained that he'd developed debilitating headaches over the past few weeks, which had gotten so bad that he was barely able to walk. A friend practically had to carry him on board the plane at Cairo airport, all the while worried that they might be stopped if someone suspected Jon's condition was caused by a communicable disease. At the time, an Ebola outbreak was raging a few countries away.

Jon had made it back to England—barely—and was now in a London hospital scheduled for exploratory brain surgery the following morning. By the time I listened to the voicemail, it was the middle of the night there, so I grabbed a few hours of fitful sleep before calling back around 6 a.m. his time, which is when the first surgical case is usually prepped. Luckily, I managed to reach him just before they wheeled him to the operating room.

He was relieved to hear from me, leaving me to hope his slurred speech was just early morning grogginess after a harrowing trip. I suspected it was more, though, and so I spared him the effort and did most of the talking. I told him I was remembering him in my prayers, even though he wasn't particularly religious. I guess that was a combination of polite expectation—after all, what else would you expect a priest to do?—and a sense that even if you didn't put too much stock in the power of prayer, it probably couldn't hurt.

"I'll see you soon," I said before hanging up.

The sabbatical that had been years in the planning now almost seemed destined. Instead of a transatlantic flight, in only twenty-four hours, I'd be just a short train ride away from Jon.

#

The trip across the ocean involved its fair share of large-family adventure, ranging from the unexpected—like the rental car shuttle mistakenly dropping us off at the Virgin America terminal at Boston's Logan Airport, only to be saved by a kind skycap who loaded an embarrassingly large number of bags as well as four already tired children onto his trolley and wheeled them all to the Virgin Atlantic gates, three terminals away—to the unpreventable, with the kids so entranced by the never-before-seen movie screens in the plane's seatbacks that they slept not a wink on the overnight flight, only to become dead weight with exhaustion upon our arrival at Heathrow.

Before Maire's call, I'd envisioned my first foray into London as seeing a West End show or having a wine-filled dinner with Bobby, the one housemate who still lived there. Instead, I headed straight to Charing Cross Hospital to see Jon, who was as gracious and kind as always, if somewhat slower in speech. His sly wit was still apparent—the sort that you knew was perpetually running in the background, waiting for the perfect moment in the conversation to offer a humorous observation—although it emerged less often.

Following weeks of misdiagnosis in Egypt, surgery had revealed a brain tumor. There are a lot of cancer terms that only oncologists understand, but every doctor knows the word glioblastoma and how hard it is to treat, especially when it's impossible—as in Jon's case—to fully resect. He remained optimistic, though, and we spent quite a bit of time talking about how great the Scottish reunion would be, even as I began to worry he might not make it there.

From the hospital, I took the Tube straight over to Bobby's flat, where he did indeed uncork a fine bottle of wine. Then I told him about Jon, and the festiveness of our welcome toast quickly faded. Thus began fortnightly trips into London to visit Jon and often also to see Bobby and his family. I'd usually bring one of my kids along, combining hospital visits with Catie's first West End show and letting five-year-old Lucy hand-deliver to Jon one of her homemade cards, featuring her favorite saying at the time: "Love is sent to you."

There was precious little I could do to help him, though, as I wasn't licensed to practice in the UK, and even if I had been, he was way out of my age range as a pediatrician. So I ended up playing some mix of advocate, counselor, and friend, listening to him as he became harder to understand, translating what the doctors were saying into terms he and Maire could comprehend, and often just sitting at his bedside, sipping a cup of his beloved English tea as I waited for him to wake up from his longer and longer naps.

In many ways, it took me back in time to when I was a parish priest, visiting congregants in the hospital or at home as they either convalesced or approached death. With no technical knowledge to fall back on or practical task to accomplish, presence was all I'd had to offer then. And now—without a prescription pad or any formal standing in that hospital—I was back to where I'd started.

#

Most academics fortunate enough to have a sabbatical work just as hard as they did back home, only in a different way (i.e., writing a book instead of teaching classes). I, too, was writing a book, but the fact that I would need four more years to complete it is a testament to the final length of that book as well as my commitment to taking the concept of sabbatical—which means a period of rest—literally. Every afternoon at precisely three, I would stop writing in order to collect the kids from school. Those drives back to our Cambridge flat are among my most precious memories because, in Vermont, my wife picked the kids up and thus heard the first recounting of that day's adventures, prompting the kids to say, "Just ask Mom," when I inquired how their days had gone after finally getting home from work. Since Pam didn't drive on the left, now it was my turn.

They came home with amazing stories about the strange customs they'd encountered, like having to wear uniforms to school or playing a mutant form of basketball known as netball. Having only known their tiny school in Vermont, they made friends from all over the world, including places they'd only recently learned about.

"He's from Georgia," my seven-year-old son, Noah, explained after describing one of his classmates. "In case you didn't know, that's a former Soviet republic." His matter of fact tone reinforced how far he'd come, when only a few weeks before the only Georgia he'd heard of had Atlanta in it and probably seemed a world away.

Thanks to frequent school vacations and inexpensive flights, we saw a lot of Western Europe, starting off with Italy's kid-friendly cuisine and getting more adventurous from there. Whatever trepidation the kids might have had at the outset quickly faded, and the three older kids didn't hesitate when Pam and I offered each of them a solo weekend trip with a parent of their choice. While Catie and Noah opted to return to cities they'd already visited and loved, five-year-old Lucy had heard cool things about a place called Barcelona. All on her own, she composed a full weekend itinerary for the two of us, visibly elated at the thought of eating lunch at four in the afternoon and dinner way past her usual bedtime. A few salient facts managed to escape her notice, though, judging from her question as we packed up our Barcelona hotel room to return to England.

"There's just one thing I can't figure out, Dad," she said. "Why do so many people around here speak Spanish?"

Meanwhile, I continued to visit Jon regularly, increasingly aware not only of all the things I couldn't do for him but also the stuff I didn't even understand. I'm a good listener and also not afraid to ask questions, but crucial information about Jon's condition seemed to be trickling out, both late and incomplete. Like when physical therapy didn't seem to be helping restore strength to one side of his body, and his doctor attributed that not to the tumor but to a stroke he'd had intraoperatively. A stroke that neither Maire nor I had ever heard of before.

It felt like, after practicing medicine for nearly two decades, the rules had suddenly changed. In America, we venerate patient autonomy, but Jon's doctors seemed to be making decisions about what treatments to administer—and not administer—based on what they deemed to be best. They told Maire only what they thought she needed to know. Heck, surgeons over there aren't even referred to as "Doctor," which I only discovered when Jon's neurosurgeon seemed moderately offended when I, in an attempt to be respectful, addressed him by (what I thought was) his formal title.

I was used to being in charge, by that point having risen to the rank of full professor. Sure, I'd spent a lot of time over the years trying to imagine how patients and families felt, having precious little control over something as important as your own health or that of someone you love. But now, for the first time, I was experiencing that first hand. Instead of writing orders and having patients and staff adapt to my schedule, I waited all day with Jon and Maire for the physicians to make their rounds, afraid to pop down to the cafeteria or even go to the loo for fear that we might miss our one chance to get some answers to an increasingly long list of questions.

How much harder must it be, I wondered, for non-medical families who don't even know which questions to ask? Even Maire—a distinguished journalist in her own right, who'd worked not only for the BBC but also Al Jazeera—often seemed lost in this strange medical world. All she wanted to do was keep Jon safe, which she referred to as her "byword" throughout his illness.

At first, I tried to stay in my lane because I knew from personal experience how difficult it can be to deal with patients' family members or friends who are also physicians. More often than not, their specialty is sufficiently distinct from whatever the patient is going through that their counsel is rooted in whatever they managed to remember from medical school, however many years (or decades) before. Only this time, my specialty was both particularly relevant to Jon's condition and notably absent from his care. He'd seen surgeons, oncologists, and physiotherapists, but not a palliative care physician.

It became increasingly clear to me that Jon was dying, and while I couldn't prevent that, at least I could influence the manner and dignity in which it occurred. So, eventually, I started to talk about things that his doctors should have brought up but didn't. Like a DNAR order and making sure Maire understood what that really meant:

ensuring that Jon had a dignified and peaceful end of life. She would say later that this explanation felt like permission to accept it, which was all part of her overarching quest to keep her husband safe.

The familiar transition in Jon's care took place as my family's time in England was nearing an end: de-escalation of treatment in the hospital, transfer to a palliative care center focused on comfort, the gradual relinquishing of dreams. He still clung to the Scottish reunion, even inquiring about cancer treatment centers within driving distance of his seaside cottage. But by the time he was transported back to his lovely apartment in Notting Hill—where I'd occasionally stayed with him over the years—he'd ceased asking about it.

It was arduous to get Jon (not to mention his hospital bed) up the steep stairs, but it was definitely worth it for him to be back in familiar surroundings. I recognized some of the photos on the walls because I displayed the same ones back home in America. Like the one from our matriculation day twenty-five years earlier with all five housemates clad in full academic attire: black suit, white bow tie, and academic robe, mortar board in hand. We smiled with a blend of anticipation and uncertainty, full of both dreams and doubts about what the future might bring. I was planning to go to medical school, although I never would have predicted I'd go into palliative care or become an Episcopal priest. Heck, at that time, I didn't even know what the word "palliative" meant and had yet to attend a single Episcopal service.

Jon was already an accomplished journalist by the time he went back for a master's degree in politics, so I don't think a prediction of a globe-trotting life—that would ultimately take him to the United Nations, the US State Department, Jordan, and Iran, before finally arriving in Egypt—would have surprised him. But none of us that day would ever have dreamed he'd be dying of cancer at fifty-five.

With the Scottish coast out of reach, the housemates—save for Henry, whose health prevented him from flying over from Canada—gathered with Maire on a summer afternoon around Jon's bed. We reminisced about Oxford days and recalled the many reunions that followed. Like the time in Boston where Bobby, who is (usually) one of the most brilliant people I've ever met, became convinced we were driving down a one-way, dead-end street. And years later, the glorious week we all spent together on the Cape, which Jon, ever the Brit, kept referring to as being "in Cod." The housemates might not remember much of what we learned in grad school, but we never forgot an embarrassing story about each other.

Maire took a bunch of photos of four old friends, including one of us raising glasses of champagne, as I held Jon's as well as my own and made sure he got as much as he wanted. Our hairlines may have receded and (at least in my case) waistlines expanded, but those smiles hadn't changed very much in a quarter century.

With the time approaching for me to return to Cambridge—where Pam and the kids were in full-on packing mode—I remember leaning over Jon's bedside. As I kissed him on his rather ample brow, we both knew it would be the last time we would see each other. I told him that I loved him, which were words Jon didn't hear very much growing up. The fact that he could eventually say them at all was a testament to the hard work he'd done over the course of his life, seeking to understand himself and the person he aspired to be.

Before leaving, I went through Jon's medication list one more time with Maire, explaining what each one did and when to administer it. Being home was right for him but also more work for her with staff no longer around to do the medical things. At the same time, it gave her something practical and profound to do for her spouse in his final days.

I was halfway through the list when Maire interrupted me. "Would you officiate at his funeral?"

I looked up from the med list at her misty eyes. The textbooks said this was another step on a family's path of acceptance: from denying the reality of their loved one's death to speaking about it to actively planning for it. I should have been grateful for such a sign of healthy coping and that Jon would have someone who cared about him officiate. I'd been to too many funerals where the minister clearly didn't know the person who died or what was truly important to them.

"It would so mean so much to Jon," she continued, "and to me. But I know it's a long tri—"

"Of course."

As I said those words, I was acutely aware that, even though I'd conducted many funeral services over my nearly two decades as a priest, pretty much all of them were for elderly parishioners. I was still young (and fortunate) enough to have never presided at a friend's. Baptisms, sure, and weddings. Celebratory occasions all. But nothing like this.

— Return to US —

Sabbatical brought many things I'd hoped for, as well as some I never expected. Returning to a country that held such sentimental meaning—especially with frequent occasions for reminiscence with Jon—reminded me of a time when the future seemed open and mortality a distant (rather than daily) consideration. And it was a source of perpetual joy to watch my kids experience a larger world while always having a loving home to return to.

It also tapped into a deep vein of regret because I never had that chance myself. With literally an ocean between me and the abuse I'd endured, and surrounded by the few people in the world whom I felt entirely safe with, I finally was able to face the pain of my past. No longer were my feelings forced to wait until it was safe to feel them, such as on the drive home from the hospital or an early morning when my wife and kids were still asleep. For a few precious months, I didn't have to brace myself for the sorrows that tomorrow might bring at work with new diagnoses and dreaded relapses. Much as a manual laborer's coarse hands will gradually soften if no longer subjected to abrasions and lacerations, my soul calluses were beginning to thin.

The return of sensation, as I came to call it, wasn't easy. In some ways, it reminded me of Tony's nerve regeneration following his bout of Guillain-Barré syndrome because the first thing I felt was pain. In the protected, empty spaces, flashbacks came on hard and strong of memory-erasing assaults and an innocence that ended far too early. Every instinct was to recoil and flee, yet I sensed how profoundly important the work of healing was. An opportunity like a sabbatical might not come again.

Rather than running away as I had so many times before, this time, I stood my ground and let the feelings wash over me. I cried my fair share of tears—which were long overdue, having dared to weep for others but never for myself—and journaled copiously. I took plenty of long walks, remembering the distant past as best I could. I hugged my kids tight and never for a moment took for granted their wide-eyed discoveries because I knew from personal experience that not everyone gets that chance. And as our time across the sea drew to a close, I counted myself incredibly blessed.

Not healed, though. At least not completely. That will take a great deal more time if it ever truly happens. But I was on a path in the right direction and immensely grateful that, instead of negotiating for a higher salary or more resources, I'd asked for time. Time to step away, ostensibly to write a book but really (as it turns out) to learn how to feel again. As I said to my kids while we were in England and have since repeated many times: "Those six months might turn out to be our best as a family." They were definitely among the best for me.

When I walked through the doors of the University of Vermont Medical Center for the first time in half a year, I felt different. More open. At a stage in one's career when some of my colleagues were building emotional barriers to protect themselves (think Dr. Williamson's "It's too fucking sad to stay in the room"), I could feel my longstanding walls coming down. The tears I'd shed that day on the tarmac after carrying Grace to her car weren't a one-off; they were a beginning.

I was ready to apply the lessons I'd learned about powerlessness—that so many patients experience and which I finally understood—to being an even better doctor. And to let the feelings come, whenever they arose and whatever they happened to be, without waiting to retreat to somewhere safe, which is something that I'd finally realized the world would never truly be for me.

#

Coming home turned out to be much harder than I could have anticipated. There was no easing back in because many of the pediatric subspecialists hadn't known the doctor from the adult team who'd covered for me during sabbatical, so they'd waited for me to get back before referring patients for palliative care. After having treated no seriously ill children for six months, suddenly I was caring for way more than I had when I left.

Every new life-threatening diagnosis was a blow that nearly knocked me to the ground. Each child who died felt like the first patient I'd lost, and every parent's grief was a gut punch that left me short of air. Even if my soul calluses had remained intact, it would have been overwhelming. Without them, it was excruciating.

I couldn't help thinking of the frog in the old fable, who was dropped in a pot of lukewarm water. The frog could have jumped out whenever he wanted, especially after a flame was lit under the pot. But because the temperature rose so slowly, the frog never noticed that he was boiling to death.

That's a pretty good description of my work over the years in palliative care as the case load increased and my emotional connection to my patients deepened. Sabbatical allowed me to escape the pot for a while, but the water never stopped boiling. And when I stepped—jumped, really—back in, there was no opportunity to acclimatize. Without the defenses that had allowed me to survive for so long, I felt the pain as I never had before.

Initially, I'd felt uniquely equipped to practice pediatric palliative care, insulated from intense suffering by my soul calluses. But only a few weeks into my return, I began to wonder if I could survive in this work and also how the people around me seemed so able to. I felt the perpetual need to slow down and process and question and rage against the injustice of what these kids were going through. But it seemed like my colleagues took those events in stride. Not that they weren't compassionate—for they were just as dedicated and professional as they had been when I left—but they weren't fazed. It was as if their lives were divided in two: work where they did an exquisite job taking care of patients and the time between the end of one work day and the beginning of the next, when their souls were light and they could enjoy life to the fullest.

For me, though, there was no longer a division. I couldn't leave work behind at the hospital because the kids I was caring for and their parents never had that option. There's no five o'clock whistle for incurable genetic conditions or weekend breaks from progressive neurological diseases. The days of seeming to observe from a distance while someone who looked like me did a respectable job caring for patients were over. For while I could never know exactly how parents of a seriously ill child felt—never having been in that position myself—I nevertheless could, for the very first time, feel that what they were going through was terribly real, down to the very last detail. It was as if someone hadn't merely colorized the black-and-white movie of my life; they'd transformed it to 3D along the way.

I must not have hidden my reactions very well because people noticed. My wonderful ethics partner, Sally—who starts every day with a smile and a question: "How can I help you today?"—expanded her inquiry to how I was *really* doing. Even the chair of pediatrics picked up on it, which is noteworthy because he had a lot of faculty to watch over. Despite his already packed schedule, he set up a regular monthly appointment for us to talk, simply to make sure I was doing okay from an emotional perspective. He was well aware of the risk of burnout in modern medicine, with palliative care among the highest risk specialties.

— Jon's funeral —

Only a few weeks into my return, as I was just trying not to let grief drown me, Maire called. I shouldn't have been surprised to learn that Jon had died, given his worsening condition when I'd left England. I hadn't really been holding out hope for a miracle, not even a modest one in the form of a few more good months. But there is no small comfort in waking up and knowing that certain people are simply alive, wherever they may be, however tenuous their connection to this world.

So I returned to the country I'd always associated with community and friendship, first in graduate school with my housemates and then with my family during sabbatical. Only now, everyone I loved was far away. Jon had died. Pam and the kids were back in Vermont. Even Bobby wasn't there, having moved to San Francisco around the same time my sabbatical ended. That left me, on the morning of the funeral, to wander the streets of Jon's old neighborhood—where he and I had browsed outdoor markets and used bookstores when I happened to pass through London—alone. I found myself wondering if that's how some of my patients' parents felt, as once-familiar sights and experiences became foreign and disorienting, for lack of the person you love beside you.

A few hours later, I climbed the pulpit of a nearby church that was filled with Jon's family and other friends, all cloaked in sorrow. In the front pew, Maire was propped up on either side by her two grown kids. Jon's elderly mother wept nearby, reminding me yet again that a parent's grief isn't dependent on the age of the child they've lost. As everyone looked up for words of comfort and perhaps even explanation, with no soul calluses to protect me, I just tried to keep my shit together.

Funeral sermons are never easy, which explains why ministers often go to extremes. The more evangelical variety harp on the heavenly bliss the departed is currently luxuriating in, making those left behind feel oddly selfish for grieving or—even more perversely—envious of where the dead person now finds themself. More honest sermons grapple with grief while spinning tender tales of the shortened life, studiously avoiding any mention of God—let alone heaven—that could elicit questions of love and justice that they can't answer.

I had struggled mightily with what to say, finally able the night before to put some words to paper. Up to that point, too many memories—of Oxford and reunions and sailing trips and weddings, his that I officiated at and mine where he ushered—competed for attention. But once I arrived in London, everything seemed simpler. I was left alone with images of Jon welcoming me to his flat on my visits over the years, grasping my hand from his hospital bed, managing a sip of champagne on one last summer day after returning home.

I described those in my homily, part of sketching the remarkable journey of Jon's life, which took him all over the world. But I also didn't shy away from the deeper questions that, of all the grieving souls there gathered, I alone was expected to address, like: *why him?* and *why now?* Instead of trying to answer them, though—which I was wholly incapable of doing—I simply named them because I knew they were on everyone's mind and heart, including my own. As people who loved Jon, we couldn't help but wonder why we were gathered in grief that day in that church without him.

"What we're really asking," I said, "is: Where is God in all of this? Jon wrestled with that question, too."

He definitely had a right to wonder and not just because of the suffering and oppression he reported on from some of the most conflictual places on earth. He, too, bore scars from his childhood, finding love rather later in life with Maire after trips down dead-end streets that, fortunately—and contrary to Bobby's memorable observation—allowed you to turn around and go back the way you came. Which laid the foundation for not a few "where is God?" conversations we had over the years, where the booze flowed freely and voices were occasionally raised.

"I don't think he ever found the answer," I said because some glib reassurance would have been untrue to my friend. "But the important thing was that he never stopped searching. Honestly. Intentionally."

Then I shared something I often say to seekers who can't seem to find God, no matter how hard they look: "God is searching for you even more." Jesus told story after story about that. A shepherd leaves his flock of ninety-nine sheep to find the one who wandered away. A woman with plenty of coins gets down on her hands and knees to search for the one she dropped. (And, upon finding it, invites all her friends to come over and celebrate.)

"I loved Jon," I said in conclusion, my voice breaking, "and I believe that God loves him even more. That won't take away our pain, but it may hurt a tiny bit less, trusting that God—who's been searching for Jon all these years, too—ultimately found him and now is there to protect and welcome him."

By the time the funeral ended, my introvertedness was really kicking in. Over the past thirty-six hours, I'd flown across the ocean, wandered familiar streets alone, written and delivered a funeral sermon for a dear friend, and wept in front of a church packed mostly with strangers. Walking into the reception and grateful that my work seemed to be done, I accepted the polite compliments of the "very nice homily, Father" variety which invariably come a priest's way because most people don't know what else to say. Interspersed among them, though, were expressions of gratitude that Jon had a friend to lay him to rest, which helped assuage the guilt I still felt for not being there when he died.

Eventually, the guests dispersed, leaving Maire and me to follow the hearse to the crematorium. There the pallbearers laid Jon's coffin on a conveyor belt leading toward the iron door of the furnace, at which point everybody turned and looked to me. Evidently, my work wasn't done quite yet.

Having never even stepped foot in such a facility—and thus utterly lacking in crematorium etiquette—I strode up to the lectern and extemporized a prayer that I hoped fit the occasion. But even after I said amen, the pallbearers still seemed to be expecting me to do something, only I didn't know what. Sensing my distress, the funeral director walked up beside me and furtively pointed at a tiny switch hidden on the inside of the lectern. The kind of switch that looks like it should turn on a light, but when I flicked it, opened the door to the furnace and activated the conveyor belt on which Jon's casket lay. I must have been daydreaming in seminary when we learned about switches like that.

While embarrassing, it also seemed strangely fitting, for I was certain that if only Jon were still alive, he'd promptly text our other housemates about how I was going to leave him to rot on the freaking conveyor belt. Yet another addition to our long list of embarrassing stories which would surely have come up at the next reunion.

If there had been one.

— Weep, and you weep alone —

While I never expected Dr. Danvers to welcome me back with open arms after I finished "gallivanting" (her preferred term) around Europe on sabbatical, I did hope it would be a time for cooling off. Instead, it turned out to be an opportunity for entrenchment. Not only was I still forced to perform evasive maneuvers in our hallway crossings, but our communication assumed a rectangular shape. Having identified something that I had done with which she disagreed, rather than walking thirty feet down the hall to my office to share her perspective, she opted to transmit this up the hierarchy to her department chair, who would laterally communicate it to mine, who would then relay it down to me. As in the childhood game of telephone that this resembled, it was often challenging to reconstruct what her original concerns were, with all attempts to engage her in direct conversation failing spectacularly.

This took a particularly heavy toll on me since palliative care is often referred to as a team sport. A lone doc can never hope to address patients' physical, emotional, social, and spiritual needs, which is why high-functioning palliative care teams have nurses and social workers and chaplains. But you also need a team for yourself because the work is so emotionally draining. After weeping with a family, it really helps to have supportive colleagues to turn to, to share your grief and help you get back on your feet.

Funding constraints, though, left the other members of the PACT team dedicated in spirit but not in time, leaving me to do many consults alone. And I always felt like the odd man out around the larger adult team as the only doctor who treated kids and—as Dr. Danvers was fond of reminding everyone—split time with clinical ethics.

Fortunately, the sense of community that was so hard to come by at my hospital was blossoming beyond its walls. I was actively involved in the American Academy of Hospice and Palliative Medicine, serving on the ethics committee and giving presentations each year at the annual meeting. Toss in the articles I was publishing—some of which would eventually become chapters in the long-awaited textbook—and you might say I'd become a C-list celebrity in the field. A-listers were usually adult docs since that was the focus of the vast majority of palliative care. Even the most prominent pediatricians—those prodigious scholars and erudite speakers who headlined national conferences, where folks like me were occasionally asked to take part in panel discussions—were generally relegated to the B-list.

But even a C-list celebrity is still a celebrity, which offered me the chance to give presentations in far-flung places like India and Wales (which went over with Dr. Danvers about as well as the sabbatical did). Those trips provided a brief reprieve from the stress of work, but my greatest support came from an unexpected place, much closer to home.

Every spring, the Hospice and Palliative Care Council of Vermont (HPCCV) holds its annual meeting at a hundred-year-old lakeside hotel that has seen precious few renovations over its lifetime. I always looked forward to that meeting, a homey affair with a silent auction offering handsewn blankets and local fruit baskets. It's blissfully free of the academic sniping of a university medical center. Few of the chaplains, social workers, nurses, and volunteers gathered there had Ivy League degrees or long strings of letters after their name, but they were too busy taking care of dying Vermonters to care. While I was composing a manuscript in my ivory tower, they'd be visiting the home of a dying patient, carefully explaining what hospice is (dignity and comfort) and isn't (giving up), making sure there's a toilet the patient can get up from and a bed they won't fall out of, witnessing a final breath, and guiding the family through next steps and blossoming grief.

Over the years, the people there had taught me so much about palliative care, and I'd tried to return the favor by leading the occasional break-out session, usually on something having to do with ethics or kids for the subset of participants who might be interested in that. But soon after I returned from sabbatical, the HPCCV director asked me to give the plenary address to the entire conference. Upon receiving the invitation, I wondered if everyone else she'd already asked had schedule conflicts. Or maybe someone had noticed—as Sally had, as well as my department chair—that big stuff was happening in my life.

C-lister that I am, I'd never given a plenary before, but the one thing I knew about it from attending a lot of conferences was that it was over fast. Barely an hour into the meeting, my work would be done, with plenty of time left over to swim in the lake or wander nearby trails. That's not as fun alone, so I decided to pull our center daughter* out of school for a road trip with Dad. I'd done the same thing with her big sister and brother when they were that age, too: old enough to appreciate the experience but young enough not to get in trouble for playing hooky.

Lucy and I spent the night before the conference splashing in the hotel pool and playing board games in our room, but while I was up at the podium, she was going to need someone to watch out for her. So, the next morning, I asked three of the older women who had helped found the Madison-Deane Initiative—an amazing community collaboration dedicated to furthering palliative care throughout Vermont— to keep an eye on her. It was a win-win-win, as I could concentrate on my talk, Lucy was showered with attention, and the ladies got to spend time with a very precocious six-year-old. Lucy had already forgotten their names by the time we were driving back home (if she'd even learned them in the first place), but for months afterward, whenever I went to work, she'd ask me to say hi to her friends.

Public speaking has always come pretty easy to me, with lots of practice early in life as Exhibit A. Not trusting that what I personally had to say was important, though, early in my career I focused on providing content. I packed in a wealth of information—syntheses of data, newly published studies—jazzed up with PowerPoint animations that were often more style than substance. Advanced entrance and exit effects, motion paths, embedded videos, and seamless YouTube links: the audience could be forgiven for not critiquing what I was saying because they were so dazzled by how I was saying it. And after years of teaching at the medical school and speaking at conferences, I had a wide range of nifty presentations saved on my hard drive, ready to be whipped out again for a new audience.

---

* Aware that our other three kids all have a unique position in the family structure—oldest, youngest, and only boy—we're very careful never to call Lucy the "middle" anything.

That didn't feel right for this occasion, though. Unlike some people I worked with, the conference attendees didn't need to be persuaded that pediatric palliative care was unique and important. They took care of both adults and kids. They also encountered moral dilemmas on a daily basis and so recognized that clinical ethics was an element of—rather than a distraction from—palliative care.

I toyed with the idea of presenting some ethical cases for discussion. Not the sexy stuff that makes newspaper headlines (such as human cloning) but the bread-and-butter issues that people deal with every day, like how to respond to a family who can't bear to let go when the patient has made it clear that they're ready. Facilitated conversations like that had gone over well during previous breakout sessions, but that year, my heart wasn't in it.

With the anniversary of our return from England approaching, I kept coming back to how much my life had changed since the return of sensation. Images of Jon filled my mind—in the hospital and back at his apartment as I raised his glass of champagne along with my own and his coffin on the conveyor belt—as did the patients I'd cared for and lost, not just in the past year but before that, too. It felt as if I was making up for lost time in the grief department, and the cumulative weight made it hard to breathe.

Who am I, I wondered, *to tell people who've spent years and sometimes decades on the front lines of hospice care how to do their business, when I'm not sure how to get through tomorrow?*

So, less out of courage than feeling like I didn't have any choice, that day in the historic inn by the lake, I traded in authority for vulnerability. Instead of charts or graphs, my PowerPoint slides displayed photos of Jon: on matriculation day, "in Cod" with our old housemates, at his wedding, and surrounding his deathbed. I described how hard it was to return to America when his time was short and what an honor it had been to officiate at his funeral, which allowed me to walk the final mile with him.

None of that came as a surprise to the people in the audience. They'd companioned a great many people down a similar road and so understood well the challenges and emotions inherent in it. They had no way of knowing that I wasn't just sharing a personal experience; I was asking for help.

The next slide showed a stanza from Ella Wheeler Wilcox's famous poem "Solitude":

> *Laugh, and the world laughs with you;*
> *Weep, and you weep alone.*
> *For the sad old earth must borrow its mirth,*
> *But has trouble enough of its own.*

I didn't have to explain to the audience what that meant. They knew how challenging it was for human beings to share what was in their hearts, even (or especially) at the end of life. Time and again, they'd seen friends and family afraid to touch a dying patient who seemed so fragile or to say what was on their heart even though they might not get another chance, because doing so would force them to face the reason those words were finally spoken: they were going to lose someone they dearly loved.

That's when the hospice worker would gently explain to the family what the patient needed and didn't need. But guiding so many people down a path that no one ever wants to walk can take a serious toll on your own spirit.

"I know how that feels," I said, omitting any mention of how recently that feeling had returned and certainly any reference to the abuse I'd suffered long ago. "So how do we keep going?"

That's the point in a lecture when you're supposed to answer your own question for the audience. Dispense wisdom and all that, anticipating objections and providing additional resources for reflection. Which is what I'd always done, up until that day.

"I don't think I know," I confessed into the microphone.

This was totally new territory for me. I was raised to never ask for help, with my father expecting Exhibit A to be disproportionately mature and invariably polite. But I'd run out of answers (or maybe I'd just started facing the really hard questions, which didn't have any). So I set down the PowerPoint clicker and just spent a few minutes wondering aloud, sorting out my thoughts in real time. I wasn't sure if my ramblings made any sense. The only thing I was sure of at that point was that if there was ever a bunch of people who wouldn't stand for someone to weep alone, I was looking out at them.

"I know we need to break down some walls," I said, recognizing that those walls were as indiscriminate as my soul calluses once had been and my vulnerability was now. "But being entirely out in the open places us at the mercy of the elements; don't we need some protection, too?"

Is it possible, I asked—and not in a rhetorical fashion—to do this important work while still having someplace to retreat to when the grief becomes too much? A refuge that would fill the void that my erstwhile soul calluses had left behind. After all, I reasoned, if we try to be there for everybody, pretty soon we won't be there for anybody.

There needed to be windows, of course, because we weren't ignoring the pain. Windows that allowed us to witness (not just watch) what was happening around us and also be seen for who we really were by the people we came in contact with. And a door that made it possible to venture forth to companion certain people—although not the whole world—on their journey.

"That door," I said, "also allows us to welcome those closest to us into our home, offer them shelter, and—in the case of my friend Jon—share a cup of tea."

Tears welled up in my eyes as I uttered his name. It was hard to believe that he'd been gone for nearly a year, especially because we'd always lived so far away from each other. When someone you frequently encounter dies, their absence feels acute. But when you only see someone every few years, the passage of time tempts you to believe they're still out there somewhere. Each reminder that he was really gone felt like grieving anew, as if all the times before hadn't been enough.

"Which brings me," I said, not so much in conclusion—since I didn't have one—but because my time was almost up, "to the one thing I think Wilcox got wrong."

I recited the final stanza of her famous poem:

Feast, and your halls are crowded;
Fast, and the world goes by.
Succeed and give, and it helps you live,
But no man can help you die.

"Everybody loves a good party," I said, "and as you know all too well, people often retreat in the face of suffering. But just because dying is hard doesn't mean that nothing can be done to make it less scary."

I went on to observe that there can even be beauty in death, which comes as a surprise to some—like Tamara, Rider's mother, before she held him as he took his last breath—and others find absurd. That morning, though, I wasn't even tempted to explain what I meant. Like many other things I was talking about, my audience understood that far better than I.

Which makes me wonder why I felt the need to say something that was obvious to my listeners. In retrospect, I can't help thinking about an adage I learned back in seminary: a minister always preaches the sermon they themself need to hear. In the midst of so much grief, maybe I needed some assurance that there was beauty—or even just some sliver of meaning—in the deaths that surrounded me. Or, at least, comfort in the community of loss that I was blessed to be surrounded by that morning.

Before concluding, a speaker is supposed to politely express gratitude to the audience for their attention. Instead, I thanked the people there (whom I was supposed to be enlightening) for teaching me most of what I knew about caring for dying kids and their families. And for inspiring me over the course of my relatively brief (compared to them) career in palliative care. And for listening to my inchoate ramblings as I searched for a path forward with precious little light to guide me.

I guess confession can be more meaningful than data-driven recommendations because I'd never gotten a standing ovation before. It felt less like a recognition of eloquence and more like an embrace. A promise that I wouldn't have to weep alone. And the fact that one of my kids was there to see it was icing on the cake, even if Lucy had long since decided that coloring with her friends was more interesting than whatever Dad was going on about up on stage.

I didn't really know how to respond, especially as someone who's never felt my best was very good. But realizing a moment like that would probably never come around again, I tried to absorb the applause for however many seconds it lasted, a feast of welcome before I returned to a world of scarcity. All the while, one thought kept running through my mind: these are my people, the ones I was just beginning to find when Dave asked me that life-changing question at the cocktail party.

I put a lot of time and energy into preparing presentations and by the time one is over, this introvert usually has barely enough gas left in the tank to politely accept a few perfunctory I-enjoyed-your-talks. That morning, though, there were a whole lot of people waiting to share stories and reflections of their own, which were as far from perfunctory as you can get. They might not all have resonated with my metaphor of a house with windows and doors. For all I knew, they might have figured out long ago how to remain fully present in the midst of suffering. But, like the first Anglicans I met back in Oxford, they respected my heartfelt searching even if they didn't agree with my conclusions. They shared incredibly personal experiences, profound insights, and sometimes just an understanding pat on the shoulder. The conduit of grief, which the return of sensation had opened, doubled as an avenue for human connection.

With my work now really done, Lucy and I spent the rest of the day playing lawn games and paddling around the lake. On that warm spring day, my soul felt lighter than it had in a long time. Not just compared to the previous year, marked as it had been with losses that pierced my heart. But extending further into the past, when my soul calluses had separated me from the world. Back then, the most I could hope for when one of my patients died was the absence of feeling. Now, though, I started to hope that, with a little help—which I'd always been taught not to ask for—I could remain open to the pain that my patients and their families were experiencing without it crushing me.

Chapter 9

Battalions of sorrows

> "When sorrows come, they come not single spies.
> But in battalions."
>
> – *Hamlet*, Act IV, Scene v

— Collin —

Cystic fibrosis (CF) is perpetually in the running for my most hated disease. Because a single channel on each cell membrane is blocked, water gets trapped inside. That causes mucus outside the cells to thicken, clogging crucial pathways in the lungs and pancreas, impairing breathing and digestion, as well as frequently causing diabetes. As a result, every day, patients need to drink multiple protein shakes, inject insulin, and swallow dozens of vitamins and digestive enzymes just to keep from losing weight. They frequently require prolonged hospitalizations for breathing treatments, antibiotics, and chest physical therapy and tracheal suctioning (which in medical parlance collectively go by the unappetizing term "pulmonary toilet"). This is all because, out of three billion nucleotides in someone's genetic code, the three responsible for that single water channel got left out.

If there's a list of recommended musical instruments for CF patients—which would include the triangle or, at most, the tambourine—Collin didn't read it. Punk rock requires a very different sort of percussion, which is obvious from the black-and-white photo on my office wall: drenched in sweat, Collin is working his ass off to maintain a double bass punk beat on the drums. The deep monochrome shadows call attention to his protruding ribs and sunken cheeks, but the expression on his face as he toured with his band is one of utter concentration and pure joy. You have to look closely to notice the clear plastic tubing in his nose, tracing back to the oxygen tank at his feet.

Statistically speaking, Collin shouldn't have had CF. Since it's an autosomal recessive condition, the odds of two carriers having a baby with the disease is one-in-four. The odds of Collin and his older sister—who was diagnosed a few months before he was born—*both* having it is that squared. Put another way, if you took sixteen, two-child families where both parents were carriers, fifteen of them would have at least one unaffected child. Bill and Deb, Collin's parents, were the sixteenth.

They didn't let that slow them down, though. Never ones to place much importance on material possessions, they shared every possible experience with their kids: concerts, camping, road trips. That's not uncommon for families grappling with serious illness, but it's usually because parents feel like time is running out. Bill and Deb, on the other hand, just thought certain things in life were awesome and wanted to share them as a family.

That explains why they'd let then sixteen-year-old Collin cut short a hospitalization—against doctors' orders—to fly to Germany to tour with his band. Bill and Deb describe that as "one of the hardest and easiest decisions" they ever made as parents, well aware of the stakes but also how much it meant to him. Collin even said the trip was so important that he was willing to die for the chance to go, and he almost came through on his promise. Eventually, too sick to finish the European tour, he barely managed to get on the plane back to New York. His parents drove six hours south to JFK airport to pick him up before turning right around and heading straight for the emergency room at our hospital in Vermont.

Other decisions were just plain hard, like whether to try for a lung transplant, which isn't as simple or as obvious as it sounds. First, you have to wait for someone with healthy lungs and the same blood type to die, and then you have to be at the top of the waiting list when that happens. Even if you do get a transplant, you're basically trading one disease for another. You need to take anti-rejection drugs to keep your immune system from attacking the foreign organs, and while the new lungs should fix CF's pulmonary issues, all the gastrointestinal and endocrine problems remain. That's why only half of CF patients who receive a lung transplant are still alive ten years later.

Considering a transplant means you have to talk about death, which almost all of us struggle with and which is infinitely harder for parents and their kids. That became clear in a landmark book from 1980 called *The Private Worlds of Dying Children* by Myra Bluebond-Langner. She interviewed children hospitalized with leukemia—which was uniformly fatal back then, although often treatable now—and discovered that no one had told any of them that they were terminally ill. All of them understood that they were dying, though, in yet another example of kids knowing way more than we grown-ups give them credit for. But the kids weren't talking about it, either, because they recognized the sadness on their parents' faces when the topic came up. Bluebond-Langner termed this "mutual pretense": parents and children both trying to protect each other, ultimately forcing everyone to carry their own version of the same burden in isolation.

There aren't many harder things in life to talk about than death. There might not be *any*, but it's still important to. That came to light in a more recent study that asked Swedish parents who'd lost a child if they'd spoken to their child about their upcoming death and whether they regretted the choice they'd made. None of the parents who talked to their child regretted doing so, but a third of those who didn't wished they had.

Even a family as close as Collin's can struggle with whether and how to talk about death, which is why his pulmonologist asked the

PACT team to get involved. Collin's father, Bill, was an engineer who reminded me of my best friend from high school: funny, easy to talk to, got your back. Deb was nearly as tall as he was, with dark hair and blue eyes that didn't look away, even when we were discussing the hardest things. Southerners who'd met as students at Clemson and then migrated north to live among us Yankees, they were used to it being them against the world, which was how it felt to talk about losing their child to an incurable disease.

They wanted to respect Collin's wishes—especially since he was almost eighteen—but also recognized how much he leaned on them for guidance. Sometimes, it was hard to tell where their sheltering him ended and Collin asking for help began. That's one of the most complex parts of pediatric palliative care: even though parents are technically the decision-makers, kids still need to be involved, especially adolescents. You have to speak in a way that they can understand, involving them to the degree that they are willing and able, all the while navigating the complexity of situations where the interests of the patient and the parents might diverge.

Fortunately, it seemed like we had some time. When CF was first identified in 1938, nearly every patient died in infancy. Thanks to medications to break up the mucus in the lungs and replace missing digestive enzymes, life expectancy increased to age ten by 1980 and the late teens a decade later. By the time I met Collin, it had risen to the late thirties.

The first thing that struck me about Collin were his kind eyes and how he laughed frequently but also a bit tentatively, waiting for others to start, as if he were holding a door out of politeness and wanted everyone else to go first. Having heard about his band and looking to establish rapport, I searched for common ground. Unfortunately, my tastes veer more toward indie folk so I didn't recognize any of the groups he loved. Strike two was pets because I'm a dog person while Collin had two cats. I was about to go down swinging when he casually mentioned the names of his cats: Giles and Willow.

"You must be a Scooby," I said, using the slang term for a fan of *Buffy the Vampire Slayer* (BtVS to the faithful).

Collin's eyes lit up. "You, too?"

If only he knew. Back when I was a parish priest—in the days before DVR—I moved the church's Tuesday night vestry meetings up a half hour to make sure I could get home in time to catch *BtVS* at 8 p.m. It was the final and climactic season, after all.

This may come as a surprise after reading the previous chapters, where I've at least tried to appear educated and erudite. On the surface, *BtVS* is about a blond cheerleader in southern California who kills vampires in her spare time. But it also happens to be an allegorical spectacle of postmodern life, a feminist challenge to gender hierarchy, and a philosophical examination of subjectivity and truth, inspiring books with titles like *Buffy the Vampire Slayer and Philosophy: Fear and Trembling in Sunnydale* (which sits on my bookshelf).

My favorite character is Giles, officially the librarian at Buffy's high school but actually her Watcher, tasked with training, protecting, and advising her. With a tweed wardrobe that's as impeccable as his British accent, Giles is perpetually puzzled by how Buffy, her best friend Willow, and the rest of the Scooby gang—a reference to the teenagers who solved mysteries on the Saturday morning cartoon *Scooby Doo*—experience angst about grades and dating even as the world is about to end, which isn't an inaccurate way of describing my life as the father of four. At one point, I harbored aspirations of upgrading my pleated-khaki-and-blue-button-down wardrobe to Gilesian dapperness, but my style challenges proved insurmountable. (It's never a good sign when you get up super early to go to the hospital, and when you return home that night, the first thing your wife says is: "Did you actually wear that to work?") So I settled for keeping a six-inch-tall action figure of Giles—a gift from Pam—on my office desk.

BtVS came up frequently in our conversations over the ensuing months, when Collin needed a break from talking about what the future held. (CF tea leaves don't need much interpretation, as your lungs will eventually fail.) It's always tempting to defer the question of transplant, but that risks turning a life-or-death decision into an *urgent* life-or-death decision, which somehow manages to make it even harder.

But that's what happened to Collin: he caught pneumonia and needed to be emergently intubated. On one level, he now seemed more at peace, no longer struggling to breathe or make impossible decisions. On another level, though, he looked so different from the Collin I'd come to know and care about. Sedation erased his easy smile, and—with a breathing tube in his throat—he couldn't have laughed even if there'd been something to laugh about.

With Collin unable to speak for himself, it was up to Bill and Deb to decide whether to try for transplant or compassionately extubate. They had the sense that Collin wasn't ready to go—not that any eighteen-year-old is ever ready—but they were afraid that might be their hearts talking and not their heads. Meanwhile, the medical team was making sure they understood that he'd need a tracheostomy to provide a secure airway just to get to the closest transplant center—nearly four hours away in Boston—where he might well die before a pair of lungs became available.

It felt like people were speaking different languages, which isn't uncommon in medicine, especially in high-stakes situations. Doctors ask patients or families to make rational decisions using the cognitive part of their brain, even though the feeling part of their brain has probably taken over and won't let go until powerful emotions are honored and processed. As a result, patients often feel misunderstood while some other physicians might wonder if patients just don't get it.

That is why I always encourage students and residents, when a patient says something that feels important, to ask themselves: *Head or heart?* Like when patients ask whether they're going to die. Sure, they might be asking for probability of survival, but more likely, they're expressing fear and uncertainty. It's always better, if you're not sure, to guess heart rather than head. That way, the worst that can happen is the patient appreciates your thoughtfulness before repeating their request for more information. If you guess wrong the other way—like by providing information when they were actually seeking empathy— you might actually make them feel more alone.

I got the sense that the PICU doctor thought we should focus on comfort. She took care of a lot of patients on long-term ventilators and wasn't even sure Collin would survive long enough to get a transplant. That depth of experience can be both informative and biasing, even in the statistics we provide. Imagine a procedure where, for every five patients who undergo it, four will survive, and one will die. A physician who thinks the procedure is a good idea might talk about an 80 percent chance of survival, while one recommending against it could reference a 20 percent chance of death. Even though those are mathematically equivalent, studies have shown that patients are more likely to decline a procedure when the risks are framed in the negative.

I don't think it's possible to eliminate personal biases. The most we can hope for is to become aware of them so that we can either try to compensate for them—like by offering positive as well as negative framing of outcomes—or simply disclose them. I have a personal belief, for instance, that lying comfortably in your parents' arms is a better death than enduring unsuccessful CPR, so I sometimes qualify a recommendation for a Do Not Attempt Resuscitation order by saying something like, "But this might be just my own values coming out here."

When it came to Collin, I was definitely wrestling with my own biases. I was going to have to say goodbye to him someday because, even if he got new lungs—and that was a big if—he would still be at risk of post-transplant complications and have to keep dealing with the non-pulmonary complications of CF. I just didn't want it to be *today*.

What eventually tipped the scales was Collin's trusted pulmonologist weighing in. He'd trained at Boston Children's Hospital and was more familiar with their lung transplant program than any of us. He felt like Collin still had a chance. Once they heard that, Bill and Deb didn't have any more questions.

#

Waiting for a transplant feels like forever. Each day could be the day until it isn't and you have to shift your hopes onto tomorrow. Your room in the ICU seems like a second home—which you'd sell in a heartbeat if even a halfway decent offer came along—and the staff like a second family with the same annoying habits that your real family has. Like the intensive care doctor in Boston who'd always say, "Hang in there," before leaving Collin's room, leaving Bill to wonder, in his words, "what the fuck *that* meant." That got to be a running joke as days of waiting for a transplant turned into weeks and then months, to the point where one of the palliative care docs made Collin a shirt that read, "Hang in there."

In an often overwhelming environment, you'd think the parents of other kids waiting for transplants would be a support because at least they could relate to how you were feeling. First, though, you had to get the details out of the way: organ and blood type. As long as one of those was different from your child's, it was okay to root for the other parents' kid to get what they needed. Otherwise, they were competition.

After six long months—which must have felt a whole lot longer to Collin, who was doing grueling physical therapy every day while shackled to a ventilator—a pair of lungs finally became available. Even though he wouldn't be out of the woods after the transplant, it started to feel like all the hard work he'd done was going to be worth it.

The ICU team was already prepping Collin for the operation when the transport helicopter landed on the hospital roof. But before he could be wheeled to the operating room, word came down from above. The transplant surgeon had finally gotten to inspect the donated lungs, and he instantly saw that they weren't viable. To this day, the sound of a helicopter makes Deb shudder.

I wondered how Collin would manage to dust himself off and keep fighting through yet another setback. It was hard to imagine him requesting that the ventilator be discontinued, which would seem to recast his hard work—all that pulmonary rehab and separation from his family because Bill and Deb's jobs required that they split time, one in Boston with Collin and one back home in Vermont—as wasted effort. But I could imagine him increasingly regretting the decision to start down this road in the first place.

Finally, after three more months, another set of lungs arrived, and this time, they were in great shape. As expected, the initial days after surgery weren't easy. Post-op pain can be pretty intense: just imagine if most of your thorax was cleared out in order to make room for replacement parts. But where once there had been no hope, a future now loomed large. Not a cure, mind you, but lots more time and much better function. If Collin had been able to play an entire punk rock gig with two CF-riddled lungs—the equivalent of fighting the heavyweight champ with one hand tied behind your back—just imagine what he could do on the drums now that he could really breathe.

A few weeks later, when he returned to Vermont, he seemed free, and not just because he was unencumbered by oxygen tubing, let alone a ventilator. Now he could go places on his own, do what he wanted, effortlessly inhale the fresh spring air. It was time to dream once again of concert tours, which this time wouldn't be cut short by near-terminal events.

That lasted a month.

The symptoms began subtly, at least compared to the terrible hacking cough he used to have. A low-grade fever initially didn't seem like that big a deal. Maybe he was tired because he was pushing himself too hard in an attempt to make up for lost time. A little Tylenol here, some extra rest there, and it would all be fine.

Then one of his docs felt a mass in his abdomen, and it didn't take an oncologist long to make the diagnosis: post-transplant lymphoproliferative disorder (PTLD). Suppressing the immune system—which is necessary in order to prevent rejection of the donated organs—allows dormant viruses to reactivate. They, in turn, can create lymphoma cells that grow unchecked like weeds in an untended field.

After all they'd gone through, Collin and his parents were in a state of shock. The sorrows were indeed coming, not as single spies but in battalions.

"We thought we'd fucking won," Bill recalls, well aware that PTLD affects only 2 percent of patients with CF who undergo lung transplant. "To have that pulled out from under you, the universe must be like, 'Fuck you, dumbass!'"

We tried to cure it, of course. A lot of cancers that were once untreatable now can often be forced into remission, at least for a while.

PTLD, unfortunately, isn't one of them. Only one in five patients with it survives. If Collin couldn't catch a break when the odds were heavily in his favor—a 75 percent chance of not having CF and then a 98 percent chance of not getting PTLD after transplant—how could any rational person expect him to catch a break when the deck was stacked against him?

But I guess I wasn't very rational when I met with his oncologist after the first round of chemo to review the latest CT scan.

"The tumor didn't grow that much," I said. "That means the chemo's doing something, right?"

She stared at me, probably wondering if I'd forgotten everything from medical school. "It's progressive."

She was right, of course. The goal of chemotherapy is to make tumors go away or at least get smaller. You don't keep giving a highly toxic medication to someone when it can't even keep the cancer stable.

At that point, the question was no longer if Collin would die from PTLD. It was when, where, and how he would die from it. Over the course of our subsequent conversations, he was clear about the general answers: as long from now as possible, at home, comfortable. He would shut down, though, when we got to the specifics.

Earlier in my career, I might have left those for another day, when Collin would hopefully be in a better place to talk. But after practicing palliative care for a while, I'd eventually recognized that there was never a good time to talk about dying, and the desire to put it off had more to do with my desire to avoid a hard discussion than from respecting the patient's wishes. That conversation needed to happen, and if I couldn't improve the timing, at least I could help Collin feel as safe as possible. That's why I drove out to his house.

When I arrived, Collin was sitting in a recliner in his living room with Giles resting on his lap. I started off by checking on his pain level to make sure we were doing all we could to keep him comfortable as the tumor continued to expand. Collin, though, preferred to talk about all the places in the world he longed to see.

I admired his realism—he recognized that his body was getting weaker, so if he didn't go now, he never would. Like we often say in palliative care: "It's always too early until it's too late." But I knew there were other things that couldn't wait.

"Would it be okay if we talked about something else?" I asked after we'd discussed his medical travel needs, remembering my training to always ask for permission before shifting a conversation to a difficult subject.

Collin nodded, his smile becoming a little more tentative. People don't ask for permission to chat about sweetness and light.

"I'm worried," I said, "that unless we make some hard decisions, you may go through stuff that won't help you and could hurt."

Worry, one of the famous "3 W's" in palliative care—the others are *wish* and *wonder*—tries to make mortality a tiny bit less scary to talk about. I was describing the state of my heart, not predicting the future. If Colin just couldn't bear to go there, he always had the option of writing me off as a worrywart.

He didn't, though. Partly because there was a lot of trust between us and partly because he sensed the truth in what I was saying. The smile faded as his eyes moistened. I remember him nodding a lot as I went into greater depth about what the future likely held for him. Less energy, more medications for pain. I kept coming back to the goals he'd shared with me about the end of his life: "at home, comfortable."

"So what exactly does that mean?" he asked.

I started off by framing things positively. "We'll focus on your comfort, all the way to the end."

That sounded so logical. Who wouldn't want to be comfortable?

He nodded again, waiting for the punchline—not the joking kind but the sort that felt like a punch in the gut.

I knew I should keep going, but it was so hard. It felt like I was letting him down. After getting a tracheostomy and diligently doing pulmonary rehab while waiting almost a year for good lungs, this would be the first thing that we ever decided not to do for him.

"If your heart stops," I said, "I don't think that CPR will help you."

That comes as a surprise to some because, on TV, most patients not only survive CPR, they typically emerge rejuvenated and refreshed.

In real life, though, only about 15 percent of hospitalized adults who undergo CPR ever leave the hospital. Out-of-hospital cardiac arrests fare even worse, given the longer response time and the variable abilities of bystanders performing CPR.

"But if that happens and no one does CPR . . ." he began, needing to be sure he understood.

"Then you would die."

There, I said it: the D-word. The one that everybody else dances around, courtesy of fancy euphemisms like "passed away," but palliative care folks are supposed to say clearly and unmistakably.

He exhaled all the way. "But isn't there . . ."

My heart was so full at that moment that, now, many years later, I can't remember what he said after that, although I can make a pretty good guess. Something like, "a chance?" or, "something else we can do?"

I could have gone over the statistics, but that's rarely helpful. Even if the odds are one-in-a-million, that's still better than none-in-a-million (which are the odds of survival without CPR if your heart stops). We weren't talking about prolonging life anymore, though. We were talking about prolonging his death.

"It won't help," I said, wondering if I should say anything about it possibly hurting, too. When done right, CPR can break ribs, which can then lacerate internal organs. If someone is already gone, though, it's not clear that they'll feel any of that. Plus, going into a lot of detail could just exacerbate a patient's fears if they opt to go through with CPR.

At that point, I wasn't sure what Collin would decide. He'd accomplished so many things that people said were impossible—he was a punk rock drummer with cystic fibrosis, for God's sake—why not expect him to do so again?

Only this time, there wasn't a lone defective body part to replace with a healthy version. The cancer was growing and spreading. Collin knew that better than anyone.

"Okay," he said softly, as he looked down and stroked Giles's fur.

#

The tumor in Collin's abdomen continued to grow, eventually causing such intense pain that he had to be readmitted to the hospital, where even intravenous opioids couldn't control it. So intense, in fact, that on one of my rare days off, the covering doctor from the adult palliative care team suggested sedating him in order keep him unconscious until he eventually died. This suggestion was not well received.

"Who *are* you?" Bill recalls thinking, although he managed to keep it to himself. "I just met you, and you want to kill my son!"

In the medical version of a Hail Mary pass in football, an epidural catheter—the kind often used for pregnant patients in labor—finally managed to get Collin's pain under control. By that point, though, he'd started spiking high fevers, leading us to wonder whether his intestine (now completely obstructed by the tumor) had perforated, allowing stool to spill out into the abdominal cavity and cause an imminently life-threatening infection. Normally, we'd do an x-ray to check, but even if there was a "perf," he'd never survive the surgery to repair it. And since you never do a test unless it's going to change management, we just started the strongest antibiotics we had and made plans to get him back home as quickly as possible.

Time was clearly getting short, and there was one last thing that we needed to talk about. Always before when he'd gotten sick—whether from trouble breathing or infection or pain—he'd return to the hospital, where we'd manage to make things better. He knew and trusted the staff there, who over the years had almost become like family to him. But given how weak he was, if he left home again, he'd probably never get back there.

This was going to be an even harder conversation than the DNAR one. That had been about if his heart stopped, but this was about where he would die.

When I entered Collin's hospital room on the day of his discharge, he was resting in bed. Bill was working on a laptop close by, and at first, he didn't recognize where the conversation was going. That was probably my fault for not introducing the topic clearly, or maybe Bill and Deb had just gotten used to doctors going on about some random test or treatment plan. When I recommended Collin not come back to the hospital, though, Bill closed the laptop and reached out to touch him on the shoulder. That's when Collin began to cry. Not just the moist eyes I'd seen before, these were real tears. The kind that pour out when the thing that you've spent your whole life staving off is close enough to touch.

Bill climbed into bed with him. Collin was about his height but much thinner, so Bill—who describes that afternoon as the second worst day of his life—could practically cradle him. It wasn't hard to imagine him doing the same thing in a different hospital room almost twenty years earlier, when Collin was a baby. With Collin's sister, Jillian, already diagnosed with CF, Bill and Deb had known that their infant son had a 25 percent chance of also having it. They'd probably held him extra close, as if trying to protect him from being struck by lightning, too, as they wondered if the universe could really be that cruel.

As he held his son, Bill nodded in my direction. Earlier in my career, I would have confirmed what that meant. "So just to be clear," I might have said, "we're not going to do chest compressions if Collin's heart stops or bring him back to the hospital or—"

So many nots. Do Not Attempt Resuscitation. Do Not Intubate. So many, in fact, that you can't blame patients for wondering if there's anything left that we *will* do for them. Instead of repeating the list of limitations, I simply reassured him that we would do everything we could to achieve his remaining goals: "at home, comfortable."

Then I returned to my office to document all that in his electronic medical record, which, technically, was the last thing I needed to do before leaving the next morning for a weeklong conference in Boston. While relieved that we had a plan in place, I also sensed that Collin wouldn't be alive when I got back. And after my return of sensation, I'd resolved not to repeat the mistakes of the past, like with Hannah, whom I hadn't dared believe I meant something to, which prevented me from ever telling her what she meant to me.

So, before heading home to pack, I grabbed the six-inch action figure that had sat on my desk for years and headed back to Collin's room. By that point, he and his dad were out of tears, and Collin was resting comfortably again. He looked up when I entered the room, a hesitant look in his eyes as if wondering whether there was something *else* we needed to talk about.

Then I held out Giles, who might be more dapper than I could ever dream of being but also dedicated his life to looking out for people he cared for, usually with the help of something he read about in a book.

"For you," I said as Collin's expression softened and I handed him the action figure, trusting that a Scooby wouldn't have any trouble connecting the dots.

#

Ever since they'd learned Collin had CF, a part of Bill and Deb had known that, one day, they would stand vigil beside their son's deathbed in a heartless reversal of how things are supposed to be. But no matter how many times people tell you something that awful is going to happen, some part of being a parent keeps you from believing it ever really will. Which is why, when that moment actually arrived two days later, Deb says they were "as shocked as if Collin had been hit by a bus." At least he was comfortable, though, thanks to intensive support from the Visiting Nurse Association's hospice division—who didn't so much visit as move in—and his oncologist, who made a fortuitous home visit and was there when Collin died.

As soon as I got the call in Boston, I stepped out of my meeting and phoned Bill and Deb. I'm not sure what I said other than that I was sorry. I probably mentioned how brave Collin was, how many lives he'd touched, and that I would miss him, too. I already did, actually, crying alone in the sterile conference center hallway for reasons that nobody around me could understand. Even being so far away, it felt like the world had changed for Collin no longer being in it.

#

Collin's memorial service was held a couple weeks later on a warm spring day in, fittingly, what had started off in the 1850s as a church but, over time, had been sequentially transformed into a toy factory, gym, and now community center. His parents wanted nothing to do with religion—not that I could really blame them, given the odds of CF impacting their family as it had—and the day felt more like a reunion of people Collin had brought together than a liturgical event. Staff from Boston Children's carpooled for the long drive north, and the doc who'd given him the "Hang in there" T-shirt flew all the way from Minnesota, where he'd recently moved.

I chatted only briefly with Bill and Deb because they had a lot of other people to greet and also because I didn't know what to say. We'd discussed so many super-important things while Collin was alive that casual conversation was foreign to us. And without him to talk about, I wasn't sure what was left. Mostly, I just tried to avoid nonsense questions like: "How are you doing?" I mean, how were parents who'd just lost their child supposed to be doing?

So I was surprised when, a couple months after the memorial, Bill and Deb called me. They wanted to debrief about Collin's final days to make sure they understood what had happened and why. When we met in my office, it quickly became apparent that they were grappling with profound self-doubt, searching for something they could—or *should*—have done differently that might have saved their son's life. So I went over everything, from the diagnosis of PTLD to its unsuccessful treatment to the decision to focus on comfort. We spent a lot of time on his pain management, especially the suggestion one doctor had made about sedating him until he died. Deb and Bill were simultaneously furious about what at the time had seemed like giving up while also wondering if they'd been selfish for not considering it.

"We weren't ready to let him go," Deb said apologetically, as if any parent ever is.

"You were there for him every step of the way," I said. "And that extra time gave you both the chance to say what you needed to say."

Judging from the way they kept shaking their heads and the number of questions they asked—all of which started with "What if?"—my attempts at reassurance were clearly coming up short. The logic was just too neat:

The job of a parent is to protect their kid.
My kid is dead.
Therefore, I failed as a parent.

When they finally ran out of questions I couldn't answer, I accompanied them down the long corridor to the main entrance of the hospital. The same path they'd walked so many times with their son—for clinic appointments and yet another admission for pulmonary toilet—that had felt so burdensome at the time but which they'd kill to have even one more of because that would mean Collin was still alive.

As we reached the revolving door, I was acutely aware of how much I wanted for them and how powerless I was to provide it. I reached out and gave Bill a firm bro-hug, searching in vain for words of solace. The void Collin left behind felt like the vacuum of outer space, making it hard to breathe.

I couldn't just let them go, though. Not carrying all that guilt, when they'd always been the most amazing of parents.

Desperately searching for words, I said softly, "Hang in there."

"Oh, c'mon!" Bill practically shouted in my ear as he pulled away.

Who could blame him? After all the books I'd read and conferences I'd attended, *that's* what I came up with? Yet even more proof that even seasoned palliative care docs—or maybe just this one—sometimes can't bear the silence of a world without answers.

"I'm sorry," I said, without specifying for what. There were so many things to choose from.

I expected to see betrayal in his eyes after all we'd been through together. You could probably forgive an intensive care doctor at *The Children's Hospital*—which is what Boston Children's used to call itself, as if there weren't any others—for saying something so vapid but not someone whose specialty was supposed to be empathic communication.

Instead of betrayal, though, there was confusion, hopefully not directed at me—who should have known better than to say something like that—but at a world without his son in it, when only a few weeks earlier an actual future had come into view and even started to shine. A moment later, Bill's expression softened, and he stepped forward and gave me another hug, longer and less manly this time.

"I know," he whispered in my ear. "We all are."

Then he and Deb turned and walked hand-in-hand out of the hospital. Miraculously, I managed to keep my mouth shut. We'd already said all there was to say, even if it wasn't nearly enough.

#

People like to say that "time heals all wounds"—which has always struck me as absurdly certain and complete—but that definitely wasn't true for Bill and Deb. In the years after Collin died, they honored him in all kinds of tender ways, like instituting an annual pilgrimage to Germany for the Wacken Open Air heavy metal music festival. While there, they'd visit clubs he'd played on his death-defying band tour, recalling how thrilled he'd been to go. Along the way, they'd reminisce about all the things they'd done together as a family, occasionally prompting one to remind the other that, no, Collin hadn't actually been with them at some recalled event. He was such an integral part of their lives, though, it was difficult to imagine him not always being there.

It was also impossible to forgive themselves for not being able to save his life.

"I had one job," Deb recalls, seven years later, "and I feel like we didn't do it."

For his part, Bill—ever the engineer—seeks solace in probabilities, especially when drawn from a movie that he and I love and Collin would have, too, if he'd lived long enough to see it. In *Avengers: Endgame*, Dr. Strange goes forward in time to envision every conceivable outcome of their impending climactic battle with the villain Thanos. He identifies 14,000,605 possibilities, prompting Iron Man to ask, "How many involve Thanos growing a weed farm on a remote planet, the Avengers attacking said farm, the weed burning up in the crossfire, us and Thanos all getting high together and decide to chill out and play Minecraft together every Sunday?"

"One," Dr. Strange somberly replies, which, of course, the Avengers manage to find because Marvel movies, unlike real life, guarantee a happy ending.

Collin faced steep odds, too. But no matter how hard Bill and Deb searched—in the decision to intubate him for pneumonia, almost a year in Boston waiting for a transplant that seemed like it would never come, and then chemo for the dreaded complication the transplant brought with it—they couldn't find a path that would save his life.

"Guess we're not superheroes!" Bill says, his self-effacing humor failing to conceal the cruelly elegant logic: *My kid is dead; therefore I failed as a parent.*

I long to relieve Bill and Deb of their guilt, which is something I have some experience with. On Sunday mornings, I raise my hand toward a kneeling congregation who've just recited the General Confession and proclaim that God has forgiven them for all their sins, the details of which I'm not privy to and, thankfully, are no longer relevant. I'd never say something like that to Bill or Deb, though, and not just because they're so passionately (and understandably) irreligious that sometimes it feels less like they overlook the fact that I'm a priest than forgive me for the company I keep on Sundays.

The real reason I'd never say that to Bill and Deb is that there's nothing to pardon them for. I learned early on in my pastoral career, when a parishioner sought me out privately for something more tangible and personal than a generic absolution, that just because someone feels guilty doesn't necessarily mean they did anything wrong. Indeed, my own first confession during seminary—which was practically an all-day affair—concluded with my confessor attributing most of my supposed transgressions to simple human imperfection.

To be sure, some people deny responsibility for real transgressions. But I think there are far more tender souls who carry burdens that are not their own. Like Bill and Deb.

As their son's doctor, I'd observed how they always did what was best for Collin. Later, as their friend, I'd told them how much I admired the love and devotion they always showed him, making the hardest decisions with integrity and self-sacrifice. They gave their son a rich and wonderful life, letting go when he needed to spread his wings and wrapping their arms around him when he dared to look down.

My voice, though, was always drowned out by the cruelly elegant logic of their dearly beloved son being gone. It made me wish that I had something more authoritative and indisputable to appeal to, which Bill and Deb couldn't help but hear and heed. If only, for one brief moment, they could set aside their anger at God—which no one, including me, would ever blame them for—and hear me, not as physician or friend but as someone who, at least on this one occasion, dared to speak with divine authority. Only, instead of reciting words from *The Book of Common Prayer*, I'd use the language of something we all loved.

"Go ahead, Dr. Strange," I'd say, "envision as many possible outcomes for Collin as you like. Don't even bother to stop at 14,000,605. You won't see a single one where Collin is still alive, even with all the Avengers fighting on his side. Bill and Deb didn't fail to find the path to survival, because it never existed.

"But you will see plenty of outcomes where Collin wasn't allowed to play the drums because of the toll they'd take on his fragile body. Where he never saw Europe or got a second chance to breathe in pure air. Where he died in the hospital or in pain or alone.

"And while you're envisioning all those even-more terrible outcomes, make sure to thank Bill and Deb. They're the reason none of those came true."

CHAPTER 10

Back when I was in medical school . . .

During my medical training, I'd often hear grizzled senior physicians mutter, "Back when I was in medical school—" before telling horror stories about how they used to be on call for thirty-six hours straight every other night.

"The only bad thing about that schedule," they'd say, trying to conceal their sleep-envy of the younger generations under a noble veneer, "is you missed out on half the patients."

Recognizing that my every fourth night call schedule as a resident had been positively decadent by comparison, when I joined the medical school faculty at the University of Vermont, I vowed never to say those words. That vow lasted all of a year until the Accreditation Council for Graduate Medical Education enacted some long-needed reforms, including abolishing all overnight call for interns. Trainees no longer being exhausted was clearly progress—both in terms of patient safety as well as physician well-being—but that didn't keep me from being a little jealous.

Work hours weren't the only things changing. Outcomes for serious disease were, too. Acute lymphoblastic leukemia, for example, went from uniformly fatal to 90 percent curable. The same was true for many genetic conditions, such as Trisomy 21 (also known as Down syndrome). Back in the 1970s, there had been several well-publicized cases of infants with Down syndrome whose parents refused the straightforward surgery needed to repair an intestinal blockage (leading to the babies' deaths from dehydration). As one mother famously said—and please pardon the offensive term, but it was the one used at the time—"It would be unfair to the other children in the household to raise them with a mongoloid." The medical establishment did not protest, with surveys revealing a large majority of pediatric surgeons (and nearly half of pediatricians) willing to honor the parents' refusal. Now, thanks to greater awareness of the quality of life that people with Down syndrome can have (even to the point of becoming TV stars or triathletes), the landscape has thankfully changed.

The next most common trisomies—on chromosome 13 (which is what Lily, whose father handcrafted her coffin, had) and 18—are much more serious than Down syndrome in terms of their impact on cognitive development (which usually peaks at the level of an eight-month-old) as well as on survival, particularly those also born with heart defects. A high percentage of affected fetuses are stillborn, with half of those born alive dying within the first week of life. These conditions are so serious, in fact, that (as mentioned in Chapter 4) for many years, the American Academy of Pediatrics (AAP) proclaimed them conditions that justified not resuscitating a newborn in the delivery room, even if the parents requested it. As a result, doctors commonly referred to trisomy 13 and 18 as "incompatible with life."

As prenatal diagnosis improved, parents could make pivotal decisions even before a baby with trisomy 13 or 18 was born. Expectant women were often told that their child (if born) would experience a life of suffering or would be a "vegetable." Nearly one-quarter of expectant mothers also reported being informed that the child would ruin their marriage and/or family. Not surprisingly, given these predictions, the disclosure of the trisomy was often followed by an inquiry as to when the parents wished to schedule the termination.

Not if. When.

That's what I was taught back when I was in medical school. And I believed it, until I met Cora.

— Cora —

Like many newly married couples, Joy and Bruce were ecstatic to be pregnant and relieved that the ultrasounds appeared normal. When their daughter was born, though, the doctors immediately realized something was wrong. Cora was very small, with rotated ears, clenched fists, a sloping forehead, and a ventricular septal defect (or VSD) in her heart: all classic signs of trisomy 18, or T18 for short. The doctors, having been taught in medical school that it was a lethal anomaly, recommended comfort care. Joy and Bruce, though, wanted everything done, including heart surgery (assuming Cora survived long enough to reach the minimum weight required). Palliative care was consulted to reconcile those conflicting goals.

I quickly learned that blond-haired Joy liked to shoot from the hip.

"We just want to give our daughter a chance," she said the day after Cora was born, as Bruce—who had a trimmed brown beard and made each word count—nodded beside her. "We've heard that some kids with trisomy 18 beat the odds."

I was about to correct her, based on what I'd learned in medical school over two decades earlier. But then it dawned on me that I'd never actually taken care of a patient with T18 before. Though the third most common trisomy, it's still an extremely rare condition. (So much so that only one child, on average, is born with it each year in the entire state of Vermont.) Out of respect for the parents' hopes—and recognizing that, without compelling data, I had little chance of reframing their decision—I pledged to do some research into these patients who supposedly beat the odds.

The first articles I found confirmed what I'd been taught about T18: median life expectancy in the US was around three days, with one outlier study reporting fourteen days. But as I read on, I soon discovered that outcomes were much better in countries where intensive treatment was routinely provided to all liveborn infants. A recent Japanese study, for instance, documented a median life expectancy of 152 days. Five months may not seem like a long time, but for parents who savor each moment, it can be. What's more, a small subset of patients survived for significantly longer: 25 percent lived to see their first birthday.

Recognizing the stark differences in life expectancy, some commentators were beginning to wonder whether the lower numbers in the US were the result of a self-fulfilling prophecy: informed that T18 was a lethal anomaly, the vast majority of parents who continued the pregnancy opted for comfort care for their baby. But babies with T18 often have congenital heart disease, which by itself requires intensive treatment to survive, even without a trisomy. That meant that T18 kids on comfort care would die assuredly and early, confirming the grim statistics and perpetuating the cycle.

Survival data got me thinking, but personal stories got me feeling. The website for the Support Organization for Trisomy 18, 13, and Related Disorders (SOFT) was replete with stories of patients who didn't match up with what I'd been taught in medical school, like a thirty-four-year-old woman with T18 who was recently a bridesmaid in her brother's wedding. My good friend, Larry Fenton, who'd treated lots of babies with trisomies as a neonatologist before shifting over to palliative care, was so intrigued by these stories that he decided to see for himself. After attending the annual SOFT convention, he wrote this moving reflection:

> How easy it is to assume we know what a good quality of life is for anyone other than ourselves. We assess the burdens of care, the impact on siblings, the impact on parental relationships, the impact on finances and the utilization of resources. But smiles and laughter need no score pad. We know what they mean. The advice we give may often be centered around our personal notions about quality of life.

What Larry had witnessed at the SOFT convention, I was now learning from Cora. Joy likes to say that her daughter's life goal is to educate and inspire, and I was her first student.

#

It's tempting to take certain things for granted with babies, like breathing and swallowing. Not for little Cora. Kids with T18 can stop breathing unexpectedly, due to a brain condition called central apnea. And swallowing is actually a complex process, requiring over fifty pairs of muscles and nerves to coordinate in perfect time in order to get food from the mouth down to the stomach. None of which is guaranteed for a kid with T18.

For the first of many times, though, Cora exceeded expectations. She breathed reliably on her own and didn't seem to mind the feeding tube through her nose down into her stomach. Her heart was doing okay for the moment, and Joy and Bruce hoped she'd gain enough weight by the time it began to fail to be eligible for surgery.

The doctors, though, weren't thinking nearly that far down the line. Sensing time was short, they were just trying to get her home.

"We were only in the NICU for a week," Joy remembers proudly, "but that was because they sent Cora home to die. Only no one told her that."

Every day came with risk. Joy and Bruce lived in Randolph Center, Vermont, population 1,466, an hour away from the nearest hospital that could handle a kid as complex as Cora. It would only take one heart arrhythmia or prolonged apnea, and Cora would never get the help she needed in time.

It turned out, though, that she didn't need much help. She was gaining weight thanks to the feeding tube, enough that the cardiac surgeons in Boston begrudgingly agreed to repair her heart. But just a few days before the planned surgery in Boston, Cora got the flu. Out of an abundance of caution, she was admitted to our PICU for oxygen and close monitoring, which ended up saving her life because there were lots of doctors around when she stopped breathing. A code was called, and it was much like what you see on TV: doctors and nurses racing into the room, a backboard slipped under Cora's tiny body, chest compressions (using just two fingers rather than both hands because she was so small), and intubation.

She clung to life, but the heart surgeons in Boston—who'd been reluctant to operate on a baby with T18 even before she coded—now outright refused to do so. They didn't think Cora would even survive the transport to Boston, let alone pull through surgery if she managed to get there. This led Dr. Williamson, the PICU director, to wonder why we were putting her through such intensive treatment.

"She's just going to die from heart failure," he reasoned, "assuming something else doesn't take her first."

I couldn't argue with his reasoning, and part of my job was to help kids die comfortably. Being hooked up to a ventilator and all manner of arterial and venous lines didn't fit that description, so I had some intense conversations in the PICU with Joy, observing that she and Bruce had already had more time with their daughter than the doctors had predicted. Good quality time, too, because, except for the feeding tube, Cora had basically been a normal kid, avoiding the overmedicalized life of many children with serious conditions.

Joy listened patiently, then proceeded to remind me that Cora was supposed to die in utero and then in the first week of life and then soon after discharge. The way Joy saw it, if Cora had exceeded every expectation so far—even the median life expectancy from the Japanese studies—why should we start doubting her now?

Joy wasn't going to let anyone give up on her daughter, and that included the doctors in Boston. She pestered (okay, *badgered*) them until they finally agreed to the transfer but only for a second opinion. Not for surgery—they made that absolutely clear.

This wasn't an uncommon plan: parents often need to be sure that every option has been tried. When *The* Children's Hospital says there's nothing more to do, there really isn't.

If Dr. Williamson had been a little disappointed that I hadn't gotten the DNR on my first palliative care consult (with Nicky), he was really disappointed now. At least Nicky's mother had eventually accepted the transition to comfort care, but Cora's mother was plowing full steam ahead. I reassured him that Joy understood the risks and benefits of proceeding and even promised to call my counterparts on the Boston PACT team and ask them to check on Cora.

That didn't appease him, though. To his thinking, what good was palliative care—even at The Children's Hospital—if it couldn't convince parents, when the burdens of treatment were great and the chance of survival small, to focus on comfort? I tried to bring up the data on improving survival for kids with T18, which might shift the balance of risks and benefits. But he wasn't interested in musings about the surprisingly good quality of life that kids like Cora potentially could have.

Surprising us once again, Cora managed to survive the transport to Boston. True to their word, the cardiac surgeons thoroughly evaluated her, ultimately concurring with Dr. Williamson's assessment that she was going to die no matter what. Having fought so hard to give her daughter a chance, Joy was crushed when they declined to operate.

But then, two days later, even as plans were being made to transfer Cora back to UVM, a cardiac surgeon Joy had never seen before walked into Cora's room. He was wearing scrubs, like the other surgeons, who'd unanimously declined to operate. What still sticks in Joy's mind, though, were his white fake-leather shoes, crusted with blood.

"I don't know anything about Trisomy 18," he admitted, "but I see a kid with a hole in her heart. I can fix *that*."

Far too savvy to mention the other surgeons' refusal, Joy remained silent. And the next morning, the doctor with the blood-crusted shoes wheeled Cora to the operating room.

Cora took care of the rest. As promised, the Boston PACT team stopped by their PICU the day after surgery to check on her, but she wasn't there. Having been extubated without complication, she'd already been transferred to the pediatric floor. Within a few days, she was back home in Randolph Center, her heart defect having shifted over one column in her medical chart from Current Problems to Past Medical History.

— Compatible with life —

Grand rounds is a big deal, the one time each week when all the faculty in the department gather together. It's usually held in the largest auditorium at the medical center, which in UVM's case is named for a long-time faculty member who was the real-life inspiration for Hawkeye Pierce, the wartime physician played by Alan Alda on *M*A*S*H*. While well-endowed hospitals have the budget to fly in external speakers, Wednesday mornings at UVM usually involve a local colleague sharing their expertise.

I usually gave grand rounds every two or three years—on issues such as prognostication and Medicaid reform—so there were a ton of topics left to choose from when the invitation came again a few months after Cora's surgery. In light of the tension I was feeling with Dr. Williamson, dating back to our difference of opinion about the ethics of brain death, the smart move would have been to go with something safe. We could all afford to buff up on symptom management, after all, or hone our communication skills.

But every time I sat down to work on the presentation, I couldn't help but think about Cora. She was so different from the description of T18 that I'd read about in textbooks, which had made it seem like kids with that condition were empty husks simply waiting to die. But Cora was active and engaged, accumulating milestones slower than other kids but growing up nevertheless, and she was deeply beloved. She would likely die prematurely—welcome to the world of pediatric palliative care—but until she did, she seemed intent on defying the self-fulfilling prophecy I'd been taught in medical school and probably had perpetuated earlier in my career. And after the HPCCV plenary, going back to purely data-driven presentations seemed like a retreat when there were so many more important (and human) things to talk about.

I sensed my shifting perspective might not go over too well, though, with the folks who couldn't believe we were doing so much—even cardiac surgery!—for a child with a lethal anomaly. (Which, as a trenchant commentary observed, isn't "an accurate clinical description; instead, it serves to convey an implicit normative view about quality of life.") But it was a lesson I wish I'd learned long ago and worried that some people might never get the chance to. So I opened a new PowerPoint presentation with plenty of blank slides—because, unlike my recent confessional plenary, this time I'd definitely need some empirical evidence to support my conclusions—and typed the title: "Compatible with Life: The Changing Face of Trisomy 18."

When my assigned Wednesday rolled around, every seat was taken, with latecomers forced to stand along the back wall. The pediatricians—including Dr. Williamson—always attended, but that morning, they were joined by a cadre of obstetricians and genetic counselors, who diagnosed T18 prenatally and counseled pregnant patients about their options. And, of course, my ethics crew wasn't going to miss a discussion of complex decision-making.

It isn't uncommon to begin grand rounds with a clinical vignette, so I started off by describing a baby with T18 and congenital heart disease. In other words: Cora. I described my long conversations with her parents, starting soon after she was born and extending into the PICU, where she'd been coded and intubated. Joy and Bruce clearly understood her prognosis as well as the burdens of intervention, including heart surgery. But they never wavered about what they felt was in the best interests of their daughter.

"Back when I was in medical school," I continued, breaking my vow yet again as I went on to summarize what I'd been taught about T18. I mentioned all the standard terms—like "incompatible with life" and "lethal anomaly"—as well as the AAP's exceptions to newborn resuscitation that I'd relied on as a resident. I also noted that, just a few years earlier, those guidelines had been revised. Instead of listing specific trisomies, the exception was now for "some congenital malformations and chromosomal abnormalities."

"Why is that?" I wondered aloud, easing into the flow of my argument. Past the point of no return, there was nowhere to go but straight ahead.

Answering my own question, I reviewed the newer data, especially from countries that routinely provided maximal treatment and thus were not at risk of self-fulfilling prophecies. Their improved outcomes—coupled with an increased emphasis on parental authority in decision-making—were leading to changes in practice. In a recent survey, for example, nearly half of American neonatologists said they would honor a parental request for resuscitation of a newborn with T18, even when the baby also had congenital heart disease.

Clearly, not everyone agreed with this shift in practice. And I wasn't just referring to Dr. Williamson, whose pained facial expression was an indication of how little he was enjoying the grand rounds. The survey authors, in concluding their article, accused the collaborating neonatologists of "abandoning the best-interest standard . . . and instead . . . adopting an 'ethic of abdication' in their approach to difficult treatment/non-treatment decisions."

"But even if you do the initial resuscitation, there have to be limits, right?" I asked, giving voice to what some people in the auditorium must have been thinking. It's one thing to provide a little extra oxygen in the delivery room; it's quite another to do open-heart surgery on a baby with limited life expectancy. Especially when the postoperative mortality for kids with T18 was nearly triple that of other children. No wonder only 8 percent of physicians would recommend repairing a VSD for a patient with T18, with an additional 30 percent being willing to do so if the parents "want everything done."

"But," I pointed out, "even if postoperative mortality is increased, the eventual risk of death without surgery is 100 percent."

I went on to quote studies showing that if a child with T18 survived surgery, they could live for quite some time. One patient, in fact, survived for eighteen years after VSD repair.

"So what does that mean for us now?" I asked.

Even though I'd intended that as a rhetorical question, a bunch of people raised their hands. Before hearing their opinions, though, I needed to emphasize that unlike some disability rights advocates who condemned any parents who chose comfort care—as if they didn't love their kid enough to fight for her—I wasn't advocating for the pendulum to swing wildly to the other side by mandating maximal treatment for every kid with T18. Even if you acknowledged that those kids can smile and laugh and clearly be loved by their parents, it was still an incredibly difficult road to walk. How gut-wrenching must it be to continue a pregnancy when you know your child—assuming they're even born alive—will have an incurable and significantly life-shortening disease? Just because we shouldn't assume that every pregnant patient would (or should) terminate a fetus diagnosed with a trisomy, that doesn't mean some pregnant patients might not request precisely that.

"Sometimes the bravest and most loving thing parents can do," I said, thinking of Tom and Mary's premature triplets, "is hold their baby for her entire life."

Essentially, I was advocating for a middle ground that both recognized the seriousness of T18 and respected the parents' decision, whether that be to prolong life (which would trigger the Williamson crowd) or prioritize comfort (which would get me disinvited from the next SOFT convention). In support of my position, I'd provided extensive empirical data, which was expected at grand rounds but that I knew was unlikely to change people's minds if they'd been made up for a while. So I shifted to a more affective—and hopefully effective—approach.

Instead of being crammed with numbers or graphs, the next slide bore only a photo of Cora from her relatively brief time in the NICU. The one after that showed her at Boston Children's following heart surgery, which she recovered from so quickly as to evade palliative care consultation. Then came a picture taken just a few weeks earlier, of nine-month-old Cora snuggled with Joy and Bruce on the couch in their living room. The next showed an article from their small hometown newspaper that starts with a question: "What do you do when your much-anticipated baby is born with a rare genetic condition that bears a 'very grim' prognosis?"

"You celebrate that baby," Joy had responded to the reporter, "as would any other parent, while doing what you can to get the care she needs, at home and at the hospital."

My final slide just said, "Thank You," at which point even more hands shot up. But while the slides might be done, the presentation wasn't. Over the course of my career, I'd attended a lot of medical conferences, learning a lot in the process from eminent scholars and polished speakers. Since switching specialties, though, I'd discovered that palliative care conferences are different because they almost always ask patients and family members to share their experiences as part of panels or question-and-answer sessions. It didn't feel right to talk about Cora when we could talk *to* Cora, so I invited Joy—who was sitting in the back row with Cora on her lap—to join me on stage.

The raised hands fell, and the room went still as Joy carried Cora up to the front of the auditorium. It suddenly dawned on me that what might be commonplace at palliative care conferences was unheard of at grand rounds. Wednesday mornings were an opportunity for physicians to talk candidly about patients, not with them. The heavy silence led me to wonder if I'd broken some unwritten rule.

Beside me on stage and nestled in Joy's arms, Cora looked as cute as any other infant (in other words, extremely). With freshly washed hair and decked out in a frilly yellow outfit, she scanned the room of white coats with epic curiosity. She had no way of knowing, of course, that she was the topic of conversation, let alone that some of the people in the audience had forecast her demise.

I knew from personal experience that Joy was plenty capable of advocating for her daughter, but it's one thing to stand up to physicians one by one and another to do so en masse. Would she hold back, I wondered, or even freeze up, standing before a sea of white in what probably felt like enemy territory?

Any concerns I had about her being intimidated by the crowd, though, receded the moment she started to tell her story.

"We've been dealing with medical discrimination since day one," she said, going on to describe how stubborn and committed she and Bruce had needed to be in order to obtain the treatments they felt Cora deserved. "But we just keep fighting, and eventually, the doctor will throw up his hands and say, 'What's the point? She's going to die anyway.'"

Nervous laughter dappled the auditorium, as if the audience wasn't sure if that was supposed to be funny or not.

"That doesn't bother me anymore," Joy continued, unsurprised by the reaction. "I nod and think to myself: *Just give her time.*"

There was no animosity in her tone, having by that point shared Cora's story with many people. "The raw, emotional aspect," Joy likes to say, "gives more of a humanitarian touch."

She was also effusive in her praise for the wonderful care Cora had received in the NICU as well as the PICU, both in Vermont and in Boston. Those hospitalizations had provided many a medical student and resident with their first chance to meet a real-life kid with T18, who clearly wasn't what they were expecting.

When she finished, I finally invited the questions that had been pent up for the last forty-five minutes. The few that came, though, were tamer than I'd expected. I guess, even if you think kids with T18 shouldn't be resuscitated, you're probably not going to come out and say that with Cora in the room. Eventually, the novelty of doctors staring at her began to wear off, and when she started to get fussy, Joy thanked everyone and carried her outside.

Now that it was "just us" again, I braced myself for hard-hitting criticism. The "incompatible with life" contingent probably thought my approach would lead to unnecessary suffering, and the SOFT crowd that it discriminated against children with disabilities. Probably the only thing the two groups have in common is that at least they know which direction the arrows will come from, whereas I—who often refer to myself as a "conservative liberal" (i.e., left of center, but not by much)—am subject to attack from both flanks. That's probably why my mentor, Dr. Orr (who described himself as a "liberal conservative") and I got along so well: we both knew firsthand how hard it was to explore nuance.

The subsequent questions, though, were thoughtful and inquisitive, mostly about altered trajectories of illness and how our preconceptions and values can play into the recommendations we give. Some rightly observed that, while T18 survival statistics were improving and Cora's story so far seemed to have a happy ending, long-term outcomes were still sobering. Dr. Williamson never raised his hand.

The audience seemed to leave with more questions than answers, which was fine with me. If the last hour had provided updated statistics and a contrarian perspective—leading them to reconsider once-safe assumptions—then I figured I'd done my job.

#

It turns out that was not a unanimous assessment, as I learned a few days later when a colleague called to warn me that Dr. Williamson was circulating a petition protesting the grand rounds. What I'd thought of as a moderate position, he evidently viewed as giving false hope to parents in a vulnerable position. He felt even the title—"Compatible with Life"—had been misleading. (Truth be told, I'd thought the title was kind of clever, maybe even unique. Judging from identically titled articles and lectures I would see advertised in the years that followed, though, I was wrong about that, too.)

I'd been prepared for impassioned disagreement and hard-hitting questions, but I never expected anyone to classify a babbling baby as having a disease that was incompatible with life. More than merely predicting Cora's inevitable death, that seemed to imply she'd never been alive in the first place.

In Dr. Williamson's defense, it's hard to let go of something once universally accepted, which had apparently served you well in practice for many years. The data I cited came from fairly small patient samples in lesser known journals, with the definitive analysis of improved T18 outcomes not appearing in a flagship medical journal for another couple of years. That analysis was accompanied by an editorial by arguably the foremost pediatric bioethicist in the country, who made the same point I'd been trying to make, only more eloquently: "If survival rates are low but not too low, neurocognitive impairment is severe but not total, and treatment is not so burdensome as to be inhumane, then parental values should drive decisions."

Dr. Williamson ultimately managed to recruit nearly a handful of grand rounds attendees to sign his petition. (At least initially, until those, like the resident who'd felt coerced into signing something he didn't fully understand, asked for his name to be withdrawn.) The petition demanded a second grand rounds on T18—in other words, twice as many as the total number of babies born in Vermont that year who suffered from that condition—in order to set the record straight.

It's hard to describe how painful that was for me. I might have differed with Dr. Williamson on several topics, but I respected his dedication to the work and to his patients. Having felt the tension between us ever since the brain death controversy, I'd reached out to him on several occasions to clear the air, only to be rebuffed. That had left me resolved to a somewhat tense working relationship, but I never anticipated the degree of antagonism reflected by his subsequent actions.

I spent countless hours wondering why he hadn't just come to me so we could discuss the management of T18, until I realized this might not be about T18 at all. Maya Angelou famously said, "People will forget what you said, people will forget what you did, but people will never forget how you made them feel." I knew firsthand how his actions made me feel—attacked, vulnerable—and I began to wonder whether the recommendations I'd made over the years or beliefs I held had felt to him not like professional disagreement but as questioning something he held sacred. Perhaps I hadn't shed the striped referee's jersey as quickly as I needed to or as consistently as I thought.

The fact that one member of the faculty had taken it upon himself to circulate a petition critical of another member did not sit well with our department chair, who from his front row seat had been impressed by the quality of my grand rounds. But there remained the practical issue that the PACT team was a consulting service, and the only way we got involved with patients in the PICU—where, along with the NICU, hospitalized children were most likely to die—was if Dr. Williamson and his team requested our assistance. Put in transactional terms, Dr. Williamson was among the most important consumers of palliative care, and the one thing he and I could probably agree on was that he wasn't buying what I was selling.

At least about T18. And brain death. Might as well start a list.

"Just take some time away from the PICU," our chair told me, as we discussed how to respond to the petition. "Let the heat die down a bit."

He's a kindhearted person and—having previously recognized the emotional toll the work was taking on me—wanted on some level to protect me. There may also have been some degree of conflict avoidance at play, which I knew from personal experience often accompanies kindheartedness. That would explain why, when I expressed my intention to invite Dr. Williamson and any remaining petitioners to join me in some honest and direct dialogue, my chair requested that I not force the matter.

"Just wait and see if the grand rounds comes up organically in conversation," he said.

Not surprisingly, it didn't. If Dr. Williamson had been willing to talk to me, he wouldn't have needed a petition.

This was the second instance of my stepping back from a conflictual situation, and it worked about as well as the sabbatical had with Dr. Danvers. Such an action can potentially defuse situations when tempers are running high but only when both sides seek reconciliation. In situations where only one party—me, in this case—does, the other party might reasonably view the stepping back as a retreat and a validation of the behavior that prompted that retreat. Subsequent reengagement won't be met with a cooler head and a hand of friendship but rather with entrenchment. It doesn't take a pediatrician to recognize that; any parent of a toddler will tell you the same thing.

Somebody else might have been able to brush off Dr. Williamson's petition as inevitable workplace conflict. After all, who doesn't have someone in their life that they don't get along with? My past, though, made it impossible for me to just accept that and go about my business. Like many survivors of child sexual abuse, threats (especially those unexpected and undeserved) provoke anxiety and hypervigilance in me. Certain aspects of the hospital environment may have long felt unfulfilling—like the lack of resources dedicated to pediatric palliative care and the indirect communication that Dr. Danvers favored—but now it was also beginning to feel unsafe. With patients and families, I could trust that if I said the wrong thing, they'd give me the benefit of the doubt because my intentions were good. (Just as Collin's father had after my infamous "hang in there" comment.) But now, at work,

I worried that I would be judged even if I said the right thing, as I believe I had at grand rounds.

I know all too well what it's like when a place that's supposed to epitomize safety comes to represent the very opposite. And while I would never equate professional squabbles at the hospital with the trauma I endured in my childhood, thematic parallels do exist, and often, that's all it takes to awaken memory and set your soul on guard. I'd already spent too many years feeling threatened to endure any more.

My almost primal reaction was to shut down and cover up, like a wounded boxer on the ropes, just as I had as a child. No longer confident of a shared purpose among colleagues, I started rereading emails three or more times before sending because if a thoughtful (though contrarian) grand rounds could provoke such outcry, how much more so might an email fragment lifted out of context? I became more tentative in recommending treatment plans based on identified patient goals, especially when the consulting doctor was expecting me to get the DNR. And I began to wonder whether Dr. Williamson might actually be right: maybe I was siding too much with patients and parents. Sure, things were working out okay (so far) for Cora, but someone like Collin might have suffered less if I hadn't allied with his parents in advocating for a transplant.

I also got back into therapy, which had been a lifeline years earlier when I first acknowledged the abuse I'd suffered. I held on extra tight to my people, like Sally and Dr. Orr. And I looked forward months in advance to annual meetings of palliative care groups, whether grand like the American Academy of Hospice and Palliative Medicine—which rotated to different parts of the country each year—or homespun like the Hospice and Palliative Care Council of Vermont, which always gathered at the historic inn by the lake. I inevitably returned from those meetings energized and encouraged by the company of kindred spirits as well as acutely aware that the next one wouldn't roll around again for a year. The fact that I felt so much more accepted and valued by palliative care colleagues beyond the walls of my institution—where I'd always dreamed of spending my entire career—made me wonder, for the first time, if there was someplace else I needed to be.

Despite all the steps I took, I still couldn't protect myself. When I was a kid, I cultivated the ability to dissociate on cue (which, in that case, was the opening click of the door to my darkened bedroom). But as sensation returned, the on/off feeling switch stopped working. Upon leaving the room of a patient who was suffering or dying, I couldn't instantly raise protective barriers against hallway collisions or accusations of providing false hope. The emotions were too strong, the reality undeniable. More than once, as I felt overwhelmed by vulnerability, I found myself thinking, *Wow, I could really use some good soul calluses right about now.*

I sometimes wonder what would have happened if I'd talked about something less contentious at grand rounds. To be sure, I would have hurt a lot less in the days (and weeks and months) that followed, but I don't think the ultimate outcome would have changed. My approach to palliative care—which involved bending rules (and boundaries) when they seemed arbitrary and unhelpful, prioritizing spiritual care, and sometimes aligning with parents around goals that I wasn't sure we could achieve—was too different from what Dr. Williamson was looking for. It was probably only a matter of time before I did or said something that prompted him to start soliciting signatures.

But even if taking the safe road for grand rounds could have spared me some pain, it wouldn't have been worth it. The audience that morning saw a side of T18 that medical school doesn't teach or at least didn't when I was a student. The next time they encountered a patient with that condition, the terms "lethal anomaly" or "incompatible with life" hopefully wouldn't come to mind and certainly not out of their mouths. Instead, they'd see a curious and beautiful little girl who might not be able to do everything that other kids could but clearly could do far more than anyone (aside from her parents) predicted she'd ever be able to.

That girl is now eleven years old, and her life has not been without its ups and downs, including some health scares and hospitalizations. She is adored by many, though, especially her parents and teachers.

Her classmates, too, one of whom happens to have tetrasomy 18—meaning that he has *four* copies of that chromosome—which I didn't even know existed. And here I thought you couldn't one-up trisomy 18.

Cora has since become a big sister, with one of her favorite pastimes being yanking little Becca's hair. And as the only person with trisomy 18 in the entire state of Iowa—where her family eventually moved—she continues to educate medical students and doctors about her condition with the humanitarian touch that facts and figures can't convey.

"Cora's accomplished more in her life than I could ever hope to," Joy mused recently, as we reminisced about that memorable grand rounds when Cora stole the show.

And more than I could ever hope to, either.

Chapter 11

The very best of friends

Before that night, I didn't know that your whole life could change in the middle of a bedtime story.

This one didn't come from a book because my so-called "mixed-up stories" are something of a family tradition. And they all come with three guarantees. First, I always start with an alliterative protagonist, ranging over the years from Peter the Platypus to—one night when I was really desperate—Ebenezer the Envelope. Second, I promise to incorporate whatever my listeners suggest, which the kids take as a challenge to come up with the most bizarre characters and nonsensical events, which may be utterly incompatible with everything that came before. And finally, the twisty and often ludicrous tale always ends with, "And they all lived happily ever after."

On that January night, the sole listener was our youngest child, Charlotte, age four, who was curled up next to me on the king size bed in our master bedroom. Some months had passed since the fateful grand rounds, during which I'd tried to make peace with a work situation that I now realized would never feel truly supportive and safe but that at least allowed me to do what I felt called to. Occasionally, there were glimmers of hope like Dr. Danvers's recent decision—stemming from her ongoing frustration at what she considered insufficient funding for the adult palliative care program—to take a job at a distant institution. Almost immediately, the hospital hallways began to feel more spacious.

A leader's departure often precipitates change. In this case, the hospital decided to consolidate the adult and pediatric teams. Having advocated for years to keep pediatrics separate, I still worried that kids were going to get overlooked. But with the decision having been made, I tried to focus on the positive. Perhaps Dr. Danvers's departure represented a fresh opportunity for community closer to home. No matter how meaningful, conversations with trusted colleagues at the occasional regional or national meeting weren't going to be enough to sustain me in doing such intense work.

— Christopher —

Cha-Cha (as she preferred to be called then) was none too pleased when a ringing phone interrupted the remarkable adventures of Ahmed the Acorn, but I assured her that the only folks who called that late were telemarketers. This would just take a second.

Picking up the handset, I was surprised to see the caller ID reading "Christopher White." He rarely called after nine, which, in Vermont, counts as late. Usually, he'd appear in person, just as our family was sitting down to dinner. Hearing a baritone "Hey you guys!" from the direction of the mudroom, one of the kids would automatically set out another plate. Then Christopher would wander in and, before pulling up a chair, slap my chest three times with an open palm and a hearty "Roberto!"

He was my best friend, and I mean that literally. I'd had other best friends at different stages of my life: elementary school, high school, med school. But inevitably, they faded into the background due to geographic distance or life developments or people simply changing over time. A therapist/friend of mine is wont to say that friendships aren't meant to last forever, but that never stopped me from hoping that they would. Until Christopher, they never had.

Witty and serious and faithful and real, he was like a brother to me. He was the kind of person you could watch really bad movies with (although his taste had, annoyingly, begun to evolve, enduring each successive *Sharknado* film more out of fraternal duty than macabre interest in just how low the franchise could go). Once the closing credits rolled, we'd debrief over much better beer, quickly moving on from the film to things that a lot of guys don't talk about: feelings, faith, family, fears. He's the kind of person who didn't just offer condolences after my father died. Instead, he offered to come with me to the memorial—six months later and hundreds of miles away—if only to watch the kids or drive the car or make it the tiniest bit easier.

We both grew up in wealthy, suburban Connecticut—six years apart, our high schools separated by the same number of miles—and contravened expectations in different ways. Instead of focusing on money, he became a Waldorf teacher and then a custom carpenter while I rebelled by moving to small-town Vermont where flannel was more relevant than status. We were also both totally devoted to our large families: his three girls were like a second trio of daughters to me, and my kids knew him as "the godfather," although it came out more like "gawdfathuh" in his awful Marlon Brando impression.

While Cha-Cha pouted over having to wait for the next twist in Ahmed's saga, I pressed the Talk button. "Hey, what's up?"

Not much, I assumed, since only two nights before I'd treated him to a blowout steak dinner to celebrate his fifty-fourth birthday.

Except it wasn't Christopher on the phone.

"There's been an emergency," his youngest daughter, Hailey, age fifteen, said breathlessly. "Dad's on the floor, and Mom's doing CPR on him. The ambulance is on the way."

The next thing I remember is saying "fuck" in front of Charlotte for the only time in my life. Then throwing on a pair of jeans and sprinting to the car, barely forming words to yell to Pam where I was going and why.

It's normally a solid twenty-minute drive from my house to his, but that night, I made it in a fraction of that. I wish I could say I prayed on the drive over there, but I didn't. I yelled: "No! No! No!"

There were also a few "This can't be happening" and the odd "Please don't let this happen," which I guess comes close to a prayer.

By the time I reached Christopher's house, the ambulance was already there. Sarah, his eighteen-year-old middle daughter, met me at the front door. Struggling not to hyperventilate, she pointed me down the hallway where one paramedic was doing chest compressions and the other was ramming an intraosseous needle into Christopher's shin, even as his wife, Karen, held his hand and whispered to him to stay with us because it wasn't his time to go. There was nothing for me to do except hug Sarah, encouraging her to breathe a little more slowly.

After the paramedics loaded Christopher's stretcher into the ambulance, Karen went with him. She knew I'd bring the girls, who were both in shock—up until an hour ago their dad had been in perfect health—and reacting in entirely different and surprising ways as we got in the car. I knew Sarah to be brilliant and fiercely independent, yet she was struggling to calm down enough to call their older sister, Anna, at college, while I rubbed her back with my free hand. From the backseat, Hailey, who was known for her silly sense of humor and breaking random bones in freak accidents, asked practical questions about what they should expect in the hospital, which I tried unsuccessfully to answer.

After pulling into the ER parking lot, I settled Sarah and Hailey in the corner of the waiting room and ran toward the trauma bay. There, a resident was performing CPR while nurses hurriedly drew up more meds.

"Stop compressions," the ER doc, Mario, ordered as Karen came over and hugged me.

"No pulse!" the resident called out.

"Then shock him again," Mario said, before turning to me. Introductions weren't necessary since we'd taught classes at the med school together. "That's number seven, along with several rounds of epi and amiodarone."

I nodded, trying to process what I was seeing. The fruits of my prayers in the car.

As the resident searched for any signs of a pulse, Mario whispered, "His pupils are fixed and dilated," which I knew meant that Christopher's brain stem was damaged from lack of oxygen.

"Still nothing," the resident said, resuming CPR without Mario needing to tell him to.

Even if he wasn't my best friend, nobody wants to make the decision to stop CPR on a healthy person in his fifties with three kids, with no explanation for why his heart had stopped. So I started to rationalize. Karen had run downstairs as soon as she'd heard a loud thud, starting CPR the instant she discovered his body slumped on the floor. The paramedics had responded promptly. A recent study had found that the longer CPR goes on, the better the chance of getting the heart beating again.

But we'd already gone way past what that study referred to as "prolonged CPR." And even if no one understood why this was happening—a massive heart attack was the most likely diagnosis—all that really mattered was that it was happening.

I felt like everyone was looking at me, which made sense. I was the director of ethics, after all. And a palliative care doc, who would certainly appreciate what fixed pupils after so many shocks meant. And who happened to know the patient as well as anybody. What more could you want in a decision-maker?

In a perverse way, it almost felt like a gift from God.

Except that you're supposed to watch movies and drink beer with your best friend, talk about your families and be there when he needs you, not tell his doctors to stop trying to save his life.

#

Time of death: 10:07 p.m.

That's what Mario declared after I said yes, we should stop. It was no longer a question of if Christopher would die; it was a matter of when he had died and when we'd bring ourselves to accept that.

Was I really telling a story to Cha-Cha an hour ago?

You might think that, my soul calluses having thinned and softened, the flood of feelings would have drowned me. But numbness can be the result of overwhelming emotion as well as the lack of it, and I had extensive experience in deferring personal collapse while there was still work to be done. Consider it the soul equivalent of muscle memory, and thankfully, it kicked in because there was a lot left to do.

Someone needed to tell Sarah and Hailey, but Karen wasn't about to leave Christopher's side. (I still can't bear to write, "Christopher's body.") So I forced myself to walk out to the waiting room, which seemed larger than I'd remembered. It felt like Sarah and Hailey—who momentarily resembled the preschoolers they were when I'd first met them—were floating adrift in the midst of a vast ocean.

There were several family rooms specifically designed for conversations like the one I needed to have, but that night, they were already occupied. The only private space I could find was a hallway to the neighboring wing with industrial carpet that's impervious to the passage of time. Hailey, already sensing what was going on, nodded expectantly as I summarized all the efforts to resuscitate Christopher, simultaneously assuring them that everything had been tried and preparing them for what I had to say next. Yet, even when broken by a professional, bad news can still be soul-crushing. When I finally used the D-word, Sarah crumpled onto the carpet whose pattern was designed to hide every stain. Sobbing, she kept shouting that this couldn't be happening, giving voice to what I was feeling inside.

I knelt down beside her and didn't even try to explain or offer words of comfort, as her cries of injustice—an almost palpable grief—filled the space. Eventually, Hailey and I helped her to her feet and walked on each side of her to the trauma bay, where we would spend the next five hours letting reality sink in, its razor edge cutting deeper with each passing minute.

Sarah went straight to the stretcher, gently lifting Christopher's head and cradling it in her lap, her only movement over the following hours being tenderly stroking his brow. Hailey sat in a chair in the corner of the room, staring blankly into space and crying a little with many more tears to come. Karen oscillated between wife and mother, her mourning for her husband interrupted only by the requisite phone calls to Christopher's dad and brothers, where she tried to describe the unfathomable. And we all worried about Anna, who was racing back from college—thankfully, her roommate had taken the wheel—and knew only that her dad had been taken to the hospital.

Unable to put it off any longer, I picked up the trauma bay phone and dialed Pam.

"He's gone," I said softly.

She'd been praying ever since I dashed out of the house, which seemed like days ago. She didn't ask any questions because I'd just answered the only one that mattered. She just started weeping, and I didn't know what else to say. I hadn't known what to say since a ringing phone interrupted Ahmed the Acorn's adventures.

Over the next few hours, I did whatever I could to help. Conversant in the ways of the hospital—and having some experience in getting patients transported back home after they die (like we did with Hope from the NICU)—I helped arrange that for Christopher, as it was a family tradition to sit vigil with the body for several days. I also ran interference for Karen and the girls when it came to good intentions, like the nurse administrator who wanted to offer a prayer that the family was *so* not ready for. Mostly, I tried to think ahead, like by removing the IV in Christopher's arm and the intraosseous needle from his shin. Used to putting those things in, I never realized how much they bleed when you take them out.

The rest of the time, I just held his hand as it got progressively colder and stiffer. Had it not been for that, I would have been tempted to believe he was sleeping, a not uncommon sight for someone who loved his afternoon naps. More than once, we'd shifted from the early show to the late to accommodate a brief lie-down before he hopped in his truck, drove over to my house, and squeezed a lime into his dark 'n stormy while I did the same for my gin and tonic. Then we'd nosh a few pistachios before heading into Burlington, which in Vermont counts as the big city despite a population of barely 40,000.

Anna arrived a little before midnight. Of all the girls, she'd had the most struggles so far in life and was also the most like Christopher (which explained why they butted heads not infrequently). That night, though, she was remarkably composed, the drive affording time to prepare herself for what, in her heart, she sensed she'd find. It was the first glimpse I had of the woman she'd become, overcoming obstacle after obstacle: dropping her nursing major in the midst of her grief over Christopher's death only to return to it later, eventually becoming a nurse, even returning to teach at her old college. And her specialty? Wouldn't you know, palliative care, with more perspective and empathy than most medical professionals twice her age.

The funeral home director arrived at two in the morning, around the same time as Christopher's younger brother. Together, we shifted Christopher over to the funeral home stretcher, and the director pulled the sheet up over his face, making everything seem more real. Not totally real, just more.

The only thing left in the trauma bay was his moth-eaten navy blue fleece, which he'd worn on so many of our boys' nights and which his head had rested on during the resuscitation. It didn't feel right to leave it behind, and I didn't think anybody would care if I kept it, while I cared a whole lot. A decade later, I still wear it all the time.

Not a single word passed between Anna and Sarah and me, as I drove the dark country roads toward their house. (Anna's college roommate and Hailey had decided to stay at ours.) We arrived before the hearse, and I asked the girls to wait in the car. The home I'd visited so many times for family dinners and birthday celebrations was littered with the detritus of resuscitation. I hurriedly collected the used latex gloves and empty syringes scattered on the floor beneath smiling family photos, struck by the dissonant blend of trauma and everyday life.

After the hearse arrived, the funeral director, Christopher's brother, and I moved Christopher onto the bed in the guestroom, which was closest to the entry hall. I wish I could say he looked peaceful, as if he'd reached the end of a long, brave struggle. But he just looked still, like a movie frozen at a random moment due to a scratched DVD, with a character in mid-sentence and no good reason why he shouldn't be allowed to finish what he'd been saying. Gently crying, Karen crawled into bed next to him.

A few hours earlier, I'd covered the distance to his house in record time, but the return drive took longer than usual. I was in no hurry to reach my destination because, after telling his three kids that their father had died, now I had to tell my four that "the gawdfathuh" was gone.

How many people have you told that someone they loved as much as anyone in the whole world has died? Probably not many, or maybe even none. If so, I'm happy for you. I really am.

I, on the other hand, was accumulating some serious experience in this area. And it sucked.

#

A few hours after a tall scotch hadn't done much to help me sleep, the sun rose. After gently rousing my kids, I asked them to sit on the couch in the family room. Pulling up a chair facing them, I could see they knew what was coming. If not from the pieces of information they already had—me racing out the door the previous night because an ambulance was called for Christopher and now being kept home from school—then from the look on my face.

They responded the way the textbooks say kids of their ages do: Catie (age eleven) wept silently, surrounded on one side by Lucy (seven) who looked like she was struggling to figure out just how she should feel—until I told her there was no right answer to that question—and Noah (nine) on the other, who cried the hardest. Of Christopher's and my seven kids, he was the only boy, and there was a unique connection there. Charlotte, by far the youngest, vacillated between sorrow, confusion, and impatience.

After a brief family prayer, the rest of the day was a jumble of sleeping, random chores that were more distraction than obligation, and mostly letting everyone do what they needed to do. For Noah, that was playing Nintendo while Catie leafed through family scrapbooks in which Christopher was pictured prominently. With nobody left for me to break soul-crushing news to, no interference to run, and no gut-wrenching decisions to make, I wasn't sure what was left. I actually longed for something (no matter how awful) to do, anything to fill the gaping and expanding void that Christopher's death had left.

When night finally fell, Cha-Cha asked me what ended up happening to Ahmed the Acorn. Despite my solemn vow to incorporate whatever came next into my stories—even if it was totally incompatible with everything that had come before—I couldn't bear to. This time there'd be no happily ever after for any of us.

"Would you like to hear," I said slowly, well aware of how important structure is to kids that age, "the story of Glowy the Glowing Wormball?"

As I launched into what was probably the least creative story I've ever told, I glanced over at the phone, tensed for it to ring. It was hard to imagine that anything could be worse than the previous night, but "At least it can't get any worse"—while intended to offer a morsel of reassurance—sounds a lot like a dare, which the universe has been known to take people up on.

#

Over the next few days, the kids eventually returned to school and I to work, although the deep ache of sadness pervaded any semblance of normalcy. I was well aware that sudden and unexpected death is more likely to cause complicated grief—as if some kinds of grief aren't complicated—but without soul calluses to shield me from the loss of my best friend, my grief was practically Gordian. My doctor-brain ticked off each associated symptom as it popped up: unrelenting sadness, insomnia, withdrawal from social interactions. My wife just says that something changed in me after Christopher died.

My ethics colleagues were wonderfully supportive. Most of them had met Christopher—perhaps at one of our kids' baptisms or a barbecue at our house—and they knew how much he meant to me. Sally and Dr. Orr are the kind of folks who don't ask, "What can I do for you?" They know that puts the onus on the grieving person and allows politeness to get in the way. They just go ahead and do stuff for you, for which I was immensely grateful.

One of the members of the newly combined palliative care team also expressed her condolences, while the rest kept plugging away at their work. I guess when you live in a world of bereavement, sometimes you don't notice a slight uptick in the population. It's not like I taped a "Lost: Best Friend" poster with Christopher's photo to my office door.

But what I did do, perhaps for the first time, was intentionally wrestle with the proverbial elephant in the room, which readers of this book have probably been wondering about since cracking it open.

Why?

Why do kids who never did anything close to deserving it die before they have a chance to really live their lives? And why, to a metaphysically lesser but personally just-as-great degree, did Christopher die when he had a whole lot more fathering—and, one day, grandfathering—and godfathering and husbanding and friending left to do? Like about three decades worth.

That's the million dollar question, isn't it? And who better to answer it, you might reasonably wonder, than a priest who also happens to be a physician that takes care of dying kids? Even better, one who wrote his master's thesis on the "problem of evil" and therefore is well-versed in the so-called "Free Will Defense," which says it's better for people to have free will and make mistakes than to be compelled only to do good.

You have to really love free will, though, for it to justify what people like Hitler and Stalin did. But you can't even try to pin the kind of evil I deal with on bad decisions or human failings. The chromosome that didn't let go as its partner tried to split off into a sperm or ovum of its own—causing a trisomy in the process—wasn't afraid to be alone. The cancer cell that reproduced uncontrollably wasn't some rebellious spirit who yearned to be free. The only person to blame for those and so many other diseases is the one who created an incredibly complex system that works miraculously well most—but definitely not all—of the time. And who for some reason chooses not to intervene when things go terribly wrong.

One thing I know for sure is that, if I were God, there are a lot of things I'd do differently. Some are lighthearted, like having hot fudge sundaes be super nutritious. Others are petty, like having Duke get upset in the first round of the NCAA basketball tournament every single year. But the first and most important thing I'd do is make sure that kids didn't suffer and definitely didn't die. What good is omnipotence if you can't even do that?

So to the million-dollar question of "why?" the best answer I've come up with—with three graduate degrees in theology from places like Oxford and Yale, followed by three decades as a physician-priest—is

In other words, I don't know. I don't know why God lets such terrible things happen, which even someone as tragically flawed as me would make absolutely sure to prevent, given a pinch of omnipotence and a nanosecond to act.

That admission might reasonably prompt someone to wonder, "So how do you love a God like that, who just watches people suffer?"

To which I'd respond: "You're asking the wrong question."

God had never been my motivation to do this work, but up until Christopher died, God had been my reassurance. Not that there was some noble purpose to the suffering of children—let alone that it had some redemptive quality, a position that long overlooked or even legitimized intense pain, usually of extremely vulnerable people—but that at least they would find balm and welcome one day. It was comforting to believe that someone a whole lot more powerful and beneficent than me was looking out for them. But now, loving God was beginning to feel like a distraction from the important work left to do (like helping kids not suffer as they died).

That's not to say that losing that reassurance—which had provided a sliver of hope on the worst days—wasn't a huge blow. It was. One that I'd have to process at some point, just not right away. Here it should be noted that I'm far from the first ostensibly religious person to struggle with the whole "loving God" thing. St. Teresa of Avila, for example, famously prayed: "Oh God, I don't love you, I don't even want to love you, but I want to want to love you." And she seems to have turned out fine: declared not only a saint but one of only thirty-six "doctors of the church" in Roman Catholic history.

I was never in danger of being declared that kind of doctor, though, because, for a long time after Christopher's death, I didn't even want to want to love God. I just wanted, in those candid moments when I paused long enough to reflect on the state of my heart, to stop hating God.

Language like that might come as a surprise, seeing as I'm a priest and thus supposedly God's representative. But while I (mostly tongue-in-cheek) asked you not to tell my bishop about my willingness to ignore the baptism requirement before marrying Harry and Carrie—or how I liberally modified the baptismal rite for pretty much

Rider's entire family—please feel free to go ahead and tell anyone you want about this priest who was trying not to hate God. Because, after watching kids (and friends) die, I definitely wasn't going to fall back on platitudes falsely attributed to Scripture—like "everything happens for a reason," which was actually coined by Marilyn Monroe and which real theologians like Kate Bowler have properly skewered—or blithely recite actual Bible verses like, "All things work together for good for those who love God." (And is there any way to recite such a verse to a grieving person other than blithely?) That would seem more the role of God's consigliere, which I want no part of.

Fortunately, there were parts of the Bible that still resonated with me. Like the psalms of lament, which blame God for the plight of the world or at least the state of the psalmist's own life. Okay, so maybe those aren't the best-known verses in the Bible (and I doubt you'll see the guy who holds up the John 3:16 sign at NFL games switch it out anytime soon for Lamentations 3:43, which reads, "You [God] have covered yourself with anger and pursued us; you have slain without pity"). That's actually a pretty common biblical sentiment, though, with laments making up nearly a third of the longest book in the Bible. Jesus himself quoted one of them as he neared death on the cross, in words that every bereaved parent I know can relate to:

> *My God, my God, why have you forsaken me?*
> *Why are you so far from saving me,*
> *from the words of my groaning?*
> *O my God, I cry by day, but you do not answer,*
> *and by night, I find no rest.*

At first, after Christopher died, I didn't pray at all, suspecting that God wasn't ready to hear what I had to say. But then I figured, "Hey, if Jesus said those words, why can't I?" So I went ahead and let loose, raging against the suffering inflicted on people I loved, which many Christians placidly accept by claiming that it must be God's will or else it wouldn't have happened that way. I truly don't understand that response because losing one's kid is the cruelest thing that I can imagine, and it deserves to be named as such in clear—and impolite—terms. Something along the lines of, "With all due respect, God, you're doing a shitty job of taking care of your children."

The way I figured it, if there really was a God out there—the sort that I was willing to believe in, not the callous and condemning variety that I'd been taught about in school—then God could take what I had to give, knowing it flowed from a broken heart. This wasn't some petty bitterness arising out of a transactional faith, where I gave God what God wanted (such as piety and contrition) and expected to have every last wish granted in return. This was about children dying. And if I didn't walk away from God after everything I (and the people I loved) had gone through, then God better damn well not walk away from me just for shooting straight.

And the simple fact that I still had *anything* to say to God meant that I hadn't turned my back on faith entirely. Having grown up in a family that was so conflict-averse that the rugs in our house practically levitated from all the hurt feelings swept under them, it took me a long time to realize that a few harsh and honest words were a stronger sign of relationship than a slew of polite ones, or even silence. As Elie Wiesel once said, "The opposite of love is not hate; it's indifference."

That is why, when parents of seriously ill children confess that they're angry at God and ask for advice about how to stop feeling that way, my reply often comes as a surprise: "Why stop?" I go on to observe that feelings are never wrong; they're just where you find yourself at the moment, so rather than changing them, the most we can hope for is to figure out what to do with them. I might also mention the good company that parent is in, from Jesus on down. But mostly, I try to reframe their question because, if any comfort is to be found in the midst of anger, it's not in trying to explain why God permits suffering but in appreciating that God knows how it feels to suffer.

That's a far cry from the God I was indoctrinated in as a child, who was more focused on a pound of flesh than an ounce of mercy. But thankfully, I went on to encounter thinkers who showed me a different side of God (or perhaps, a different god entirely). The great Jewish theologian, Abraham Heschel, movingly describes the divine *pathos*, where God doesn't just hear but suffers with the Hebrew prophets as they cry out, "O Lord, how long shall I cry for help, and thou wilt not hear?" Raised to believe that Jesus was sacrificed to appease the demands of a rigid and aloof God, it was a revelation for me to hear the Reformed theologian Jurgen Möltmann say that "in the suffering of Christ, God himself suffers." Which might hold out some hope to bereaved mothers and fathers, if not for answers, then at least companionship because "a parent losing a child" is a pretty apt description of the Christian salvation narrative.

That sense of companionship in grief didn't make all the pain go away, but at least it helped me feel less alone. Faithwise, I still felt mired in a haze of anger and confusion, but thankfully, there were occasional glimpses of something worth clinging to, like on those rare Sundays when I forced myself to go to church. The prayers seemed rote and the creeds primeval, but if I could just endure the words that no longer made sense, at the end, I'd get to reach across the altar rail, shoulder-to-shoulder with friends and strangers, for something our souls desperately needed, even if we weren't sure exactly what that was.

And if I was really lucky, the organist might play a favorite hymn, the familiar notes somehow skirting the swirl of doubt in my brain and directly penetrating my heart. Sometimes it felt like a heavenly chorus was transporting me back to simpler times, before the losses piled up and the childhood memories resurfaced. Reminding me why I came to faith in the first place and felt called to be a priest.

Especially so for the hymn that filled the cathedral the day I was ordained, which has always brought tears to my eyes. Back then, it was the familiar early verses—which are set against the dominant melody and wax poetic about binding unto oneself everything from the "sun's life-giving ray" to the "whirling wind's tempestuous shocks"—that spoke to me. Now, though, my soul gravitates to the sixth verse, an outlier in the midst of grandeur, where the music temporarily becomes simpler and the words more intimate, jettisoning flowery language to get right down to what a wounded soul needs to hear:

> *Christ beneath me, Christ above me,*
> *Christ in quiet, Christ in danger,*
> *Christ in hearts of all that love me,*
> *Christ in mouth of friend and stranger.*

Those words are so contrary to the reality I see in my life and work that the fact I'm even tempted to believe them makes me wonder if they might actually be true. Beautiful as they are, though, they still don't explain why we sometimes lose the people we love. There has to be something more, which, hopefully, I'll discover someday.

I still pray, though not as often I once did and not nearly as politely. When I read the Bible, it's less to conform—or perhaps "contort" is a better word—to whatever the text says but rather to grapple and sometimes reject and occasionally rage. That's engagement, though. That's still a relationship with God or at least the willingness to consider one.

The way I see it, leaving a blank page is less an admission of defeat than a meager sign of faith, daring to hope that there really is an answer out there, even if I haven't found it yet.

#

Christopher's memorial service took place about a week later in a packed sanctuary with panoramic windows looking out over Lake Champlain. After a few other close friends offered their remembrances, I opened mine with a concept that everyone there was familiar with: "Christopher time." He was perpetually late for everything, which is why, when he had the temerity one year to arrive punctually at our house for Christmas dinner—catching us when we assumed we had a solid half hour left to finish meal prep—it seemed almost rude. The only time he was ever early was when you needed him, like Noah's seventh birthday party when the horde of second graders had grown bored with *The Empire Strikes Back*, which was supposed to keep them occupied until cake and presents. Just when I'd run out of game ideas (as well as patience), "the godfather" miraculously appeared and filled the vacuum with lightsaber battles and Yoda-inspired scavenger hunts.

I could have gone on for hours with Christopher stories, but I didn't just want to talk about him. I needed to talk *with* him, as if he were still here with us, which, in many ways, it felt as if he was. I informed him that I was now officially a University of Virginia fan, not because it was his father's alma mater or because their basketball team happened to be undefeated at the moment—although that helped—but in honor of his faded Cavaliers cap (which I pulled out of my back pocket and proceeded to don) that he'd forgotten at our house so often that it came to feel like communal property. I also promised to trade in my beloved gin and tonics for his signature dark 'n stormy and vowed never again to use bottled lime juice (which he considered sacrilege).

Then I turned to Anna, Sarah, and Hailey, acutely aware that Christopher and I had spent a lot of time talking about him taking care of my kids if I was gone—that's the worst-case-scenario part of my personality coming out, although subsequent events would prove that I lacked sufficient imagination—but never about the reverse. Until that moment.

Looking into their tear-streaked faces, I told them I recognized that they weren't my kids, but I loved them as if they were. And I would always try to be there for them, whether it was giving advice, showing up at graduations, or making damn sure that prospective suitors treated them with honor and respect. They smiled at that, well aware of my long-stated plan—intended to compensate for my pathological niceness—of breaking out full clerical attire when greeting my daughters' future dates at the door, and inviting (okay, *ordering*) them to sit on the tiny plastic stepstool that my kids used to use to reach the silverware drawer so that I would loom over them as I demanded to know if their intentions were honorable.

I especially wanted Christopher to hear that last bit because I like to think I'll see him again in the same way that Daniel and Miriam dream of seeing Lily. If there really is a heaven—which sometimes I just have to believe in to make it through the hardest of days—it must be populated by the people we love who went before us. I'll look for him as soon as I arrive. I like to think he'll find me first, and I'll answer his most pressing question before he even has the chance to ask it.

"I took good care of them," I hope I'll be able to say.

I finished up with a quote from *Top Gun,* which even Christopher had deemed too awful to watch, let alone re-watch as many times as I have. The quote comes after Tom Cruise's copilot, Goose, is killed in a plane crash.

"God, he loved flying with you, Maverick," Goose's widow says to Tom Cruise. "But he'd have flown anyway, without you. He'd have hated it, but he would have done it."

I tipped my Cavaliers cap to the heavens and said, "I loved flying with you, man. You're the best friend I ever had. The best friend I'll *ever* have. And I will always, always miss you."

People sometimes talk about funerals bringing closure, which sounds so neat and clean. As if this were some proper conclusion, equal parts inevitable and satisfying. But as I left the sanctuary, there was only a terrible sense of an ending. I couldn't believe this was goodbye.

#

I feel like I just broke a rule. This book was supposed to be about families facing the serious illness of a child, with my story serving merely as a scaffold to provide narrative structure. But in devoting an entire chapter to the loss of a friend, however dear, it might seem like I'm equating my own grief to that of bereaved parents.

So I need to be absolutely clear: if this were a competition about whose suffering is greater—and what a terrible competition that would be—bereaved parents would "win" hands down. They've had enough sorrow for a million lifetimes, which is why many people aren't sure what to say to someone who's lost a child. To which I respond, as an experienced palliative care physician, "Join the club." Grief—especially the raw kind that bereaved parents say never heals—is scary and unnerving. There's no magic incantation that will make it better, let alone go away.

But even if there's no one right thing to say, there are a few wrong things, like, "Hang in there," even if you see that on a kid's T-shirt in the ICU or overhear a supposed palliative care expert blurt that out in a desperate moment. And vapid aphorisms like, "God needed another angel in heaven," because who'd even want to speak to—let alone hang out forever with—a god who'd take a kid away from their family because of their own needs? And if you start a sentence with "But at least . . ." you probably shouldn't finish it, because any attempt to draw some measure of goodness out of a child's death is doomed to fail.

The mother of all things you shouldn't say, though, is, "I know how you feel." Don't ever say that, because you don't, and trust me, you don't want to. My soul is singed just by coming near what bereaved parents are experiencing. But I do think, especially after Christopher died, that I know how "it" feels, if by "it" you mean losing someone you love. And I'm pretty sure bereaved parents wouldn't mind my saying that because every one I know has a deep river of empathy carved into their soul for anybody who's in pain of whatever duration or degree. Their concern is not that everyone else acknowledge the superiority of their suffering but simply that suffering itself be stopped or at least lessened a little bit, if not their own, then other people's.

While you wouldn't think I'd need yet another reminder of the cruel unpredictability of life—which is practically the *raison d'être* of pediatric palliative care—Christopher's sudden death prompted me not to leave anything important unsaid. That's why, soon after the funeral, I wrote a very long letter to my ninety-four-year-old mother, listing all the things I appreciated about her. Okay, maybe not all—that would have required multiple volumes—but the ones that leapt to mind, ranging from hitting me countless grounders in the backyard until I finally grew brave enough to get my body in front of the baseball, to accepting my friends without any judgment and my past girlfriends with only a little, and (after I left home) mailing me newspaper or magazine clippings that she thought I'd find interesting, which I often did but always appreciated her thinking of me more.

I have absolutely no doubt that, if she'd ever had even an inkling of what I was enduring as a child, she would have intervened immediately to stop it, which is why I never told her about the memories that were gradually returning. (And why I only started writing this book after she had died.) History can't be rewritten, and there's already enough regret in the world without piling more on the people you love the most.

I also treated Dr. Orr to lunch at the same Indian restaurant across the street from the hospital, where, fifteen years earlier, he'd persuaded the chair of the ethics committee to take a chance on some young doc who'd written out of the blue, asking for a job. It was remarkable to think back to how many stars needed to align for me to get where I was that day: if a drought hadn't cut short Pam's and my kayak trip or if someone else at the B&B had hogged the one copy of the *Burlington Free Press* or if the editors hadn't chosen that precise day to print an editorial on the ethics of feeding tubes, who knows where Pam and I would have ended up or what job I'd be doing. Without Dr. Orr, I wouldn't have even known there was such a thing as a clinical ethicist—let alone become one on the way to focusing on palliative care—or found a home in Vermont.

I was pretty sure he knew how much his friendship, counsel, and being "Grandbob" to the kids meant to me. But after Christopher's death, "pretty sure" was no longer good enough.

"You know," I said, after we'd finished reminiscing about the remarkable events that had brought us together, "you're like a father to me."

Having helped countless patients navigate the hardest decisions over a long career as a family doc and then clinical ethicist, he wasn't often overcome with emotion. But the curry wasn't spicy enough to cause the tears in his eyes.

"And you're like a son to me," he replied softly.

Christopher's death also forced me, once and for all, to relinquish my dream of a perfect life. The fact that I still harbored such a dream may seem absurd in light of what I endured as a kid. Back then, I'd been told, over and over again, what a wonderful life I had, reality notwithstanding. It took a massive amount of work to acknowledge my Bizarro World for what it was because, once you admit that something isn't absolutely perfect, everything comes into question, and you might just be forced to admit it was actually tragic.

Dreams don't die easily, though, and even if the first part of my life had been scarred, that didn't prevent me from aspiring to perfection from that point forward. Beyond seemingly assuring my own happiness, that would also have made it crystal clear to my abuser that they couldn't break my spirit. At the very least, it would draw some good out of the precise opposite, applying the resiliency I'd developed in order to survive in the service of a noble cause.

The building blocks of an idyllic life had been in place: wonderful wife, healthy kids, the very best of friends, fulfilling job. We lived beside Lake Champlain in what we called our "forever home," each afternoon stopping whatever we might be doing when someone called out, "Sunset alert!" in order to gather on the deck and watch the sun drift behind the Adirondacks on the distant shore, the fading light filtering through the branches of the lone tree in the backyard: a majestic five-hundred-year-old burr oak. Over a decade into my tenure at the University of Vermont, another twenty years would bring me to retirement age, at which point I'd ride off into the sunset as the beloved *paterfamilias* of ethics and pediatric palliative care.

Then the phone rang on a cold January night, shattering my perfect plan for (the rest of) my life. I would spend years grieving that, even as I began to wonder whether I was clinging to some things simply because they contributed to that idyllic vision rather than leading me where I needed to go.

CHAPTER 12

Doing to and doing for

— Emerson —

I'm sure there must be some young, kind, and innocent couples out there who don't have children with life-threatening diseases, but I mostly hang with the ones who do. Like Sarah and Steve, whose beautiful daughter, Emerson, had a rare genetic condition called Gaucher's disease, where the absence of one particular enzyme leads to the buildup of toxic substances in multiple organs, including the brain. Enzyme replacement can slow the progression in some types of Gaucher's, but Emerson had the most severe form. The only thing left was supportive care, which basically meant trying to prevent foreseeable complications (like seizures and bleeding) and making sure she was comfortable.

    Having recently moved from the Pacific Northwest to a small town in Vermont, Sarah and Steve were far away from friends and family. Fortunately, they found a virtual community in the Courageous Parents Network (CPN), a remarkable organization, founded by a bereaved parent named Blyth Lord, that provides education and support for parents caring for (and mourning) seriously ill children. That's where they heard about something called palliative care, prompting them to reach out to our PACT team for assistance.

Listening to them describe their situation on the phone, I could practically feel their sense of isolation. So—vividly recalling how much more at ease Collin had seemed, sitting in his favorite chair with Giles nestled in his lap—instead of offering Sarah and Steve an appointment time in the clinic, I offered to go to them.

It's always struck me as odd that, when someone feels bad, we ask them to leave the comforts of home and go to the last place in the world they probably want to be (i.e., the hospital). So, while house calls may seem like the stuff of a bygone era, many pediatric palliative care teams offer them. You can get to know a family on a much deeper level by seeing the photos on their wall and not being in a hurry to see the next waiting patient.

When I arrived at their house on a snowy winter morning, Steve answered the door. Quiet, with a light brown beard flecked with gray, he was simultaneously welcoming and vaguely suspicious, whether about palliative care in general or a house call in particular, I couldn't be sure. His wife, Sarah, was soft-spoken with an open face and a smile that equally accommodated laughter and tears. She was holding eight-month-old Emerson, who had piercing blue eyes and clearly didn't suffer from stranger anxiety.

We sat in the living room, steam rising from my cup of coffee as sunlight glinted off the hard-packed snow outside. I usually open initial visits with get-to-know-you questions like what parents do for a living and how they met. But before I could begin, Sarah and Steve had a bunch of questions of their own.

> *Palliative care is what, again?*
> *That's nice, but what exactly do you do?*
> *Isn't that the same thing as hospice?*

After I'd answered what over time had become familiar questions, we circled back around to Sarah and Steve, who were well-versed in Gaucher's, the few treatments available, and the inexorable progression of the disease. They described wanting Emerson to have a full life and being willing to fight as hard as they could to achieve that goal.

I'd heard that many times before from parents who understandably felt cheated that, instead of watching their child grow up and become an adult and perhaps a parent themselves, they might only have a few years together. Or even less.

"She's a fighter," parents often say.

And they're right. The kids I work with have overcome more obstacles—and have shown a greater depth of courage in doing so—than I ever will. And even for the most terrible diseases, there are usually a few patients who defy the odds. Who could ever blame a parent for wondering, *Why shouldn't that be my kid?*

It gradually became clear to me, though, that when Sarah and Steve referred to a full life, they didn't mean duration. They'd always felt that Emerson was an old soul, with whatever time the three of them had together (even if all too brief) being the last leg of her journey. And that, hopefully, would include a full arc of diverse experiences and discoveries, like playing in the snow and eating solid food for the first time.

That's what they were fighting for, even if some people didn't think they were fighting as hard as they should or for the right thing. Some other families of kids with Gaucher's had opted for feeding tubes and ventilators to prolong their child's life, reasoning that just because there isn't a cure today doesn't mean one might not be discovered tomorrow.

Having identified Sarah and Steve's human hopes, now it was my turn to translate those into a medical plan. At first, that might not seem very hard since it was clear that invasive procedures didn't align with their goals. All I had to do was put some orders in place. Do not insert feeding tube. Do not intubate. Do not attempt resuscitation. So many "nots" that it's little wonder less palliative-minded physicians often frame treatment choices in binary terms: "The other option is to do nothing."

That is precisely what Sarah and Steve were struggling with. At that point, Emerson was still able to do the things she loved: banging on drums and cymbals, trying new foods, dropping things on the floor and watching the nearest adult dutifully pick them up. When the time came that she couldn't do those things anymore, Sarah and Steve didn't want her to suffer. But they also couldn't bear the thought of just standing idly by.

"It goes against every instinct in me to not do anything!" Sarah said with added force if not volume.

I empathized with that feeling while also trying to draw a distinction between doing something for someone and doing it *to* them. A feeding tube that keeps someone strong enough to keep living a life they feel is of good quality: that's doing something good for them. But simply sustaining necessary physiological functions—which often requires invasive procedures that can cause significant discomfort and potential complications—is doing things to the patient.

Although Sarah and Steve were nodding, that distinction hadn't seemed to give them what they were looking for. I paused for a second, aware of the bright sunshine streaming through the windows—which if you didn't pay attention to the snow cover might make you think it was balmy out there—and the intense love in that room. There was an almost palpable sense of parental protection surrounding Emerson, the primal mama/papa-bear instinct that Sarah had mentioned.

I wish I could claim that everything I say is well thought out, formulated after considered preparation, and based on all available evidence. But that wouldn't be true, as you already know from my boneheaded "hang in there" comment to Bill, Collin's dad. Sometimes I just say whatever pops into my head, which often resonates, as the idea of holding your children for their entire lives did with Tom and Mary. Other times it falls flat, perhaps because the family isn't in a place to hear that right now, or I misread the situation, or—like in saying goodbye to Bill—I wasn't brave enough to endure the silence. Saying what comes to mind isn't a sign of impetuousness but rather of my belief that, if your heart is in the right place, more often than not, whatever you say will have some positive meaning. Even when it doesn't, Grace had taught me that the patient or family is likely to cut you some slack because you were honestly trying to help.

A classic example I often share with students comes from Melvin Konner's wonderful memoir, *Becoming a Doctor*. Already a recognized anthropologist on the Harvard faculty when he went back to medical school, Konner relays the story of a young doctor placing his stethoscope on the chest of a patient who was in remission from lung cancer. What the doctor heard told him that the cancer had returned, and he thought, "Oh, shit."

Except he didn't just think it. He muttered it under his breath with the patient's ear inches away.

So much for firing a warning shot to prepare the patient for bad news to come. The doctor had committed a massive breach of decorum, one that seemingly threatened the rapport and trust he was seeking to build. But the patient—who had long prepared himself for the possibility of recurrence—saw it differently.

"That's okay," he said reassuringly. "It's nice to know you care."

What I said next to Sarah and Steve was neither as spontaneous nor irreverent as Konner's comment, but it felt risky nevertheless.

"In medicine, there are a lot of things that we can do to keep a body alive, and we'll keep doing those things until someone tells us to stop."

Sarah and Steve nodded. Other docs had already reviewed their options for when Emerson's condition declined. And I had to be careful not to overemphasize the potential burdens of intensive life-prolonging treatment, which risked compounding grief with guilt if they decided that was in their daughter's best interest.

"If those aren't right for Emerson," I said, leaning forward, "then preventing them *is* actually doing something. It's protecting her from things that will only bring her harm."

Bioethics has long taught that medical decisions should be made in the child's best interest, but that feels awfully calculated to me. I now can see, in retrospect, that more by instinct than insight, with Steve and Sarah I'd stumbled onto something just as primal as parents wanting to do something for their child: their need to protect that child.

Put another way, parents are just trying to be good parents to their ill child, which studies show takes two basic forms: making informed decisions about medical interventions and ensuring that the child feels loved. Both are important to every parent, of course, and there is significant overlap in specific hopes and goals. The categories simply describe the primary understanding of what a good parent should focus on. Not surprisingly, as their child's disease progresses and cure ceases to be a possibility, about one-third of parents in the informed group transition to the loved group.

Steve and Sarah didn't have to make that transition because they were already there. After working diligently to understand Emerson's condition and explore every option, they knew what was important for their daughter. And reassured that protecting her from burdensome procedures was doing something quite profound, they spent the final months of her life savoring each and every moment.

—Ethics and palliative care —

It's often said that "if you've seen one palliative care program, you've seen one palliative care program." At some medical centers, palliative care is a section within a division (frequently oncology), while at others, it is a stand-alone division within a department (often internal medicine or family medicine). On some teams, all the physicians split time between palliative care and their primary specialty—with that diversity viewed as making the team stronger—while on others, physicians only do palliative care with uniformity engendering acceptance.

As long as either everyone is doing things a certain way or no one is, the system seems to work well. But when almost everybody on a team focuses exclusively on palliative care for adults, it can leave the one person who only treats kids (and splits time with another specialty) feeling like a square peg trying to fit in a round hole. Which is why I tried really hard to assimilate into the newly combined palliative care team—led on an interim basis by Dr. Danvers's former second-in-command, whom I'll call Dr. Kelly—like by stepping up when there was a last minute need, whether it be facilitating the weekly educational conference or covering a holiday weekend.

It really didn't help, though, that my other specialty was clinical ethics. You'd think that palliative care and ethics would get along famously—because who isn't a fan of relieving suffering and helping patients make choices aligned with their values?—but those two have a history. Back before palliative care was even a specialty, ethicists were the people you called to help patients make end-of-life decisions. It's not hard to see why some ethicists get a little prickly about being replaced by the new kid on the block, especially one that can bill for its services—unlike ethicists, to the frustration of hospital bean counters—and has more star power, with Atul Gawande writing a glowing article about palliative care in *The New Yorker*, which he later expanded into a bestselling book.

For their part, some palliative care folks feel like they already have ethics covered, given how often they encounter moral dilemmas in their work. I saw that frequently at my hospital where, as an ethicist, I often recommended involving palliative care, too—like for an adult patient with untreated symptoms—but when someone suggested to the palliative care team that ethics also be consulted, their usual response was, "Why do we need them?" Granted, palliative care folks have more experience with moral dilemmas than many other physicians, but that still doesn't make them trained ethicists.

Tired of everyone sweeping the tension between the two disciplines under the rug—and being the only person at the University of Vermont who practiced both—I kept searching for a collaborative way forward. A golden opportunity seemed to present itself when I was invited back the following year for a return engagement at the annual meeting of the Hospice and Palliative Care Council of Vermont. The members of the formerly adult-only palliative care team, though, didn't view it as golden. Why, they wondered, would someone who only did palliative care part-time be invited to give the plenary? Again!

Recognizing, though, that I'd be in familiar and friendly territory—and that many in the audience, due to the rural setting, did double duty in both ethics and palliative care—I forged ahead, titling my talk "Behind frenemy lines: Optimizing the crucial relationship between ethics and palliative care." I started off that morning by describing what the two fields have in common, like helping patients and families make crucial decisions. That includes an overlap of personnel—palliative care clinicians often serve on ethics committees, and some ethics consultants are also palliative care docs, which I was living proof of—to the point where some universities even have combined departments of ethics and palliative care. I also made sure to highlight the areas where only one specialty was relevant, such as symptom management for palliative care and organizational issues unrelated to serious illness for ethics.

I spent most of the talk, though, describing how distinct approaches can be complementary. Ethics provides a specific, impartial opinion, whereas palliative care builds alliances with patients and families through longitudinal relationships. There are times when the two services can work together in the service of the patient, especially in high-stakes situations (such as those involving prolonged hospital stays or forgoing life-sustaining treatment) where there may have been a breakdown of therapeutic alliances. Rather than viewing the other as an enemy pretending to be a friend, it's more productive to opt for the other definition of a frenemy: someone who really is a friend but sometimes also a rival.

More informational and less personal than the previous year's plenary—and this time, sadly, without Lucy along for the ride—the talk was still well-received. The question-and-answer period went over time, ranging from age-old questions (like how to treat a patient who'd lost decision-making capacity) to newer ones (like policies regarding Medical Aid in Dying, which Vermont had recently become the third state to legalize). And I was reminded once again of the generosity and dedication of the people on the front lines who toiled long hours without much recognition.

"Very interesting," Dr. Kelly said, once the Q&A finally ended. "I look forward to discussing this with you further."

That's what I assumed she wanted to talk about when she summoned me to her office a few weeks later. Instead, she slid a brochure across her desk toward me.

"Can you explain this?" she asked.

I recognized the cover. "That's for a continuing medical education conference in October in Stowe."

To attract doctors, CME conferences are usually held in idyllic settings at the optimal time of year. In January, you can escape the cold in Hawaii or Cancun, but October is when all the "peepers"—as in leaf peepers—visit Vermont.

"And you're speaking at it," she said.

It was more of a statement than a question since I was listed on the brochure as one of the presenters.

"A friend of mine runs it," I explained, "and every couple of years, he asks me to give a talk."

"And you're talking about," she said, opening the brochure to the Saturday morning agenda, "palliative care?"

I nodded, struggling to connect the dots between the brochure and what felt like anger in the room.

"But it's not *pediatric* palliative care, is it?" she asked, in the tone of a prosecuting attorney.

I shook my head, wondering when we were going to get around to how palliative care and ethics could work together.

"And," she continued, "you really think you're qualified to speak on that topic?"

I tried not to get defensive as I observed that—since there was no specifically pediatric palliative care certification—I'd passed the same board exam that she had, which covered both adults and kids. Heck, I currently served on the eight-member committee that wrote the questions for that exam. I also pointed out that my session fell on a weekend when I wasn't on call, in case she thought I was taking a day off from work to do it.

"You should have run this by me first," she said.

"I didn't know I was suppos—"

"That's how this team works. When somebody requests a talk on a topic, we discuss it together and decide who'll do it."

It would have been nice if someone had told me that. But now that I knew, I said I was fine if someone else from the team wanted to give the talk. It seemed like a win-win: someone else would have the chance to speak, and I'd get my weekend back.

"That won't fly," she said. "Your name is already on the program."

"Then I can team up with someone, and they can do most of the talk."

She shook her head. "No one else on the team is available that day."

It took me a second to comprehend those words. Was she really saying that it was better for the conference to avoid discussing palliative care than have me talk about it?

"I didn't intend to offend anybody," I said. "I can explain to the team that I just didn't know about the rule."

"I'm not so sure about that."

I took a deep breath. Impaired communication was one thing, unrealistic expectations another. But this was something else.

I have my fair share of character flaws, having been accused over the years—sometimes with good reason—of being holier-than-thou, messy, poor at follow-up, and a horrendous singer. (To give you a little context, a person next to me at church once tapped me on the shoulder to ask if I was on the right hymn, which I was.) I've worked hard to change the things I can and prayed for serenity when it comes to my singing, which my daughter Lucy has compared to "the sound of a pregnant whale in labor." One thing I'd never been accused of, though, was dishonesty.

Always before, in a confrontational situation like that, my pathological niceness would kick in, and it didn't take Sigmund Freud—or even Dr. Phil—to figure out why. Even if you knew deep down in your soul that it was terribly wrong, what passed for love in your childhood might be as close to the real thing as you were going to get. You didn't dare risk losing it, so you got über-nice and definitely didn't speak your mind. All the while, you never stopped hoping that, just maybe, if you returned evil with love instead of fighting back, then that person would finally see how much you were hurting—even if they couldn't recognize that what they were doing was wrong—and stop.

Dr. Kelly, of course, wasn't responsible for my history, but the conversation with her was the moment I stopped trying to "nice" my way out of conflict. Not so much because I recognized in my head that it hadn't ever worked but because my heart would no longer let me. Life was too short, as my work kept reminding me. And with my dream of a perfect rest-of-life having died with my best friend, I was less concerned with preserving a fragile vision that I could now see wasn't bringing me joy.

"I feel like my character is being questioned," I said, which most people wouldn't recognize as the courageous statement that, for me, it was.

Dr. Kelly denied that was her intent—and I took her at her word—but seemed to recognize that may yet have been the impact. Even though we were clearly on different pages, the ensuing conversation was sufficiently frank that it gave me hope that at least we were reading from the same book. I left her office a little proud of myself for taking a stand and harboring a measure of hope for increasingly direct conversations in the future.

Which is why I was surprised, a few days later, when her department chair knocked on my door. (It's never a good sign as a faculty member when a chair comes to you.) After a little perfunctory chit-chat, he got down to business.

"Dr. Kelly came to see me," he said somberly, going on to describe how distressed she was about the conference speaking opportunity.

I couldn't believe what I was hearing. I'd been willing to cut Dr. Kelly some slack, attributing her initial reaction to a combination of misunderstanding, stress, and lingering distrust from the Dr. Danvers days. I'd even dared hope that this would be a fresh start for us on the road to open communication.

For her to run to her department chair, though—and for him to come knocking on my door—made me wonder if rectangular communication should be listed as a core competency of the palliative care division. I wanted to leap out of my chair and yell, "Don't you get that there are patients up there (pointing at the inpatient floors above my ground-level office) and out there (gesturing toward the window, where a rural state with precious little palliative care awaited) who are suffering? But instead of figuring out how we can all work together to help them, we're dithering about who should give a Saturday morning talk at some conference that people are probably attending for the pretty leaves?"

You don't speak like that to anyone's chair, though, at least if you still want to have an academic job in the morning. But having been honest and direct with Dr. Kelly, I wasn't going to turn back now. So I described to her chair how it felt to be judged for violating an unspoken rule, as well as confirming my willingness—one might even say eagerness—to have someone else speak in my place, except no one was able to. I also described my hopes for more direct communication on the team and less emphasis on who got to claim a presentation at a local conference for their curriculum vitae.

He listened intently, then paused long enough for me to hope for candor and a renewed commitment to collaboration. Then he encouraged me to be more sensitive to my colleagues' academic aspirations. Even if rising from his chair hadn't clearly signaled that the conversation was over, I wouldn't have had any words in response. How could getting promoted to a higher rank of professor take precedence over the suffering of kids and families? As my office door closed behind him, all I could think about was the famous observation that the "the politics of the university are so intense because the stakes are so low."

I knew all too well what it felt like to live in a Bizarro World, having grown up in one where I was told over and over again in myriad ways that wrong was right and manipulation was love. Long ago, I discovered that it was easier to abide the contradictions than question even a few of them, which would have thrown my worldview into chaos and forced me to confront a level of pain and violation that my young self—or, indeed, any child—was incapable of grasping. So I came to defer to the assessment of others, which, if nothing else, was consistent.

It's important, though, not to risk equating an abusive childhood with a challenging work environment. It wasn't like I was perfect and the rest of the palliative care team was wrong. Swinging from the masochism of "it's all my fault" to the self-protection of placing all the blame on others is no improvement. It would be more honest—and less binary—to admit that the problem was us, in some combination of needs and expectations, strengths and weaknesses.

Perhaps a better analogy, then, than a Bizarro World is to a "Class M" planet on *Star Trek*, a show I adored as a child—so much so that I formed a Star Trek club with kids in my neighborhood and actually thought William Shatner was a great actor.* Every weeknight at six, I could count on the *Enterprise* establishing orbit around an unfamiliar world, where Mr. Spock would promptly scan the atmosphere to see if it had sufficient oxygen to sustain humanoid life. Fortunately for the crew—not to mention the production budget—nearly every planet they encountered happened to be Class M, akin to Earth. Other classes of planets weren't bad; they just supported different forms of life.

Metaphorically speaking, the oxygen I needed in my work environment was direct and honest communication and a recognition that seriously ill kids deserved outstanding palliative care that honored their unique needs. And while I loved so many things about Vermont—like its slow pace, three degrees of separation, and our beautiful home where every afternoon brought a sunset alert—I began to wonder whether I could survive in a place that perseverated on a speaking gig while patients suffered and their families grieved. Put another way, in a world where I couldn't breathe.

— Emerson: Part two —

Just as Tamara hadn't thought death could be beautiful—until Rider showed her how—Sarah and Steve logically assumed that if you knew your child was going to die, it would be impossible to experience fun or joy. Yet having reframed their concept of good parents from doers to protectors, they found themselves free to savor every moment with their daughter. While obviously deprived of countless other memories they should have accumulated, they never felt robbed during the time they did have with her. And precisely because she endured so few medical interventions, Emerson got to be a little kid.

"When she died," Sarah recalls, "she was still here."

---

* I do recognize that references to *Avengers* and *Star Trek*—when taken together with my philosophical appreciation of *Buffy the Vampire Slayer*—make me look like a major nerd.

While brief in absolute terms, those final days seemed to stretch out with sacred memories filling the space. Like when Sarah frosted Steve's birthday carrot cake with cream cheese, and Emerson was immediately smitten. From that point on, any time she saw carrot cake, she'd bang her spoon and demand her fair share (or more). It got so bad that Sarah took to hiding the cake in a cupboard in order to avoid a confrontation. In the weeks after Emerson's death, Steve and Sarah would often reminisce about all the times they'd made Emerson's beloved carrot cake for her. Only much later did it occur to them that Emerson had died only five days after Steve's birthday.

She died in the hospital, which in the adult palliative care world is often viewed as a failure, since most adults prefer to die at home. But kids with serious illnesses spend so much time in the clinic and the hospital that the staff often comes to feel like a second family, who, in the final hours, allow parents to focus on being Mom and Dad rather than worrying about their child's medical needs. The staff's dedication was intensely meaningful to Sarah and Steve, but also foreshadowed another loss: with Emerson gone, there was no longer an occasion to see the people who'd been such a support to them.

I was enduring a meeting on the far side of campus when my pager went off with the news. I hurried back to the hospital, not that there was anything I could do at that moment. Just as I had on my very first palliative care consult over a decade before, I simply tried to "stay awake" in the midst of sorrow, hoping that tearful if wordless companionship might mean something to Sarah and Steve.

So many conversations and feelings had gone into planning for a moment that had now occurred. The impish grin might be gone, but Emerson still looked like her beautiful self, sheltered in Sarah's arms. (Parents never stop protecting their kids.) Sometime later that day—not when Sarah and Steve were ready, because no parent ever is—they'd walk out of the hospital for the first time without their daughter.

For all I knew, I might never see them again since the person who had brought us together was now gone. So I asked them if it would be okay if I gave Emerson a kiss before I left. Sarah and Steve—who obviously didn't know about my soul calluses or devastating self-doubt or the "phone call" from Hannah that I wasn't brave enough to return—might have assumed that was my standard response to a patient's death. But it was actually the first time I'd ever asked that question, which a few years earlier never would have crossed my mind to ask.

After Sarah nodded, I kissed Emerson lightly on her still-warm forehead, silently offering a prayer of gratitude for the lives she'd touched and thanking her for letting me be a very small part of her journey.

— After a child dies —

When I tell people I practice pediatric palliative care, their minds immediately jump to three things: kids, cancer, and death. While that explains their need for a stiff drink, only the "kid" part is actually true. Cancer might be the most frequent reason adults need palliative care, but in pediatrics, both genetic (think: Lily, Collin, Cora, and Emerson) and neuromuscular (think: Rider) conditions are more common. And even though many kids who receive palliative care ultimately die, there's hopefully still a whole lot of living to be done.

So, too, for their parents, after their child is gone. Parents have to figure out how to get out of bed the next morning and make it through an entire day until another sleepless night rolls around. They still have obligations—like to their other children (if they have any) and to their work—as well as questions to answer. Some are immediate, like setting the date and format of a memorial service. Others are farther down the road, like whether to try having more children (which is especially complex if their child died of an inherited condition).

Listening to parents' survival stories, it seems like there are two parts to their lives. In the same way that the Western calendar is divided in two based on someone's birth (i.e., before Jesus was born, followed by *Anno Domini*), bereaved parents' lives are divided by someone's death: when their child was alive and all that comes later. The difference doesn't just involve what the parents do or how they live but also who they are.

"The me before Emerson," as Steve observes, "is not the me after Emerson."

It feels like that second portion of a bereaved parent's life falls into three stages, the first of which might be described as "coming to terms." It's not coming to peace because there really is no such thing when you've lost your child. It's not even acceptance because that feels dangerously close to capitulation about something that will never be okay and also ignores the half-waking state each morning when you dare to believe that this was all just a dream that, thank God, you just woke up from.

"Coming to terms" refers to a truce, with neither side accepting responsibility but acknowledging that continued war is in no one's best interests. It also describes a journey toward words that eventually will describe the loss of a child, which are necessary because other people expect them. For instance, "Do you have any kids?" is a common question with no simple answer. Not including the child who died seems a denial of their very existence, but the alternative risks generating awkward questions for which the inquirer is surely unprepared.

"I actually feel worse for them," Steve says. "This is our life, but I want to help them through it."

Some people stop asking questions at that point, having gotten far more than they bargained for. A few, though, keep going. Children, especially, who thankfully don't know any better. Like the five-year-old who saw Emerson's tombstone and remarked, "Well, at least it's big enough that if your next child dies, you can put their name on it, too." What seems uncouth can actually be freeing to talk about, since how could Sarah and Steve, on some level, not have considered the possibility of losing another child? If it happened once, it could happen again.

Like the very young, the very old are often willing to engage. Having gone through enough in their own lives to no longer fear tragedy, they might—upon hearing that Sarah and Steve lost a daughter—dare to ask what her name was. And just once in the years after Emerson died, ask what she was like, which in every other context would be a casual question, but it brought tears to Sarah's eyes.

The only people in the middle who don't run away are the ones who understand what it feels like to lose a child, who are a big part of the second stage: keeping on. Again, the word choice is important; no parent really moves on because the child they lost is never far from their minds. If the last chapter of a child's life stretched out—creating the sense that Emerson had always enjoyed carrot cake and not merely in her last five days—the time since gets compressed to the same degree.

Collin's mom, Deb, describes it this way: "Whether it's five years or five days since he died, it feels like no time at all."

With almost nobody able to relate to what they'd gone through, Sarah and Steve understandably gravitated toward the few who could. Online materials like those provided by CPN were a big help, as were other bereaved parents they met through grief groups and weekend retreats. Clearly, I belong in the category of "can't relate to what they'd gone through" because I always thought (and taught my students) that it's better to start with commonplace topics like jobs or the weather in order to lay the foundation for bigger things, like making big decisions and processing grief. That's precisely how I'd intended to begin the first conversation with Sarah and Steve—before they hit me with a volley of frank inquiries—but over time, they would help me understand that when grieving parents are in the company of the few people on earth unlucky enough to truly understand how they feel, the conversations often go in reverse order. Like the campfire chat at Faith's Lodge—a retreat center for people working through grief—which started off with a discussion of what kind of headstone to buy for your child.

"When you can share stuff like headstones," Sarah says, "it makes it easier to talk about what sports team you root for."

Another part of keeping on is deciding whether to become parents again. Sarah and Steve longed for another child but wanted to make absolutely sure that baby wouldn't inherit Gaucher's, too. Two and a half years of unsuccessful in vitro fertilization wasn't as hard as Emerson dying—*What could be?*—but it was, in Sarah's words, "more desolate." Both past the age of forty by this point, she and Steve were considering egg donation when they discovered that they were already pregnant the old-fashioned (read: genetically random) way.

The odds were in their favor—only a 25 percent chance of the baby having Gaucher's, which is autosomal recessive—but they'd been in Emerson's favor, too. Sarah and Steve needed to know for sure, and being told to wait two weeks for genetic results felt like an eternity. Then they learned that the initial test was inconclusive and had to be run again. Another two weeks, which somehow seemed even longer.

"That period of time was really hard," Sarah says, reminding me yet again that bereaved parents are professionals at understatement, maybe because it's impossible to overstate what they've gone through.

Yet even when the test results finally came back, confirming that baby Margot did not have Gaucher's, Sarah and Steve didn't make any assumptions. They didn't paint the nursery or buy any outfits for Margot, for instance, until Sarah was practically giving birth. And when they finally did, it wasn't a sign of trust that everything would be okay. Sarah and Steve so cherished Emerson's things—the clothes she wore and toys she played with—that they didn't want to be left without anything physical of Margot's to hold onto in case she died, too.

"Thinking about the possibility of death isn't a good thing," Steve admits, "but it's part of our life."

You might think that would turn Sarah and Steve into the world's worst helicopter parents, but it didn't. Faced with the random—some might say capricious—nature of a universe where awful things just happen, they found freedom in simply doing the best they could.

"Margot will probably be fine," Sarah says, the "probably" a sign that certainty no longer exists in their world.

Margot, as it turns out, is more than fine, prompting well-meaning folks to conclude that everything is finally good. They're more likely to ask about Emerson now, too, because it feels like there will be a happy ending, after all.

The folks from Faith's Lodge know better. "I'm sure this brings up a lot of complex feelings," one said to Sarah, out of personal experience, after Margot was born. To which Sarah nodded, similarly aware that it's possible to be sad and happy at the same time, maybe even all the time.

After coming to terms and in the process of keeping on, a lot of bereaved parents also choose to give back. They aren't so much trying to draw a morsel of goodness out of tragedy as simply acknowledging how painful and solitary some journeys can be. They go where they're needed, which is a place most people prefer to believe doesn't exist. Which is why, after her daughter, Hope, died, Kate didn't stop pumping breast milk. She kept going for months, eventually donating ninety-eight bottles to a woman in Kentucky with an adopted son, whom she was matched up with online. (When she and Spencer think back on that, they often find themselves humming the tune of "99 Bottles of Beer on the Wall.") It's also why Sarah and Steve got involved with CPN.

They started off by sharing their story—including the part about how protecting your child is a huge part of being a good parent—which became part of the network's growing video library that had been such a comfort to them as they navigated Emerson's illness. Sarah also joined the parental advisory council and later added content manager to her growing role. These days, you can find her and Blyth Lord, the founder, tag-teaming podcasts and grand rounds at various medical centers, sharing a perspective that healthcare professionals desperately need to hear. I often encourage students and residents, if they have a few spare minutes, to watch the CPN videos about how parents decide about resuscitation or tracheostomy or where their child will die because that's what our patients' parents are going through right now.

For bereaved parents, though, giving back runs deeper than simply doing a good deed. For while their lives may be divided into the me before their child died and the current me, there isn't a clean break between the two. Something of the past always remains, which offers a bridge between the life they knew and the one they now have. That bridge is their child, and every contribution they make to other families in need—which they wouldn't have known how to do if they'd even thought to try had their child not died—is a way of making sure that the world never forgets one very special kid.

Chapter 13

My people

Facing your own mortality—what in palliative care is known as "advance care planning"—is an act of moral courage. It's incredibly tempting to deny that a day will ever come when your health is imperiled, which explains why only about one-third of Americans have completed an advance directive. Yet, however frightening it is to anticipate your own death, it's far worse to contemplate your child's with no morsel of comfort to be derived from a rich, long life. The entire natural order is inverted and distorted as parents are asked to acknowledge the unthinkable. Yet some parents—like Dave and Julie—dare to do just that in order to spare their child pain and ensure that they will have the fullest life possible.

— Ella —

"Our pediatrician said you could help us plan ahead," Julie said, her radiant smile momentarily fading. Dave—muscular and slim like the college basketball star he once was—sat beside her, holding five-year-old Ella, who had long, curly hair like her mom, with wide eyes that never seemed to blink.

"I can try," I said, glancing over at their pediatrician—who is among the kindest and most dedicated physicians I've ever known—in whose office we'd all gathered. "But first, tell me about Ella."

As a group, we physicians aren't very good listeners. Despite being taught in medical school to ask open-ended questions, we tend to assume that we already know what the problem is. Understandably eager to solve it—and move on to the next one because there's always another patient waiting—we permit patients to speak, on average, for eleven seconds before interrupting them. In palliative care, though, we encourage patients and families to take the conversation wherever they want. What initially seems like a tangent might just bring us to a place of meaning—a sacred hope, a hidden fear—which I would have had no way of anticipating, let alone asking about.

Dave and Julie started at the beginning, when Ella was born at a birthing center in Baltimore. That she was purple and not breathing should have prompted immediate intervention, but instead, the midwife encouraged Julie to talk to Ella and rub her back. Dave could tell that something was terribly wrong, though, so he immediately called 911. Unfortunately, the closest NICU was clear across town, and by the time Ella arrived there, she was already having seizures from the initial lack of oxygen. The doctors said she'd never do a lot of things that kids are supposed to do, like eat, drink, walk, and talk. A few days later—during which Dave and Julie repeatedly made it clear they weren't ready to give up—the hospital sent Ella home with a feeding tube in her nostril and instructions to return in three weeks for surgery to place a permanent one through her abdominal wall.

Dave and Julie's story deeply resonated with me because our oldest child, Catie, had also had some breathing issues when she was born. Nothing as severe as Ella's, just "transient tachypnea of the newborn" which, as the name suggests, gets better on its own after a few hours. She probably would have been fine without intensive care, but as a precaution, she was wheeled to the nearest NICU, which happened to be one floor up, not on the other side of town.

Fortunately for Ella, Dave and Julie aren't very good at doing what they're told. They found a speech therapist with an amazing track record of helping babies nurse, who showed them oral massage exercises that they faithfully performed on Ella every three hours. With the help of a special needs bottle, Ella was sucking like a champ by the date of her surgery, which now clearly wasn't necessary.

That was only the beginning. Hyperbaric oxygen therapy, acupuncture, yoga, and physical and occupational therapy followed, in the hope that Ella would defy the doctors' grim predictions. Dave was so dedicated to his daughter that he withdrew from training to be a physical therapist in order to be Ella's paraeducator throughout her schooling. Their efforts paid off: by the time I met her, Ella had already done a lot of things that most folks put on their bucket list and never get around to doing, from traveling the world to swimming with dolphins to writing poetry.

"Poetry?" I asked, wondering how a nonverbal kid could pull that off.

Julie explained they'd discovered a communications computer that allowed Ella to choose letters with her eyes, making possible verses like this:

> *Dolphins are fabulous*
> *Fun and slimy*
> *They are really smart and not too grimy*
> *I love dolphins*

Just because life is miraculous doesn't make it idyllic, though. Day in and day out, Dave and Julie would grind and blend Ella's food, freezing some and spending hours patiently spooning the rest into her mouth. On many nights, she couldn't settle down, forcing Dave and Julie to tag-team sleeping as the other one held Ella in a position where she could finally get comfortable, causing their backs to ache and throb. Most parents are familiar with long nights leading to exhaustion and despair, but the anticipation of their child ultimately growing out of it keeps them going. Dave and Julie had no such comfort yet still described those sleepless nights as "the best, hardest thing we've ever done."

Many parents of seriously ill children are reluctant to engage with palliative care—because that forces them to admit that the doctor's prognostications might actually come true—and finally do so quite late in a kid's disease course. Dave and Julie, on the other hand, reached out to palliative care long before any decisions needed to be made. They wanted to be prepared for the future and also recognized that they weren't exactly on the same page about what to do when it arrived. Julie felt that some procedures would be too much while Dave was more all-or-nothing, favoring steps that were necessary to keep Ella alive.

"There really aren't any good choices," Dave sighed, prompting me to ask if I could make a recommendation.

That might not seem revolutionary because, for most of the history of western medicine, physicians didn't make recommendations. They just went ahead and did what they thought was right. But the pendulum swung to the other extreme in the twentieth century, with such concern about infringing on patient autonomy that some ethicists urged physicians to avoid making any recommendation, even though that's one of the most important elements that patients consider when making a medical decision. Those ethicists might have a point if the recommendation is based on the physician's values, but the reason palliative care docs spend so much time listening is to understand the *patient's* goals. An image I sometimes use is the patient (or the parent, in the case of a child) as the captain of the ship—who gets to determine the destination—while the palliative care team is the navigator, whose job is to figure out the safest and most reliable way to get there.

With Dave and Julie's permission, I recommended that we continue with treatments that were high-benefit and low-burden, like antibiotics for an infection. But if Ella's condition declined to the point that she needed painful interventions that were unlikely to get her back to writing and swimming and smiling, those didn't seem to make sense in light of Dave and Julie's goals for her.

"Not everything," I said, "but also not nothing. Sort of like a middle road."

"I guess that sounds okay," Dave said softly.

Just okay and definitely not good because nobody ever wants to think about their child dying. But at least Dave and Julie knew a plan was there when they needed it, which allowed them to enjoy each day as a family.

— Ella: Part two —

I didn't see them again until six years later, which is probably a record in pediatric palliative care as well as a testament to the exquisite care Dave and Julie provided. Ella had just been admitted to the hospital following a recent cascade of complications: gastroesophageal reflux, thrush, pneumonia, and clotting problems that required platelet transfusions, raising the possibility of leukemia. After reviewing the long list, I told Dave and Julie that I thought we'd reached the end of the middle road. What was once the best of both worlds—giving Ella more time without compromising her quality of life—now felt like the worst, assuring neither her comfort nor her survival. We'd reached a fork: either pursue intensive interventions (likely requiring transfer to the ICU) or focus on comfort.

Dave was initially surprised to hear that, as he'd thought this was just Ella's new normal. Julie, on the other hand, felt like this was what we'd started preparing for years earlier. Except back then, everything had been theoretical—"If we get to that point, then we won't . . ." But acting on that plan now would mean actually saying goodbye to Ella. And that was infinitely harder than any hypothetical, as I knew from the adult patients I'd consulted on over the years who'd taken the courageous step of completing an advance directive which said, "I don't want to live if I can't ___," including things like take care of myself or recognize the people I love. Years later, though, when they eventually lost that crucial ability, life might not seem as bad as they'd anticipated, at least compared to no life at all. While some patients kept to the original plan, others reconsidered.

That night was as restless as many that preceded it, but somehow, this one seemed different to Dave. Maybe it was being in the hospital—which had come to feel almost as familiar as home—or not having further adventures to look forward to. Whatever the reason, in that sacred solo-parent time while the rest of the world was asleep, he recalled a moment when he just knew that the plan we'd made long ago, to let Ella go if she could no longer do the things she loved, was still right for her.

It's a strange and sacred thing to sit beside a child whose parents are about to take her home to die. If you dare to be quiet for long enough—which, trust me, is an incredibly difficult thing to do, when every fiber of your being wants to flee the piercing sadness—you're overwhelmed by the jumble of emotions. Sadness and relief. Memory and shattered hope. A deep yearning that, in those precious seconds eleven years before, oxygen could have reached Ella's brain in the same way that it had Catie's. Although, judging from Ella's poetry, she might not have shared my yearning:

> *I chose this body*
> *These limitations*
> *These circumstances*
> *Do you think that was Love?*
> *You better believe it!*

As Dave and Julie waited for the discharge paperwork to be completed, there wasn't much left for us to talk about: the hospital staff had said their goodbyes, hospice was lined up, and Ella—who was still so small that Julie said she never seemed like more than a baby to her—was resting comfortably, too weak even to smile. But leave it to Dave and Julie in the midst of their own unquenchable sorrow to be interested in other people.

"So what's your story, Bob?" he asked.

In some ways, it was an overdue question. Over a long period of time, we'd talked about some of the most important things in life: love, commitment, sacrifice. But medicine is an asymmetric discipline, with doctors asking intensely personal questions while usually revealing little in return. After all the three of us had been through, though, it didn't feel right to hold back.

"We had this sense there was something spiritual about you," Julie said after I mentioned my other job.

I took that as a compliment because it's always struck me as odd that so many folks feel the need to tell others that they are Christian, when it seems to me that other people should be able to tell you're a faithful person by how you act. But when Julie asked if I'd preside at Ella's memorial service, I have to admit I was surprised. Unlike baptisms—which need to have at least a little God in them—memorials can be anything you want, from prescriptive religious services to God-free community gatherings like Collin's. I knew that Dave and Julie had an eclectic spirituality, which made their request the reverse of what I'd experienced in the past: instead of someone simply needing a priest but not knowing any, Dave and Julie were just looking for someone who loved Ella and also "had something spiritual" about them. The ordained thing was an unexpected bonus.

"I'd be honored," I replied without hesitation.

Dave and Julie didn't need to hear about my on-again/off-again relationship with God, which after Christopher's death was currently in the off position. They weren't looking for some liturgical event full of rote prayers that begged for forgiveness for, what? Self-sacrifice? Heartbreak experienced? Injustice endured? No, they just wanted someone they trusted to proclaim that if there was a god out there—which at the moment seemed like a big *if*—that they would welcome Ella and watch over her now that her parents no longer could.

Eventually, it was time for Dave and Julie to, as they put it, "walk the long mile out of the hospital" that had mended Ella so many times. The instant they stepped foot in their house, though, they were confronted by how much their world had changed. Instinctively heading straight for the kitchen to prepare Ella's food as they had each day for over a decade, it began to sink in that her body was shutting down, and she would never eat again. Feeding her was the first of many things that they would soon realize were past for them.

Over the next four days, all the stuff the textbooks say happens when someone is dying happened to Ella. Sleeping more. Urinating less because there was less fluid in her body. Eventually, her pulse became weak and her hands cold as her breathing slowed. All the while, Dave and Julie never left her side as people stopped by to say goodbye. Over two hundred of them by Dave and Julie's estimate, bringing food or offering to help. The last one left at 4 p.m. on a Sunday—which happened to be Mother's Day—offering Dave and

Julie what would be the last half hour of Ella's life to spend alone with her.

Ella was resting in Dave's arms when she died, as Julie held her feet. Julie says she "felt her leave her body," even as Dave was having a vision. He describes seeing a veil drop and being welcomed by three beings of light in what was simultaneously the most still and celebratory experience of his life.

"It felt like a graduation," he recalls. "Like a job well done."

And so he began to whisper, over and over again in gratitude and grief, "We did a good job. We did a good job."

Long ago, I learned that bereaved parents are professionals at understatement. I always attributed that to years mourning their child, which gradually made things that would rock anyone else's world seem mild by comparison. But maybe time doesn't have anything to do with it. Maybe it's the experience of loss itself and all the love and tears and sacrifice and confusion that lead up to one unavoidable moment.

Dave had only been bereaved for a few minutes, and yet describing the job he and Julie did as "good" might be the biggest understatement I've ever heard.

Their pediatrician made a house call to "pronounce" Ella, and I stopped by a few days later—once the influx of family and friends had eased—to go over the details of what Dave and Julie were calling the "Celebration of Ella the Great." We spent several hours in tender conversation, flanked by poster boards of photos of Ella doing what she loved to do: rafting, paddle boarding, and swimming with dolphins. Recalling those sacred times, they described the empty silence of a home without her, especially in the moments right after she died. Even the birds who frequented the backyard feeder stayed away that day, thankfully returning the next—and each one since—as if having devoted sufficient time to mourning.

— For the first time in forever —

Catie met me at the door when I returned home, where the contrast seemed almost palpable. Long ago, a baby who didn't really require intensive care had it nearby, while another who desperately needed it couldn't reach a NICU in time. It wasn't as if Ella had done something wrong, and Catie was too young to do anything right. I guess years of not having found a reason why kids get sick wasn't a good enough reason for me to stop searching.

Despite not knowing where I'd been—not to mention being only twelve years old—Catie immediately sensed something was very wrong. She invited me to come inside and tell her all about it, which sounded like what a parent should be saying to their child, not the other way around. I talked in between bites of an oversized lunch of comfort food beside a vase of Mother's Day flowers that still had a little life left in them.

After I told her about my visit with Dave and Julie, we wandered out to the back deck to watch her two younger sisters play in the yard on one of the first really warm days of spring. Hidden amid the blooming leaves of our ancient oak tree, birds chirped—never having had a reason to stop—as Catie leaned her head on my shoulder, which allowed me, in turn, to rest my head on hers.

As the realization of life's fragility washed over me, I felt—perhaps for the first time fully—how much the emotional toll of my medical work was impacting my most important work: being a father. I'm acutely aware of how quickly childhood goes by, even assuming that a kid gets to live through all of it (which, given my specialty, definitely feels like a risky assumption). But with each patient's death cutting me to the core, threatened by Dr. Williamson, and feeling isolated in the palliative care division—which ran much deeper than the few examples I've included here—I wasn't as present as a dad as I used to be. Sure, I managed to maintain my weekly rituals, like doing aikido with Noah on Tuesdays and then going out for pizza, and taking Lucy to the library after school on Wednesdays. But part of my brain was always somewhere else, struggling to identify something I could do differently that might make the hospital feel like a safer place. So much so that when the kids begged for a mixed-up story—once a family tradition, also cherished by their friends who'd join us by the lakeside campfire—I'd either fall back on well-used characters and humdrum plots or simply say, "Maybe later." Over time, they began to ask more politely and less often. I felt like a window was closing.

Fortunately, there seemed to be a light at the end of the tunnel. Dr. Danvers was gone, and while Dr. Kelly was filling in, the hospital searched for a permanent section chief of palliative care. Few people applied for the job, but one happened to be an accomplished researcher in the field. Just before the hospital offered the job to Dr. Selzer (as I'll call him), a local philanthropist—who just so happened to be one of Lucy's friends from the Hospice and Palliative Care Council of Vermont meeting—made an incredibly generous donation to upgrade the position to an endowed chair. Positions like that are pretty rare (even more so in pediatric palliative care, with only two in the whole country at the time) and a sign of the community's commitment to the work.

Even better, I thought of Dr. Selzer as a friend. Not the sort with a capital "F" who has stuck with you through thick and thin but someone whom I'd had good conversations with at national meetings and whose articles I'd read with interest. Which is why, shortly before he began his new position, I put everything on the table in a long conversation over a beer at the annual assembly of the American Academy of Hospice and Palliative Medicine. I described everything that you've read up until this point and more, reviewing the successes—like creating the PACT team, passing the state Medicaid waiver, and most of all helping patients and families—as well as the rookie mistakes I'd made and my pathological niceness with Dr. Danvers when a crucial conversation had been called for.

Talk about radical candor; I was becoming the Abbie Hoffman of honesty. In some ways, though, it didn't feel like I had any choice. Long after most other people probably would have, I'd finally reached the conclusion that the status quo was unsustainable. Having witnessed the toll the work environment was taking on my spirit, my wife even wondered whether I should just go back to doing ethics full time, which in many ways made a lot of sense. Until I found palliative care, after all, I'd thought ethics was the perfect blend of the things I was trained—and felt called—to do. My partner, Sally, wasn't just the best coworker I'll ever have; she's the best coworker anyone will ever have, not to mention a dear friend. My mentor, Dr. Orr, had succeeded at pretty much everything in life except, thankfully, fully retiring.

But so much had happened since I hung out the shingle for the PACT team and not just in terms of the experience and knowledge I'd acquired. I had changed with the return of sensation and the growing courage to believe in myself and what I felt to be true.

"I really love palliative care," I explained to Pam one day, in one of our increasingly frequent conversations about the challenges at work.

I didn't need to elaborate; she'd not only heard it all before, she'd seen it in me over the past decade.

"If not here, though," she asked, "where would you do it?"

That might appear to be merely a logical follow-up question, but it was far more profound. A full-fledged pediatric palliative care program requires three things: passionate philanthropic support (because pediatric palliative care will never pay for itself), mission-driven leadership, and a large enough patient population to justify a true interprofessional team, meaning at least a medium-sized city. Vermont had the first, might be getting the second, and would never have the third. So that meant moving away.

Again, a pretty common event. According to the US Census Bureau, the average American will move 11.7 times. But my wife and I had both exceeded our lifetime allotment as children, and that's not what we wanted for our family. Over our fifteen years in Vermont, we'd laid down deep roots, both in a network of dear friends and being blessed to live in what we called our "Forever Home," complete with the venerable oak tree—witness to explorers and revolutionaries, provider of shade on hot summer afternoons, and still fertile (judging from the acorns dotting the lawn) after all these years—which my wife referred to as her true north. That's why I'd always said no to the more prestigious jobs that occasionally came calling because, up until then, I'd loved where I was.

But now that we were actually considering other opportunities, the process of elimination didn't take long. The closest pediatric palliative care program was Boston Children's Hospital, and while I loved the team there—the director of which had become a valued mentor—I didn't think the city would be the best fit for our family, even assuming there was a job open and they offered it to me. It didn't take long to cross other regions off the list: my wife grew up in the Midwest and I'd lived in the South, and neither of us was eager to return. Some years earlier, I was recruited for a position in southern California, but the cultural dissonance was palpable.

"Maybe the Pacific Northwest," I mused, based on my extensive experience there: a fortnight sailing the San Juan Islands with Pam and Jon and a couple of other friends fifteen years earlier. "I guess that would mean either Seattle or Portland, but Seattle seems kind of big. And I don't know if Portland even has a children's hospital."

I wasn't sure if narrowing your choice down to a state you'd never set foot in—that might not even have the kind of hospital you need—counted as progress. But that's where we left it.

In the meantime, my family kept me going, often without even realizing it. I remember one weekend afternoon in particular when I was trying to take a nap. With four kids and two dogs in the house, it shouldn't have been surprising that I failed in my attempt. Normally that would have prompted some suppressed frustration, except this time the sound keeping me awake was our center daughter singing.

Lucy has an amazing voice and plenty of courage to go with it. At the ripe old age of eight, she entered a talent competition—of her own volition, with very little guidance from Pam or me—and sang "One Small Voice" up on stage all by herself in front of a darkened crowd at the largest music hall in Burlington. A cappella!

And boy does she love to sing. December meant "Silver Bells" on repeat. And thanks to the movie *Frozen*, "Let It Go" had interrupted many a previous nap. Every elementary-school student probably knew those lyrics, but Lucy had memorized the rest of the soundtrack, too. The song that happened to wake me up that afternoon was "For the First Time in Forever," which felt like an answer to a prayer that I hadn't even uttered.

> *For the first time in forever*
> *There'll be magic, there'll be fun*

That took me back to carefree times when mixed-up stories had rolled off my tongue, instead of deflecting kids' requests by claiming to be too tired. I recalled sleeping through the night and actually looking forward to going to the hospital—where I'd envisioned spending the rest of my career—instead of having a somber cloud descend on Sunday afternoons because, in a few hours, I'd have to go back "there," where I no longer felt safe. It wasn't hard to relate to Elsa's refrain from the movie, which Lucy regaled the house with that afternoon:

> *Don't let them in, don't let them see...*
> *Conceal, don't feel*
> *Put on a show*
> *Make one wrong move and everyone will know*

What had my life come to, I wondered, when a Disney princess was describing the state of my heart? But it was less Elsa than my beautiful Lucy, who delighted in the mixed-up stories I told and didn't begrudge the ones I couldn't bring myself to compose. Who sang out loud without concern for who might be listening or what they might think. Who had no way of knowing how much her songs warmed my heart.

> *'Cause for the first time in forever*
> *I finally understand*
> *For the first time in forever*
> *We can fix this hand in hand*

For a few precious moments, as I hovered in that liminal space between sleep and waking, where dreams and reality feel the same, I let myself imagine the world she was singing about, where the worst thing that could happen was another kid not wanting to sit with you at lunch or play with you at recess. Kids didn't die in that world, and good intentions took you a long way. Truly resting for the first time in a long while—much more so than in my usual fitful sleep—I was so very grateful for that one small voice, which, to me, wasn't small at all.

— Ella: Part three —

The "Ellabration" took place in a beautiful park on the shores of Lake Champlain. The buffet tables were set up—ready to be crammed with whatever yummy food the attendees might bring—and I'd prepared a brief reflection. Beyond that, though, not much was certain. Dave and Julie were originally from Baltimore, where a separate service for family would be held two weeks later. Only local friends would be attending this one, assuming that they'd heard through the grapevine when and where it was being held and could finagle a weekday off of work. In just a few minutes, the service was scheduled to start, but only a handful of people had shown up.

This isn't what Ella would have wanted, I thought as I scanned the empty tables waiting for food that might never arrive. I glanced back yet again at the parking lot, by that point willing to settle for even a few more people, just enough so that the open lawn wouldn't seem so vast. I turned to Julie to suggest pushing back the starting time, but she was looking in a different direction. Following her gaze, I saw what she would later describe as "a sea of pink and purple coming over the hill." They'd all turned out—doctors, nurses, hospice workers, teachers, and friends galore, many carried or pushed in their wheelchairs by parents who had walked a similar path as Dave and Julie—for Ella. Grace, it turns out, often comes not in the direction you're looking or in the form you expect.

Amid the floral skirts and pink boas, there was but one black suit in sight: mine. Dave and Julie had liked the idea of me wearing my clerical collar, which seemed to offer the best of both worlds: a dash of tradition but without all the baggage of a Bible-laden funeral. Evidently, our middle road still had a few miles to go.

While the crowd set up their lawn chairs, speakers were booming out upbeat Latin rhythms, because dirges were definitely not Ella's style. The once-empty field now seemed filled to capacity, and I welcomed everyone to the Ellabration. A few friends of Dave and Julie then offered remembrances, describing how Ella inspired them and changed their lives. Finally, it was my turn.

I've given a lot of homilies in my time—at baptisms, weddings, funerals, and for years every Sunday as a parish priest. Some are meant to teach, a few to confront. Nearly 10 percent of my rural congregation walked out, in fact, during my first sermon after the outbreak of the 2003 Iraq War, when I described cuddling my baby daughter the previous night and wondering how an Iraqi dad might feel if he was doing the same while bombs rained down from the sky. Thankfully, the exodus returned the following Sunday and stayed.

An Ellabration was not the occasion for challenge or religious instruction, assuming I could have pulled off either. I just wanted to offer the people gathered a morsel of comfort, so setting aside the theology I'd spent so many years studying—which didn't take much effort, given my current crisis of faith—I went back to the basics: the words of Jesus. Specifically, a story that I thought Ella would have loved.

"Jesus was no stranger to tough love," I began, going on to explain that, instead of trying to appease the religious leaders of his day, he warned them that they'd be humbled for their pride. Like the rich young ruler who thought he was doing great because he followed all ten commandments until Jesus told him he better sell everything he had and give that money to the poor if he really wanted a shot at eternal life. And the leader of the synagogue, whom Jesus proclaimed a hypocrite after he condemned Jesus for healing a crippled woman on the Sabbath. Sure, Jesus could have waited until the next day so as not to ruffle any feathers, but hadn't she suffered long enough?

There was one group, though, that Jesus never judged: kids. He called them the "greatest in the kingdom of heaven," and warned people that it would be better to "be drowned in the depths of the sea" than cause a kid to stumble. The Bible says that the first person he resurrected was a twelve-year-old girl, even if the subsequent raising of Lazarus is better known.

"Let the little children come to me," Jesus said, after the disciples tried to shoo away parents who were bringing their babies to him to be healed. "Truly I tell you, whoever does not receive the kingdom of God as a little child will never enter it."

And who, I wondered aloud to the resplendent crowd, better exemplified receiving the kingdom of God as a little child than Ella, whose joy and honesty touched the hearts of everyone she came in contact with. Whose life was equal parts leaning on people to help her get what she really needed and showing them that they might not need everything they thought they did.

I clearly have no compunction about using someone else's words, especially when they say things better than I ever could. So far in this book, I've drawn from sources as eclectic as Maya Angelou, Elie Wiesel, and *Top Gun*. That afternoon, having started off quoting Jesus, it felt right to end with one of Ella's own poems. It was her party, after all, and she deserved to be center stage:

> *Love hides in each of us*
> *Waiting to emerge*
> *To be seen in an action*
> *To be heard in a whisper*
> *To be felt as a touch*
> *It is in us because*
> *It is us.*

There was definitely a whole lot of love emerging that day, and I couldn't help but think that—for all the aphorisms like "Palliative care, it's about how you live" and "Hope for the best and prepare for the worst"—this was what pediatric palliative care was really about: people of all ages and abilities, from every walk of life, sporting pink boas and the random amethyst tutu, coming together on a sunny day beside the lake to celebrate a child they loved and who changed them for the better. To share their memories and their tears, to support parents whose grief was only matched by their gratitude. This is precisely what drew me to palliative care, and it is what I was feeling far more deeply in a grassy park than inside the walls of the hospital.

Episcopal services always conclude with a postlude, typically a meditative organ solo by someone like Bach or Haydn. But that afternoon, the postlude was a hip-hop anthem by Outkast. "Hey Ya" just seemed so Ella, and as the service concluded and the feasting was about to begin, the purple-clad congregation danced to the rhythm and sang along as one:

> *Now all the Beyonce's, and Lucy Liu's, and baby dolls*
> *Get on tha floor get on tha floor!*
> *Shake it like a Polaroid picture!*
> *Oh, you! oh, you!*
> *Hey ya! Hey ya!*

People stayed for a long time after the service and not just for the delicious food and drink. They shared stories and memories, vacillating freely between joy and sadness, and eventually departed with a gift: packets of seeds that would eventually yield vibrant sunflowers, photos of which guests still send to Dave and Julie in remembrance of that special day, now years ago.

My work done, I ate my fill and chatted with the many folks I knew: Ella's pediatrician, nurses from the hospital, hospice workers I'd collaborated with on other cases. The same thought kept occurring to me as at that cocktail party years ago, when Dave's incisive curiosity set me off on a path of discovery, and at the HPCCV annual meeting at the historic lakeside inn: *These are my people.*

People I admire and respect. Who inspire and teach me. Who are doing this work for the same reasons I am and are open about their hopes and sorrows and mistakes and frustration, expecting others to be as well.

Leave it to Ella to bring us all together and to show me that I shouldn't have to wait for an Ellabration—or some organization's annual meeting—to feel at home. Life was too short to spend most of my working hours struggling to breathe in an inhospitable world (pardon the pun). My people were out there; now I just had to figure out a way to surround myself with them.

Chapter 14

Irrigation and debridement

I envy surgeons, who get to remove tumors and stop hemorrhages and mend broken bones. Put simply, they cure people.

Palliative care, on the other hand, gets its name from the Latin *pallium*, meaning "to cover." In other words, we don't solve problems; we just make them less obvious, less burdensome. Now, don't get me wrong: that can still make a huge difference in people's lives. If it didn't, my last fifteen years of work wouldn't be worth much. But even as I've tried my best to comfort and companion, I never stopped dreaming of cure.

Becoming a surgeon was never really an option for me, anyway, since my dexterity is more intellectual than manual. I might never have stepped foot in an operating room, in fact, had medical school not mandated one surgical rotation. I put that off as long as possible, but eventually, graduation loomed, and in an act of mild desperation, I hit up my classmates (who'd long ago completed that requirement) for advice. One offered this pearl: "Whatever you do, don't contaminate anything in the OR. So if you're not sure what to do with something, just drop it on the floor."

I kept repeating that under my breath as I performed the mandatory five-minute hand wash before entering the operating room for the first time, where the scrub nurse handed me a sterile towel. As I dried my hands, I made sure not to brush up against anything, especially the table of gleaming instruments—scalpels, clamps, and random gizmos whose names I never learned—over which she stood guard.

The anesthesiologist had just intubated the patient and the surgical residents were prepping the operative site when the scrub nurse thrust out a sterile glove for me to insert my hand into. The only problem was I was still holding the towel. Unsure what to do—and so focused on not contaminating anything that I didn't notice the nearby bin for used towels—I followed my classmate's advice and just dropped mine on the floor.

This was not well-received.

"Am I supposed to pick that up?" the scrub nurse yelled at me. "Do I look like your mother?"

My head shook like a jackhammer. I wasn't really sure what she looked like because she was wearing a mask, but I was quite certain she bore no resemblance to Mom.

The rest of the rotation went downhill from there, but I still remember something I learned about treating a deep laceration. It's not enough to wipe off the outside and put a bandage over it. You have to make sure there's no dirt or debris left in there, which is why you irrigate the wound with normal saline (which happens to be the concentration of human tears). A classic rookie mistake is going light on the saline, for even a tiny speck left behind can cause a serious infection.

Dead tissue will also keep a wound from healing. So after irrigating, you scrape away layer after layer until you get to living tissue, which is known as "debriding." You know you've gone deep enough when you see a trickle of blood because dead tissue (conveniently as well as metaphorically) doesn't bleed.

Irrigation and debridement—which surgeons refer to simply as I&D—is the only way to give whatever has survived a chance to heal. It also happens to be a pretty good way of describing the preceding few years of my life: recognizing what drew me to pediatric palliative care, sensation returning while on sabbatical, and now weathering the flood of emotions that attended the deaths of patients like Collin and a friend like Christopher. Through a lot of tears and steadily scraping away at the soul calluses—a sort of psychic I&D—my channels of feeling had reopened.

While surely a sign of healing, it also brought an overwhelming sense of vulnerability that I was all too familiar with from my past. The losses I was experiencing would have been difficult to navigate in even the most nurturing of environments, but the palliative care division was never going to be nominated for "Most Supportive Workplace." Without those soul calluses to protect me—and experiencing the pain around me even more acutely—I wasn't sure how to keep going.

I dared to hope that Dr. Selzer, the incoming leader of the palliative care team, would positively influence the environment at work. I hoped Dr. Selzer would acknowledge the unique needs kids and their families had and recognize that diverse skills—like pediatric training and expertise in ethics—could be assets to the team rather than cause for suspicion.

But instead of transforming the workplace culture, he codified it.

"It's critical," he announced on his first day on the job, "that people only do palliative care *or* ethics, never both. Every major medical center has a firewall between the two."

I knew that wasn't true, having extensively researched the topic for my recent talk at the state hospice meeting. Regardless of what other hospitals were doing, though, he had the authority to determine the path ours would take. And while I enjoyed doing clinical ethics, my heart was really with palliative care. If that meant giving up ethics, I was willing.

"We also can't have people only seeing children," Dr. Selzer continued. "Everyone will do both adult and pediatric palliative care."*

It didn't take a great deal of insight to figure out which people he was referring to, since I was the only person who—up to that point,

---

* It's worth noting that a few years later, UVM restored the independence of the PACT team, which is now led by two wonderful pediatricians.

at least—only treated kids. So much for my hope that he'd embrace diversity rather than enshrine uniformity.

But at least he'd made expectations clear so I wouldn't be in danger of violating unwritten rules (like Dr. Kelly's "When somebody requests a talk on a topic, we discuss it together and decide who'll do it"). And I was actually looking forward to treating grownups, having worked extensively with adults in my ethics role. Writing questions for the palliative care board exam had also required me to keep up with all the medical literature, not just pediatrics.

In that respect, it seemed like I was better off than the other members of the team, some of whom had zero experience—and often the same amount of interest—in working with children. To be sure, adult skills can translate pretty well to an adolescent, but most pediatric deaths occur in infancy (and two-thirds of those take place in the first month of life). I promptly started collating materials and resources for the rest of the team to help bring them up to speed on pediatrics in general and the unique world of the NICU in particular.

Dr. Selzer, however, didn't share my concern.

"I've actually never done a pediatric palliative care consult," he casually admitted a few days later, "but I actually think that'll be an advantage. At least I won't be tempted to make treatment recommendations."

His comment reminded me of a band I listened to in high school who claimed they didn't practice because it ruined their style. But Dr. Selzer wasn't referring to recommendations per se—which we both recognized as an integral part of palliative care—as much as the sort that I made. The kind that too often took the side of patients and parents, even in supposedly straightforward situations like brain death or conditions that were once deemed "incompatible with life."

My approach to palliative care clearly resonated in certain circles—like AAHPM, to whose board of directors I'd just been elected—but within our small division, it felt like I'd always be the odd person out, no matter what sacrifices I was willing to make. And while I might have been willing to accept children not being the main priority, I couldn't work in an environment that was going to treat them like little adults. That denied that kids were special.

This felt like the day I'd been waiting for, ever since my very first palliative care consult with Nicky. In the meantime, my soul calluses might have healed and my self-doubt begun to dissipate, but the third long-term effect of my childhood abuse remained: a profound sense of helplessness. No matter how hard I'd tried as a child, nothing I did or said had made any difference. The world around me carried on, indifferent to what I was enduring, which led me to stop daring to believe that I could actually change anything.

In much the same way, I never really expected to succeed in palliative care; I only felt called to try. That's why, despite all the children and families helped by the PACT team over the past decade, part of me was always waiting for someone to say, "We appreciate your effort" or, "Some people aren't cut out for this." Who knows, when Nicky's mom returned with cookies for the staff, if she'd said something other than what she did—or maybe just hadn't said anything at all, leaving me to wonder if all I'd managed to do was not make anything worse—I might have hung it up right there. But her encouragement (and that of other parents along the way) had kept me going. Until now.

Maybe Pam was right. Maybe it was time to go back to ethics, where perhaps I should have been the whole time. At least there, surrounded by Dr. Orr and Sally and the wonderful ethics team, I could breathe.

I even considered a career change, if that's what it would take to stay in Vermont, ranging from high school teaching jobs to maybe even retraining as a psychotherapist. (I'd been through quite a bit of therapy by that point, so I figured I must have picked up a few pearls along the way.)

There was just one problem. By that point, I'd begun to do something truly foreign: I'd started to believe in myself. Sure, I hadn't done a formal fellowship, but all the books I'd read and rookie mistakes I'd made and things I'd blurted out—ranging from the inspired

("Hold your babies for their entire lives") to the misguided ("Hang in there")—seemed to be adding up to a little bit of wisdom.

My initial stated reason for working in palliative care had been an unmet need whose attendant suffering I was able to withstand thanks to the insulation around my soul. But now, I was beginning to wonder if my childhood trauma didn't only provide the *motivation* to prevent other children from suffering as I had. Could it be that my own experience as a kid—now acknowledged and fully felt—actually allowed me to connect with my patients in a way that someone spared of pain never could?

That question called to mind a famous passage from the Gospel of Thomas, which is considered apocryphal yet seems more full of truth to me these days than some of the canonical gospels: "If you bring forth what is within you, what you bring forth will save you. If you do not bring forth what is within you, what you do not bring forth will destroy you." If true, then not at least trying to ease a child's suffering had ceased to be an option.

I'm definitely not God's gift to palliative care because there are some families I don't connect deeply with, and I can rattle off a long list of colleagues at other institutions who know more than I do and are far more empathic. If I had to choose a palliative care doctor for my children, I'd pick any of them over me in a heartbeat. But just because you're not the best at something doesn't mean you can't still make a contribution, especially in a field that most people prefer to think doesn't exist and that precious few choose to work in. And, luckily for me, those same colleagues proved a huge support while I struggled with a terrible choice. Should I give up the work I loved or leave the place that my family called home?

Usually, in academic medicine, you invite someone to give a talk at your institution because you really want to hear them speak on a specific topic. Custom and courtesy obligate you to take them out to dinner the evening before and spring for a hotel for the night. This time around, though, the reasoning worked backward. Recognizing what a challenging time it was for me, friends in places from Texas to Tennessee looked for an excuse for us to get together. Grand rounds seemed an ideal excuse, so they leveraged a one-hour talk—on whatever topic I felt like covering, with travel costs covered by their university—into a couple days of shared meals with their spouses and kids and deep conversations about why we did what we did (and how we managed to keep doing it). As skilled palliative care docs and even better friends, they acknowledged what a hard decision lay ahead of me while always encouraging me to follow my heart.

I'd just returned from one of those trips when a job announcement popped up in my inbox. That was not an uncommon occurrence, given the number of mailing lists I was on, and in the past, I would automatically hit delete. But when your work situation was like mine, you started paying attention to want ads.

This one definitely caught my eye because it described the creation of a new leadership position, which would allow someone to craft a culture rather than be dictated by one. It wasn't just any leadership position. It was an endowed chair in pediatric palliative care, only the third one in the country, in fact. It just happened to be at Oregon Health and Science University.

I guess Portland does have a children's hospital, I remember thinking.

After the conversation Pam and I recently had about where we might go if we ever left Vermont, I couldn't not throw my hat into that ring. We didn't really discuss the job, though, because with endowed chairs coming around so rarely—especially in places cool enough to have their own TV show—a ton of people were sure to apply. My colleagues at other institutions thought I had a decent chance with some going so far as to say that I was "made for that job." But these were my friends talking, and I was so bruised from my current work environment that I doubted I'd even make the first cut.

I never expected, a few weeks later, to receive an invitation to visit Portland for an interview. Things were getting a little more real, so Pam and I had to decide whether to say anything to the kids. We opted not to because why inject uncertainty into their stable lives when this almost surely wouldn't amount to anything? I just explained that I was going out west to give a talk, which—if you count my so-called "audition lecture"—was technically true.

Having always been very open with them, though, keeping it to ourselves wasn't easy. Especially the night before I flew to Oregon for the first time, when I took Catie (then almost fourteen) to see the national tour of *Rent*. I'd first seen that show on its initial Broadway run in the 1990s, back when I was doing my residency. Even though it focused on adults in Manhattan coping with HIV—which would take Angel's life and threaten Mimi's—the themes of loss and family also applied to the kids I was treating (and in some cases losing) for the first time. That night with Catie, I especially resonated with Mimi's boyfriend, Roger, who fled his sorrow by moving across the country.

"I hear there are great restaurants out west," sings Mark, his soon-to-be ex-roommate.

"Some of the best," Roger replies softly.

As Catie and I listened to their dear friend (and Angel's lover), Tom Collins, sing the familiar refrain:

> *I can't believe he's gone*
> *I can't believe you're going*
> *I can't believe this family must die*

I thought of the non-biological family we'd created for ourselves in Vermont. If Christopher hadn't died, I'm not sure I ever would have considered moving, no matter how painful my work situation was. Yet, even with him gone, leaving Vermont would still mean saying goodbye to his wife, Karen; their kids; Grandbob and Grandma Joyce; Sally; and others.

I closed my eyes and listened to Angel's boyfriend's last, bewildered line in the song: "I can't believe this is goodbye." So many of my patients' parents have expressed that same sentiment that it was the intended title of this book until my center daughter rejected it as "way too depressing" and my oldest daughter came up with a better idea, drawn from another musical, which she and I first saw together.

About to get on a plane for a place I'd never seen, I grappled with the possibility that I might have to leave my forever home. And on the eve of a potentially life-changing job interview, I still clung to a fading hope that something unexpected and wonderful might occur at UVM. Or perhaps I wouldn't click with the folks in Portland, or my audition lecture would fall flat.

After all, at the end of *Rent*, Mimi makes a miraculous recovery, and Roger moves back east. Maybe I wouldn't have to say goodbye after all.

#

November is justifiably called "stick season" in Vermont, as the trees are bare and brown, their leaves long fallen and the ground frozen firm. That's why I was so struck by the lush, green Oregon landscape as my plane broke through the clouds over Portland the following afternoon. Mild temperatures and consistent (to put a positive spin on the matter) rainfall in Oregon clearly make a big difference.

Everything also seemed so new compared to the northeast where I'd lived nearly all my life. While our beloved oak tree was witnessing Revolutionary War battles on Lake Champlain, Lewis and Clark were still three decades away from reaching the Pacific. Compared to UVM—the seventh-oldest medical school in the country—OHSU was a new kid on the block, less than a century old and not sufficiently set in its ways for "we just don't do things like that" to be an acceptable response. Case in point: when OHSU ran out of room to expand on the hilltop where it was founded, it purchased a second campus down by the Willamette River, less than a mile away as the crow flies but a good fifteen minutes in street traffic. Recognizing that the commute would be impractical for patients and staff, someone came up with the wild idea of constructing an aerial tram over the city—connecting just the two OHSU campuses—which is now the iconic image of the university.

At the same time, Oregon and Vermont have a lot of things in common. Both are rural, red states with a big blue city tucked in the top left corner. They each have a proud countercultural vibe where T-shirts are frequently seen exhorting people to "Keep Vermont Weird" or "Keep Portland Weird," depending on your coast. And they harbor claims of greatness in the same crucial metrics, often having to do with beer. For instance, Oregon ranks among the top ten states in total number of microbreweries, while Vermont tops the list on a per capita basis, with its meager "capita" making for a helpfully tiny denominator. With six times its eastern sibling's population, Oregon has justifiably been called "Vermont on steroids."

In preparation for a long day of interviews, I'd done my research on OHSU and its pediatric palliative care program, which had been providing outstanding care for many years and now was at an inflection point, about to significantly expand thanks to a major philanthropic gift from the Cambia Health Foundation. More importantly, I made a vow to myself: I wasn't going tell anybody what they wanted to hear (assuming I even knew what that was). Having had my fill of indirect communication and academic politics, I just wanted to show everyone who I was, warts and all. They could draw their own conclusions.

I got my first chance at the opening breakfast interview with the president of the Cambia Health Foundation. Expecting some polite chitchat while we waited for the coffee to arrive, I quickly discovered that Peggy Maguire isn't the sort of person to waste time.

"So why palliative care?" she asked before we'd even sat down.

Years earlier at a cocktail party in Boston, Dave had asked me the same question. Back then, I'd started off with a list of practical reasons—ranging from my desire to be involved in crucial moments in childrens' lives and the current lack of an established program at my hospital—which would have worked just fine at a job interview. In fact, that probably was what Peggy was looking for. But after spending the last decade struggling to understand what my final answer to Dave really meant, after he'd kept digging and pried loose the truth, I wasn't going to retreat now.

"Because," I replied, "I don't want anyone else to hurt the way I did when I was a kid."

If Peggy was surprised by the personal nature of my answer, she didn't show it. She also didn't ask me to elaborate, probably recognizing that was already as deep as someone can go. She just moved on to her next question about mistakes I'd made—from which there were plenty to choose—and what I'd learned as a result.

"And what's your personal mission statement?" she asked, not even countenancing the possibility that someone applying for this job wouldn't have one.

Where the heck's the coffee? I thought.

Peggy was waiting on an answer, though, so I riffed.

"To do the best I can with what I have," I said, hoping that my past experience with bad judgment really had led to good judgment. All the while I was thinking, *I might really like these people.* Sure, these were probably just Peggy's standard interview questions—not personally tailored to hit me square in the heart—but she obviously cared about things other than glitzy names like Yale and Johns Hopkins on a résumé. She cared about the why as much as the what, making me wonder if the rest of the people at OHSU would, too.

She was just about to ask the next question on what would turn out to be a long list, when I realized I'd left out something important.

"And also," I added, "to follow through on my most sacred commitments."

That was for my family back in Vermont because this wasn't just some job interview. Whatever came of it might change not only my life but those of the five people I loved most in the world. If it was best for us as a family to stay put, then that's what I would do, no matter how hard it might be for me.

More interviews followed, each of which reminded me how wonderful it was to be back in a freestanding children's hospital where I didn't have to explain why kids deserved to have their unique needs met. Recalling how meaningful my first HPCCV plenary had been—when I'd forsaken fancy animations for immediacy and vulnerability—for my audition lecture, I didn't just simplify my PowerPoint slides; I left them back in Vermont. And in lieu of a predetermined topic, I just asked the audience what they'd like to talk about.

The first person to raise their hand described a recent case of a child who was clearly dying but whose parents continued to request intensive treatment because they believed God would perform a miracle. Lucky for me, I knew a fair amount about that topic (from both the medical and theological sides), and Dr. Williamson—in whom such a query might well have precipitated a grand mal seizure—was on the other side of the country. Rather than spouting off about what I thought, though, instead, I invited insights and suggestions from the audience.

Long ago, I'd come to the conclusion that there are few truly unique ideas in life and that the primary role of educators is to incorporate communal wisdom into a workable framework. Fortunately, a friend of mine had done exactly that in a recent journal article about miracles, providing an apt and easily remembered mnemonic for how to respond to a patient or family's request to continue treatment while waiting for divine intervention. Not surprisingly, the people in the audience that day came up with each recommended step on their own: be clear about our professional obligations, honor the family's beliefs, never abandon the patient or family, and—perhaps most controversially but also profoundly human—don't be afraid to admit that you hope for a miracle, too. All that was left for me was to reorder their suggestions on the auditorium's white board with slightly modified language, eliciting not a few expressions of "Wow!"

> **A**ffirm the family's belief
> **M**eet the family where they are in terms of hoping for a miracle
> **E**ducate from your role as a medical provider
> **N**o matter what, stand by the patient and family

The audience—whose evaluations would play a role in whether I got offered the job—may have thought me insightful and brilliant, not realizing that all it took was a willingness to listen and a good enough memory to recall the four-part AMEN protocol. (I should note that I did give proper attribution at the end of the lecture, but the impressing had already been accomplished.)

Days like that always conclude with the requisite interview dinner, which might be more important than all the formal conversations that preceded it. It certainly was for me because I recognized that I couldn't do the work that I loved without being part of a supportive team. With our ties loosened after a long day—and tongues loosened by Oregon's justifiably famous pinot noir—I discovered that the people around the table were not only dedicated professionals but down-to-earth and big-hearted human beings. From morning to evening, I'd gone from *I might* to *I do* really like these people.

By the time the festive dinner concluded, it was too late to catch a flight back east. So I just had to stay over another day, which happened to be the Portland Book Festival (at that time known as Wordstock). I already knew that Portland had Powell's, the largest independent bookstore in the country, but I hadn't appreciated how much people there loved books until I saw the line for a panel of three authors—only one of whom I'd even heard of—trail out the door of a church, down the block, and around the next block, too. And when someone came up to me in the line and said how much he'd enjoyed my talk at OHSU the day before, the city didn't feel nearly as big as the official census said it was. Maybe more than Vermont's three degrees of separation, but not quite six.

#

A great trip where I got to meet wonderful people and explore a cool new city: that's all I figured it would amount to. Which is why, a few weeks later, I was so surprised to get an invitation to return for the second (and final) round of interviews. This was getting serious, so Pam came along to see things for herself. I happened to mention the opportunity to my old housemate, Bobby, whom I hadn't seen since the afternoon three years earlier when we said goodbye to Jon in London.

"How about I meet you there?" he said, proceeding to fly up from San Francisco to celebrate me having recently joined him in the fifty-year-old club.

He even took me out for a Russian feast to celebrate, where we consumed a thoroughly unwise quantity of vodka for the eve of a potentially life-changing interview.

The following morning, while Bobby chugged coffee back in his hotel room while waiting for the aspirin to kick in, I met with people I liked even more the second time around, describing my vision of a program that emphasized direct communication and embraced a diversity of skills. As I did, the mental image I kept returning to was one of an open palm. Rather than clinging to something that might or might not be good for me and my family, I wanted to be open to whatever the future would bring. As I said to my potential future boss, Dr. Braner—the chair of pediatrics, who has a huge heart and a deep commitment to palliative care for kids—at the end of the day, "My worst fear isn't that you don't offer me this job. It's that you offer me the job and I take it and move my family out here, only to discover it's not right, either for me or for you."

The other finalist was an extremely accomplished and gifted physician, so Pam and I stuck to our plan of not putting the kids through potentially unnecessary angst. If OHSU offered me the job, then she and I would have a very serious conversation. And if we decided we might want to take it, then—and only then—would we tell the kids. Those were two very, very big ifs.

The plan was working fine until one night over Christmas break. The two younger kids were already in bed, but I stayed up late with Catie and Noah (now almost twelve) to watch an episode of *Stranger Things*. Without my noticing, Catie picked up my cell phone to check the next day's weather.

"Hey Dad," she said, holding the screen out for me to see, "why is there an ad for a house for sale in Oregon?"

Not telling the kids was one thing, but lying to them was never an option.

"Let's talk," I said, plopping down on the ottoman while they sat cross-legged on the shag carpet, as if I was going to tell another mixed-up story. What I proceeded to say probably sounded just as far-fetched to the two of them, who had been born and raised in Vermont and—at least in Noah's case—probably thought they'd never leave. This story, though, carried no guarantee of a happy ending.

"Work has been really hard," I said, which didn't come as a surprise to them. They knew what I did for a living and had also heard me describe my work environment.

I expected Catie to be offended that Pam and I hadn't mentioned the possibility of leaving Vermont—our kids seem to believe our family is a democracy rather than a benevolent dictatorship—but she accepted our rationale for not wanting to worry her.

"It must be really bad if you're thinking of moving," she said.

After years of trying not to weigh them down with things that kids shouldn't have to worry about, I needed them to understand what would make me consider leaving everything we knew and everyone we loved. So for the first time, I went into more detail about some of the hardest moments. Not what happened to me as a child—because unless this book ever gets published, my kids might never know about that—but what was happening every day now: grieving so intensely for the kids I was treating that I could barely defend myself against the attacks of some coworkers.

I'd just described that as feeling "flayed open" when the most amazing thing happened. Noah got up on his knees, reached out, and held me. I'm not talking hugging here, which tends to be rather brief. He *held* me, tight, unflinching, for what must have been close to a minute. A couple of times I let go a little bit, as if to give him permission to stop, but he never did.

Noah, you have to realize, is a super-smart kid who knew full well what moving across the country would mean: leaving his school, his godmother Karen, his surrogate grandparents, and especially his friends, including his best friend since he was three years old. But he also could sense how much the last few years had wounded me and wanted my pain to stop.

I'm pretty good with words—I do have an MFA in writing, after all—but I don't have any to express how much that moment meant to me. As a child, I was trained to believe other peoples' version of reality at the expense of my own heartfelt intuition and to accept what felt horribly wrong if that's what it took for someone else—someone I trusted implicitly—to get what they were seeking. Since then, I'd had some wonderful experiences where another person cared about me in a selfless way so that, for a moment, I didn't need to worry about them and their needs.

But this was a generosity of spirit that I'd never experienced before, if I even realized it existed at all. When I was Noah's age, I'd been deprived of things that every child has a right to receive—care and protection—and here he was providing me with something that no parent has a right to expect: feeling my pain so profoundly that he would do anything in his power and make whatever sacrifice to take it away. After fifteen years of marriage, a cumulative thirty-seven child-years of parenting, and some really amazing friends—I'm talking about you, Christopher—I can safely say that I'd never felt more loved than I did in that moment, being held by my son.

Then came the waiting since the other finalist's interview followed mine. Finally, after what seemed like years—but was really only a couple of weeks—my office phone rang with the caller ID showing the area code for Portland. Before picking up the receiver, I took a deep breath. The next few minutes would either close a door or raise a lot of potentially life-changing questions.

It was Dr. Braner, who asked me how I was doing and to which I replied in kind. I was really hoping that was all for the pleasantries, but he went on to inquire about the weather in Vermont—which, in January, leaves little to the imagination—and proceeded to tell me about the rain they'd been getting in Portland.

Is he just letting me down easy? I wondered. *If so, I wish he'd just put me out of my misery.*

"Well, Bob," he said, before taking what felt like the longest inhalation in history, "we'd love it if you would join our team at OHSU."

I don't recall what I said in response, although gratitude was certainly involved. I do remember setting the phone down gently and resting my head on the laminate desk that had once been Dr. Orr's, expecting a flood of tears after all I'd been through over the past few years. But only a trickle came out because Pam and I now had a huge decision to make. No more hypotheticals about if I would like the position—I loved it—or if they would offer it to me. We needed to decide whether to stay or go.

We both had always said that nothing is more important than each other and the kids. Having endured such pain and isolation over the past few years—and feeling called more than ever to do whatever I could to keep other kids from suffering the way I once had—I felt like we should go west. The way I figured it, the six of us would still be together, only in a different place. I couldn't help but think of the biblical story of Naomi who, upon the death of her husband as well as both her sons, instructed her two daughters-in-law to return to their respective homelands. One, Orpah, did just that, but the more famous one refused.

"Where you go, I will go," Ruth said to Naomi. "Where you lodge, I will lodge. Your people shall be my people."

I was saying something very close to that to Pam: *If you loved me, you wouldn't want me to stay in this environment.* But as an Ivy League grad who'd worked as a foreign correspondent in the Far East for over a decade, moving purely for her husband's work felt stereotypical and wrong. What I viewed as portable—the people who would always be family no matter where we were—she viewed as central, taking precedence over any job.

If we stayed in Vermont, then our kids would never have to pause, as she and I did, when someone asked them where they were from. They wouldn't have to start over again, as she and I had so many times at their age. Where our kids' lives began, so there would ours end, with Pam—in the kind of advance care planning that does a palliative care doc proud—being very clear about where her remains would one day go.

"Under the tree," she'd often say, referring to the five-hundred-year-old oak in the back yard. "Under *our* tree."

I'd asked Pam to be my Ruth by moving with me, but she was actually taking the comparison one step further and reversing the roles. In the verse after the one quoted above, Ruth goes on to say to Naomi: "Where you die, I will die, and there will I be buried."

In our seventeen years together, whenever Pam and I had disagreed about something, we'd been able to reach out and our hands would meet, perhaps not in a place either of us wished to be, but at least we could feel the other's touch. The mere knowledge that a meeting place existed—even if neither of us could bear to stay there for long—sustained us. Only this time, we were so far apart that no matter how far we stretched, the other remained beyond our fingertips.

Sometimes it wasn't really clear that the other person was reaching out at all.

We talked about the potential move a lot, then agreed not to mention it for a while, even as I slogged away at work, wondering how long I could keep going there.

A door was closing, though, because OHSU needed an answer. In the end, Pam and I didn't reach a decision at the end of some huge heartfelt conversation. Heck, we weren't even in the same place.

One Saturday morning, I'd driven our six-year-old to Smuggler's Notch, hoping to squeeze in a little work while she was in ski school. Jeffersonville (population 783) isn't exactly teeming with coffee shops, so after dropping Cha-Cha off, I grabbed a table at the first one I saw and opened my laptop. A couple of dark roast refills later, I called to check in with Pam.

I'm not sure how the conversation came around to Portland since that was the one thing we weren't going to talk about. But somehow, we still ended up there.

"You know what this feels like?" she asked.

I shook my head, even though she couldn't see me. I knew what so many things felt like but maybe not the one she was talking about.

"It feels like you have brain cancer," she explained.

"Gee, thanks."

"And," she continued, as if I hadn't said anything, "you could probably manage to live with it if we stayed here. At least for a while."

I nodded, aware that "manage to live with it" is what palliative care is all about. But even though I wasn't cut out to be a surgeon, I'd never stopped hoping for cure.

"Or," Pam said softly, "we could find a cure in Oregon."

I took a deep breath, needing to make sure that I'd heard her correctly. "It sounds like we're going."

However long she paused, it was enough time for the café to go silent, if not for the world to stand still.

"Yes," she said, "I think we are."

After being flayed open at work, sabbatical and therapy and journaling and friends' conversations and kids' songs and hugs had steadily scraped away at the soul calluses and other dead tissue that needed to go if I was ever going to heal. But it was Pam who finally released my tears and not the polite ones I'd shed at my desk when the job offer came through.

I covered my face with my hands as my shoulders heaved, clearly not about to repeat my rookie mistake of going easy on the saline. Snot was definitely involved. Talk about irrigation and debridement.

The other people in the café were polite enough to keep staring down at their cups of coffee, but I still turned away toward the window. At first I gazed out at the mountains in the distance, wondering which one of those weaving specks on a white background was my youngest daughter. Then my gaze fell on the sign hanging just a few feet away, which I'd failed to notice upon entering. It was a curved wooden beam—the sort that prevents beasts of burden from escaping and forces them to stare straight ahead—with a crack down the center. And on it was written the perfect name for a breakfast spot, especially one where I felt set free: The Broken Yoke.

#

Pursuing one dream often means letting go of another. I'd long clung to the dream of a perfect (rest of my) life: living in our forever home, hanging with my best friend, and riding off into the sunset after a long and distinguished career at UVM. One part of that died with Christopher, and now it was time to let the other parts go, too.

As I thought about how to say goodbye to so many people I'd come to care deeply for over fifteen years at UVM, I kept thinking back to the last day of my pediatric internship. I'd woken up—metaphorically, at least, since I hadn't gotten any sleep on call the previous night—to the greater latitude and responsibility of a second-year resident. But whereas I had so much to look forward to, the supervising senior resident I'd been partnered with the night before had just graduated. Her pager, which for three years had kept her up at night while also assuring her that she was needed, now belonged to a newly minted intern in the revolving door of medical education. As the rest of us scurried around from floor to floor, continuing to take care of patients, she wandered alone toward the exit and disappeared from sight, if not also from memory.

I never wanted to fade away like that with people at UVM wondering, *Hey, whatever happened to that guy?* I also didn't want my friends to learn of my departure through some generic all-users email from my boss with template thanks and well-wishes. So I made a list of about thirty people who meant the most to me and reached out individually to every one of them. "Do you have a minute to chat? How about coffee? When's good? I'll come to you."

I didn't go into detail about my reasons for leaving because it was obvious to anyone who knew how much I loved pediatric palliative care. A handful recognized how miserable I'd been, and to them, it was enough for me to say something like, "I would have taken good here over great somewhere else, but I can't take bad over great."

Those were wonderful conversations, recalling distant memories and reminiscing about tough cases we'd worked on together. As such, they bore resemblance to another kind of farewell. Ira Byock, one of my palliative care heroes, talks about the things that people need to say before they die: "I forgive you. Will you forgive me? Thank you. I love you. Goodbye." I didn't often say the first two but always the last three and heard the same in return.

I also needed to say goodbye to the medical students who had been such a big part of my life. My mom was a teacher and always thought I'd be a good one, too, but I didn't get the chance to find out until I joined the faculty at UVM. Having been frustrated in grad school by ethics discussions that didn't lead anywhere, I resolved to make things practical and real. So for the last decade, on the first day of medical school, I'd shown the incoming class a clip from the television show *ER*, which depicts a married couple involved in a serious car accident. The husband is bleeding internally and will die without surgery, but he refuses to leave his wife even though she likely is brain dead. Not wanting to lose him, too, the doctor surreptitiously detaches one of her EKG leads, making it appear that her heart has stopped. Before being whisked off to surgery, the husband expresses his gratitude for being allowed to stay with his wife while she "died."

The students who'd walked into the lecture hall revering truth-telling and patient autonomy had to grapple with the thought of losing two patients instead of one, while the ones who wanted to save anyone they could were left wondering how far they were willing to go in pursuit of that noble goal. For many, the subsequent discussion was their first—though certainly not last—experience of searching for (and ultimately making peace with) the least bad option.

All the students knew me, although some might not have forgiven me for assigning the only essays they had to write in medical school. I let them know I was leaving and thanked them for allowing me to be a small part of their journey over a barbecue at my house for the ethics special interest group and, of necessity, by a personal email to the rest. All I had left to do was take down fifteen years' worth of my kids' drawings from my office walls, chit-chat with colleagues who stopped by the traditional cheese-cube-and-celery-stick farewell reception, and linger at a last-day lunch with Sally and another friend before walking out of the medical center for what I thought would be the final time.

#

The last part of my dream to let go of was our forever home, which also profoundly affected Pam and the kids. Having been raised in a family where children were meant to be seen and not heard, I always wanted mine to form their own opinions and feel free to speak their minds. Sometimes I wonder if that might have been a mistake.

Upon learning of our intended move, Lucy traded in the cabaret for a printing press. The lead article in the inaugural edition of our home newspaper, *The Macauley Times*, might have benefited from a spellcheck, but the fact that she got my last name—which also happens to be hers—wrong left no doubt as to the depth of her feelings:

> Robert Macaulay and Pamela Burton-Macaulay (in support of the move) have decided to move to Portland, Oregon after less than two months of deciding. They decided to move because of Robert Macaulay's terrible work situation. Anger and sadness arose across the whole family. *Guess Vermont isn't our forever home!*

Noah was more succinct in his response. A few weeks later, as he and I noshed pizza after our Tuesday night aikido class, I observed that he was a little quiet.

"When someone's about to ruin your life," he replied, "sometimes you don't feel like talking to them."

I didn't blame him for that nor appreciate any less him holding me that memorable night. He was a huge-hearted twelve-year-old, not Gandhi. He had a right to his feelings, and I was glad he was telling me about them. Even if it was mostly as an explanation for why he didn't want to share anything more.

Pam and I tried our best to ease the kids' transition, like by planning cool trips with their friends to places like Boston and New York City. I even designed custom purple wristbands (Lucy's favorite color) that read *Macauley Strong*, decorated by our family's sacred symbols including a violin (since three of the kids play stringed instruments), a lotus flower (since Pam is a yoga instructor), and Yoda (for Noah, of course).

Cortez might have burned his ships upon arriving at the "New World" in order to motivate his crew, but knowing how much our Vermont house meant to Pam, especially, we decided not to sell it but rather rent it out, which meant we could reserve a couple of weeks for our family each summer. That way we could come back and see friends and also not close a door on the future. Pam was moving away because I needed to, and I will gladly return one day if she needs to. Like Ruth said to Naomi: "Where you lodge, I will lodge."

It still felt like goodbye, though. Noah and Lucy had learned to ride two-wheelers in that driveway, Baby Cha-Cha came home there from the hospital, and many a night, Christopher had wandered in to join us around the dinner table. But preparing a house for other people to live in means taking down the family photos and boxing up the scrapbooks. If "settling in" has an opposite—settling out?—that's what we were doing as we packed box after box, silently wondering whether the kids' paintings or annual family portraits would be enough to make our new house in Portland ever feel like home.

Amidst all the packing and with tender hearts, we tried to enjoy our final summer there. That's a magical time of year in Vermont, with county fairs and tractor pulls, wildflowers and fireflies. Each night found us dining at the picnic table under our beloved tree in the company of friends, including those we'd been meaning to get together with for a while and now wouldn't have another chance. And no matter what any of us were doing, when someone called out, "Sunset alert!" we would all stop and gather to watch the sun descend over the Adirondacks so far to the north that it sometimes felt as if the whole world was off balance and, maybe one day, the sun would keep going and never come back.

CHAPTER 15

Redemption

After all the sacrifices Pam was making, for the transcontinental trip, it only seemed right that she get to fly with the girls, which left the Macauley males (i.e., Noah, the two dogs, and me) to drive. In preparation, I spent hours identifying signature things he and I could do along the way—chicken wings in Buffalo, deep dish pizza in Chicago, Mt. Rushmore and the Badlands in South Dakota—and hoped that time and distance would give him a chance to adjust. Of all our kids, he valued familiarity the most, and walking onto a plane in Vermont and getting off in Oregon seemed a perfect recipe for him hating our new home.

Finally, with boxes packed and plans forged, the Lake Champlain ferry pulled away from the Vermont shore. Sitting in the driver's seat of our crammed-to-the-gills Buick, I caught a glimpse of our oak tree in the distance and couldn't stop thinking about a joke I once heard:

"What did the fashion model[*] do when they heard that the majority of car accidents happen within five miles of home?"

They moved.

---

[*] "Fashion model" can be replaced with any other profession—not to mention hair color or sports team allegiance—that one wishes to cast as unintelligent (and inevitably will offend by telling the joke).

The reason the joke is funny, of course, is that accidents are more likely to occur near wherever you live, due to the frequency of driving in that area and failure to pay attention to familiar surroundings. In moving across the country, it was entirely possible I was acting like the butt of the joke. What if the problem wasn't my old work environment—whose hallways had been the site of multiple collisions, ideological and occasionally even physical—but something about me that would be just as big a problem in my new one? As my imposter syndrome flared up again, I wondered if this might be the shortest tenure of an endowed chair in modern memory.

I kept those fears to myself, of course, as I drove Noah and the dogs across the country and in my initial days of work. I'd read enough books on leadership to know that team members need confidence and enthusiasm from their new director.

The welcome at work proved to be extremely warm and the learning curve just as steep. I hadn't realized how comfortable it is to know who everybody is and how everything works, as I did after fifteen years in Vermont. Yet, even as I struggled to learn a different system and meet loads of people, I was surprised by how great it felt to be the new guy. After so many years at UVM, I could practically hear folks there thinking, *Oh, that's just Bob,* when I asked students, "Head or heart?" after a patient wondered aloud whether they were dying or after I ticked off the many differences between adult and pediatric palliative care. Most of them had heard my schtick plenty of times before.

What had felt like old hat to them, though, seemed to strike my new colleagues as fresh and fascinating. I'd say the same stuff I've been saying for a long time, and people would reply with a "Whoa!" that would put Keanu Reeves to shame. I knew, eventually, that stuff would become familiar to them, too, but I was happy to ride this wave all the way into shore.

There were a few moments, though, when I thought I might wipe out. Like my first grand rounds since the fateful one at UVM. I probably should have heeded Santayana's famous dictum about learning from history so as not to repeat it, but I was done filtering what I believed. Forgoing a safe topic, I made the case that, instead of asking patients whether they wanted to be resuscitated, doctors should tell patients what their code status should be. (I did emphasize that the conversation should start with the patient's goals, which the physician could then translate into a medical plan, including code status.)

I considered it a nuanced argument filled with real-life examples, but I'd thought the same about the presentation on trisomy 18. That's why my pulse skyrocketed when I noticed a couple of intensive care doctors waiting around to talk to me afterward. Evidently, three thousand miles and four years wasn't enough to erase the memories of petitions past.

"That might have been the best grand rounds I've ever heard," one of them said. She was junior faculty, though, so probably hadn't heard that many grand rounds before.

"It was recorded, right?" the other one asked. "Because I think we should include it in the in-service for our nurses."

Which indeed occurred, making me feel both appreciated but also sorry for those nurses required to sit through it. In-services happen every year, so they'd have the dubious distinction of reaching the "Oh, that's just Bob" stage before everybody else.

#

I was still getting settled into my new job when the past came calling. Sifting through reams of emails one afternoon, I was surprised to find one from UVM. Thinking that chapter of my life was over, I assumed that—as former faculty—my name must have been added to some extensive mailing list. Expecting a form letter, the opening line seemed almost nonsensical, forcing me to read it over several times before I finally grasped its meaning.

> It is our honor to write to you on behalf of the University of Vermont College of Medicine Class of 2018 to humbly request your presence and delivery of the commencement address at our 217th Commencement Ceremony.

I sat back in my chair and took a cavernous breath. My last few months at UVM had felt like one long, tender goodbye to the institution that over many years had formed me as a physician and as a person. Leaving the hospital on my final day of work, I'd thought I would never return. The email felt like much more than an invitation to give a short speech; it was reassurance that UVM was missing me a little, too.

And now I'd have the chance to say a proper goodbye alongside the students who'd meant so much to me. We had started together—they gave me the chance to be a teacher, and I delivered their first lecture in medical school—and now we would leave the same way. That parallelism had clearly also occurred to the class president, judging from the last line of their email:

> We realize you would be coming from a long distance, having just experienced many transitions of your own. As we, too, journey in our new clinical roles, it seems incredibly apt to hear from you again, grounding us in the truth of the intimate, profound purpose that is the physician's calling.

Even as I began to wonder how I could possibly express what was in my heart—for a place and people that meant so much to me for so long—in the allotted ten minutes or less, I was reminded of the more recent and painful past at UVM. Not long after the graduation invitation popped up in my inbox so did a request from the parents of a patient to no longer interact with a specific member of our pediatric palliative care team at OHSU, based on their perception that the team member wasn't really listening to them.

Where I used to work, that's the sort of thing that would incite a rush to judgment with recriminations about lack of commitment or even integrity. But I didn't have to play by someone else's unwritten rules anymore. Now I could write my own, fostering a culture that I would want to work within, creating an atmosphere where we all could breathe.

So instead of metaphorically sliding a conference brochure across the desk—as an angry Dr. Kelly once had with me—and demanding an explanation, I invited the team member to help me see the situation through their eyes. What was their sense of what happened? What was their side of the story? I wish I could say I responded that way because that's what all those books I'd read about crucial conversations tell you to do, but really it was because I knew firsthand how awful it felt to have someone assume the worst about you rather than engage in direct conversation. I didn't want anyone else to feel the way I so often had.

It was an honest and heartfelt dialogue and a reminder of what an intensely human endeavor palliative care is. For every patient you totally click with, there's another you don't really connect to. So I assured the team member—and in the process reminded myself—that just because someone doesn't resonate with what you say doesn't mean you did a bad job, the same way that someone thinking you're great doesn't mean you did a good one.

As we identified some things to pay attention to in the future, I thought again of how palliative care is often called a team sport. With the rest of the Vermont PACT team "dedicated in spirit but not in time"—and the adult team not exactly jazzed about having a pediatrician/ethicist in their midst—I'd spent a decade essentially flying solo. Trying to address patients' emotional and spiritual needs as well as their physical ones, I'd failed in some areas and been judged for a few I'd actually managed to succeed in, as evidenced by Dr. Williamson's response to my rare sacramental involvement.

That's why it felt so amazing to finally be part of a true interprofessional and supportive palliative care team. The first consult I did at OHSU, flanked by a skilled nurse, social worker, and chaplain, was positively transformative. I didn't have to (try to) attend to every need of the patient and family because there were gifted professionals beside me who did that exceedingly well. And instead of feeling like I had to protect myself from those around me, I started to believe I could lean on them.

— Kharma —

That was especially the case with Kharma, who up until a few days before we met had been your average twelve-year-old. (And, remember, in the palliative world, "average" is something to be envied.) With long blond hair and an incandescent smile, she always seemed to brighten the room, so I wasn't surprised to learn her parents' nickname for her was "Sunshine."

Her family lived in rural southern Oregon, where her two younger brothers loved being outside as much as she did. So much so, in fact, that Kharma and her dad, Tim (whose thin braid of a beard hung down to his chest), hatched a plan to buy an RV for family road trips. The only hitch was that the practical one in the family—that would be her mother, Erin, who had long straight hair and could have starred in an Ivory soap commercial—wanted to make sure it paid for itself. So together, Tim and Kharma came up with the logo, slogan, and colors of "Our Journey RV Rentals," which started off with one camper that Kharma christened *Sweet Pea*. Over the next couple of years, they added four more rental vehicles to what became the family business, which Tim envisioned Kharma taking over one day.

After some shorter forays, the family was finally able to carve out three weeks for a real summer vacation in *Sweet Pea* to several national parks: Yosemite, Yellowstone, Glacier. Just before they left, though, Kharma came down with what they thought was a cold. Only instead of getting better, it started affecting her appetite and energy level. When she started having trouble breathing, too, she was life-flighted to OHSU, where a CT scan revealed a tumor in her chest.

Before a child gets seriously ill, there are usually warning signs like subtle weight loss or a fever that just doesn't go away. Even if the gradual trajectory doesn't ultimately impact the amount of grief the parents experience—assuming such a thing can be measured—those signs offer time to comprehend the new reality or stockpile a few more treasured memories. Like Ella, who in the process of setting my personal record for the longest time between receiving pediatric palliative care consultations (six years) had written beautiful poems and swam with dolphins. Kharma, though, didn't even get six weeks.

A biopsy showed her tumor had metastasized from somewhere, but the origin didn't matter as much as the type: two distinct variants of an extremely rare cancer, each of which had only been reported in two other people in history and never together. Tim wasn't exaggerating when he said that Kharma had a "cancer that no one's ever had before."

It was also essentially impossible to treat. That is why the parent support group on the oncology floor actually managed to make Tim and Erin feel more alone. Everyone else was discussing chemotherapy, while their only option was hospice.

"We didn't even have hope," Tim remembers. "We were done."

In contrast to every other patient mentioned in this book, I didn't actually spend much time with Kharma. The pediatric oncology team had diagnosed her and was offering the meager treatments available, and the child life specialists were helping her understand what was happening to her body. She already knew a little about cancer because the family dog, Levi, had died from it a couple of years earlier.

With so many bases covered, the danger was not deficiency but redundancy, so I focused on the few things that someone else wasn't already doing much better than I could. One was clarifying goals of care, which was especially challenging because what most parents experience as a steady evolution over months or even years—from denying the diagnosis to striving for cure to hoping for a decent amount of time to being willing to accept anything that might actually be achievable—Tim and Erin had to navigate quickly. All the same emotions came up, like anger and confusion and grief, only this time rapid-fire and in no particular order, contrary to what the textbooks say. And like many other parents, they coped in slightly different ways.

Tim was a pharmacist and took it upon himself to explore treatment options, understandably reluctant to take the word of doctors he'd only just met that his daughter was going to die. Erin, though, seemed to intuitively sense what Tim needed empirical proof of. Despite their distinct approaches, they somehow managed to walk the well-worn path of palliative care—from maximal treatment to forgoing burdensome treatments (like CPR) to focusing entirely on comfort—hand-in-hand, with little time to rest after making one decision before being confronted with another.

Back when my soul calluses still provided a buffer between the world and me, I'd tried to imagine how I would feel if one of my kids got seriously ill in order to empathize with what the parents I was working with were experiencing. Upon hearing that, a wise old friend of mine (who happens to be psychotherapist) had ordered me to stop immediately.

"That's a fool's errand," he'd explained because, no matter how hard I tried, I'd never truly comprehend what those families were going through.

And even if I managed to come close, over the course of a career, the cumulative toll would be too great. We humans aren't designed to lose our children; we aren't even designed to *think* about losing our children, especially on a daily basis and in rare and unexpected ways.

Initially, I'd heeded his advice, but with the return of sensation, I no longer had to try to imagine. The connections would just happen, especially when there were similarities like the breathing problems Ella and my oldest daughter, Catie, both experienced. So, too, with Kharma, who was the same age as my center daughter, Lucy. Whereas Catie wants to understand and explain (and ultimately control) everything around her, Lucy doesn't care about the rules of the world because she doesn't play by them. On the soccer field—which she ventures onto only under duress—she's content to twirl her curly black hair and gaze up at the clouds while the ball rolls by. And she has simple tastes: given a sketchpad or the ingredients for baking chocolate chip cookies, she likely won't be heard from all afternoon.

With that comes an innocence, stemming from some unspoken (and ultimately unreliable) agreement that if she leaves the rest of the world alone, it will return the favor. Were she ever to fall seriously ill, her first reaction wouldn't be rage but rather bewilderment. *How could this happen? Tomorrow will still be there for me, right?* Twelve is a perilous in-between time, old enough to sense the importance of what she's told but too young to know how to cope with it.

Kharma loved to draw, too, although she preferred spending time with her cat, Coco, to baking cookies. I didn't need to try to imagine how Tim felt as his daughter looked up to him—ever before her protector—and asked him for something he'd give his very life to provide her, if only he were given the chance.

If that were Lucy, I'd need to do *something* to help her. So, recognizing Tim's expertise in symptom management, I invited him into medication decisions in a way I never had with a parent before. After all, he understood more about opioid pharmacology than I did. I explained the reasoning for each of my recommendations, down to the choice of medication and the number of milligrams.

Each night we walked the same tightrope that I had with Grace in New York City, using enough analgesia to control the pain but not so much as to make her too sleepy. Each day seemed to bring another hope to relinquish—like a longed-for family trip to the coast, leaving only getting home to Coco to shoot for—and a complication that made me feel like the universe had gone beyond crass indifference and now was just piling on. Like one of Kharma's brothers developing appendicitis, and the best we could do was let him stay on the oncology unit after surgery so that his parents could merely shuttle room to room, rather than floor to floor.

I longed to help, but at that point, I might not have even pulled off making a shitty situation less shitty (as a parent of a former patient had once summarized my job). So I resorted to hugs, which aren't as simple as they sound. I'm cognizant of boundaries, and the last thing I'd want is a parent to feel uncomfortable. And it's not just a male/female thing. Some dads are huggers, but it gets weird real fast if you reach out to embrace one who's not.

Despite the complexities, sometimes it feels wrong not to try. A handshake is fine at the fifty-yard line before kickoff but not in a confined hospital room after discussing what a good death might look like for someone's kid. So, after revising Kharma's pain plan for the umpteenth time following yet another setback and before giving Erin a hug as usual, I turned to Tim, my fellow dad. My hesitation was verging on awkward when Erin saved the day.

"He's a hugger," she whispered to me.

So I put my arms around him, and when Erin joined in, I dared to hope that what they say about three-legged stools not falling over was true.

With Kharma stuck in the hospital—because Tim and Erin weren't going to leave any of their kids behind—and Coco back home, we found ourselves in a classic "Mohammed and the mountain" situation. Fortunately, Make-A-Wish is the MacGyver of palliative care, and they came through once again. Thanks to their generosity, Tim was able to fly home alone the next morning and back that afternoon with a feline companion, who was barred by multiple health and safety codes from entering the hospital. Yet for some reason, a sign mysteriously appeared on Kharma's door: "Check with nurse before opening. Elopement risk."

Finally, after what seemed like countless ups and downs, Kharma was as stable as we could get her, and her brother was ready for discharge. Hospice would meet them at home the following afternoon. She might not have much time there, but—as Collin taught me in his final days—for those who long to be in familiar surroundings with their family (both human and feline), even a little while is worth the effort.

— Return to Vermont —

All of this was happening at the close of summer, which had begun with the UVM graduation. Vermont felt both intimately familiar—seeing old friends and wandering the paths that, every day for fifteen years, I'd taken to teach classes, attend meetings, or simply walk to my office—and also strangely foreign with Pam and the kids back on the other side of the country. A great deal had happened in my life over the past year that my former colleagues knew nothing about and vice versa. It felt like I'd entered a liminal space where I no longer formally belonged, but I had left recently enough that I still knew most everyone and understood the unwritten rules. Acutely aware that the sense of separation would only grow as time went on, I resolved to savor that moment when I still felt more like family than a guest.

In contrast to the soon-to-be graduates' first day of medical school, on their final day I didn't show them any video clips from *ER* or nifty PowerPoint animations. I didn't even use notes, because I knew by heart what I wanted to say.

"Back when I was in medical school," I said as I came out from behind the lectern to stand on the edge of the stage, "I remember being so excited—and relieved—to finally graduate. And I'll definitely never forget the night before I started my residency when I did something I'd never done before."

The students were probably expecting something truly sage, coming from the guy who'd delivered every ethics lecture they'd heard in medical school. One had confided that when he and his classmates were confronted with an impossible question, they'd ask themselves WWMD? (As in, "What would Macauley do?") But that sunny May afternoon, they were in for a surprise.

"I drove the wrong way down a one-way street," I confessed to scattered laughter.

In my defense, I'd just moved to Baltimore, and the street I was driving on was one of those weird ones that starts off one-way and becomes two-way, which worked out fine on the drive to the residency welcome dinner but proved problematic on the way back. Especially when I saw the flashing lights of a police car behind me.

Before the officer even had a chance to ask for my license and registration, I started blubbering. "I'm really sorry. So, so sorry. But I'm a doctor, or at least I'm going to be a doctor. Tomorrow, actually. And there are going to be a lot of kids—"

When he cut me off, I figured he was going to give me either a ticket or a breathalyzer. (I hadn't been drinking, but from my behavior, he could have been forgiven for wondering if I had.) Instead, he offered some free advice.

"Take it slow, buddy," he said, "and pay attention to the signs. And, please, try not to hurt anyone."

Then he walked back to his car, leaving me to drive home slowly and (this time) in the right direction. I couldn't believe he'd let me go when I was so clearly guilty. Nor could I stop thinking about what he'd said.

"Those words have stuck with me ever since," I said, "because they have direct application to our work."

It's hard to take it slow, I told the audience, because there's always too much to do: patients to evaluate, procedures to perform, orders to write, knowledge to acquire. So much that we have no choice but to multitask, which the younger generation—with their smart phones and multiple computer monitors—was not only skilled at but eminently comfortable with.

"Sometimes, though," I said, "we need to slow down and focus on just one thing."

Like when a patient is talking about what they long for or are frightened of. Or when they can't sleep because hospital nights seem to last forever, and they just need to know they're not alone in the world.

"We also need to pay attention to the signs and not just the red ones that say, 'Wrong Way.' Which clearly I didn't that night."

Neither had I paid attention, recalling the analogy of the frog in the pot of water, to the temperature rising around me in a world of suffering and all-too-frequent loss. Only when I finally had a chance to escape for a while did sensation return, both allowing me to recognize everything that I'd endured so far and compelling me to find a way to survive in that world going forward.

I reminded the graduates that some signs in life are subtle, like fatigue, despondency, and insomnia. But if we overlook them, we'll end up either creating a barrier that prevents us from truly empathizing with our patients or crumbling under the weight of sorrow and have nothing left to give.

"Trust me," I said, "I know firsthand how dangerous both of those can be."

The officer's final bit of advice to "try not to hurt anyone" probably sounded familiar to the graduates. "First, do no harm" is the fundamental rule of medicine and an especially important one to remember when—after so many years of study and observation—these newly minted doctors finally got the chance to actually do something. I encouraged them, though, to always keep in mind the distinction between doing things for a patient and merely doing things *to* a patient. Because, for every patient who needs a prescription or a procedure, there's at least one other patient who just needs someone to listen to them, to stand by them when things get hard, and to companion them on the final leg of their journey.

"Because you're not called to simply avoid harming people. You're called to heal them."

I don't think I used the word "grace" in describing what that cop said to me all those years ago, but it kept popping into my head—just as it had during my conversation with thrice-orphaned Shirley, not quite as many years ago—as I relayed his final advice to the graduates. What I deserved that night in Baltimore was a moving violation, yet instead, he'd offered wise counsel (which I was still quoting over two decades later). Even more than that, though, he showed me mercy.

This, in turn, brought me back around to the Parable of the Prodigal Son—which I'd long said was a favorite but only recently had begun to understand—where the undeserving younger son was welcomed, not with judgment but celebration. Having spent much of my life emulating the judgy elder son in that story, only to have Dr. Danvers provide me with an opportunity to see things from the other side, I finally recognized that what ultimately brings you home is more important than whatever took you away in the first place. But it took a Baltimore cop, whose name I never caught, to remind me that there's a third character in the parable, which I now realize is more about grace than deservedness. That's why I now refer to that story by its alternate title: the Parable of the Loving Father.

By that point, I'd reached my assigned time limit, but I couldn't leave out the most important thing of all.

"Thank you," I said softly into the lapel mic, "for allowing me to be a part of your journey on both the first day of medical school as well as the last. I wouldn't be the teacher—or the person—I am if it weren't for you. Now go out there and heal some folks."

As I turned back toward my chair, I was amazed that I'd managed to hold it together with so many emotions coursing through me: thanksgiving, wonder, affection, hope. My UVM story—like that of each of the graduates in the audience—was coming to an end. Not in the way I'd long dreamed of, riding off into retirement as the elder statesman of ethics and palliative care but in a totally unexpected fashion that was no less wonderful.

It was only after I was seated that I noticed none of the students were. They were standing and clapping, and a second later, everyone else in the audience was, too. Things started to get awkward when the faculty members on stage stood up, too, leaving me the only person out of the thousand present still in his chair. I couldn't just sit there, blushing, until they decided to stop, so I stood and bowed my head toward the students, resting my palm over my heart in gratitude. They just kept going, though, so without really thinking about what I was doing—only that I needed to do something—I started clapping, too, this time for the graduates. That created a tender crossfire of applause which prompted the audience both to smile and sit back down so we could get on to the real business of the day.

One by one, the graduates were called up on stage to receive their diplomas and have their chosen faculty member drape a hard-earned doctoral hood across their shoulders. I had the privilege of congratulating each one as they exited the stage and to hood my favorite medical student over my entire tenure at UVM (and now a friend), who just happened to be graduating that year.

The formal recession brought us out into bright sunshine on the college green where the air practically crackled with relief over the end of four long years of written tests, clinical assessments, early morning rounds, and national board exams. Proud parents took photos of "the doctor in the family" as alumni welcomed the newest members of our fraternity.

Looking around at the beaming students, I couldn't help but think of another old joke: "What do you call the person who graduated last in their class from medical school?"

Doctor.

That might be faint reassurance to patients, but it conveys an important lesson. Logically speaking, somebody there must have graduated last in the class, struggling along the way with the material or their self-image or parts of life—relationships, family—that medical school doesn't pause to honor. That student made it, though, and will be a licensed physician one day, likely an excellent one, with the academic precipice they once teetered on long forgotten. There are far more important qualities of a doctor than class rank, speaking as someone who's never excelled at standardized tests.

I hope it meant something to the graduates to discover that someone who now appeared to know so much that he deserved his very own bracelet-ready abbreviation (WWMD) had once been so afraid that he didn't belong that he'd driven the wrong way down a one-way street. I hope this book will serve as a gentle reminder not to assume, just because someone seems like they've got it all together—Ivy League-educated doctor, endowed chair, fucking brilliant wife,* and four awesome kids—that they aced their boards and were universally respected (just talk to Dr. Williamson). Heck, for all you know, not too long ago, that person might have been considering leaving medicine altogether if that's what it took for their family to be okay and for them to be able to breathe again. And going back even farther, that person might have suffered a hell of a lot in ways that they're only beginning to understand, making it nothing short of a miracle that they ended up where they are today. As Robin Williams, who we now know was speaking from profound experience, said, "Everyone you meet is fighting a battle you know nothing about."

Celebratory group photos taken, the graduates and their families started walking toward the student center for the formal reception. Even if I hadn't needed to catch a plane, I wouldn't have been tempted to follow. I'd seen the people I'd come there to see and said the words that were on my heart. This was the graduates' day, not mine. The chance to wish them well on the next stage of their journey—and thank them for being such a huge part of mine on what was our last day at UVM—allowed me to close the book on a sacred chapter of my life rather than simply fade away.

#

---

* Earlier in the book, I described my wife as "smart and wonderful," but my first and best reader—who I also happened to be married to—offered this elaboration.

Later that summer, I returned to Vermont again, this time with my family. It felt so familiar to be in our old house, where we slipped back into cherished routines: picnics under our majestic tree, sacred pauses upon each afternoon's sunset alert, roasting s'mores over a lakeside fire. After having struggled over the past year to integrate into a new community, it was a blessing to lose track of who was coming over and when. We'd leapt to the top of everyone's priority list because that was the only chance all year we'd get to spend time together. (Noah's best friend didn't so much visit as move in.) If there's such a thing as rock stars in rural Vermont, for two weeks it was us.

So idyllic was our return that I'd be lying if I said I didn't occasionally muse about what life would have been like if we'd stayed. But I realized that there was more to UVM than graduations and to Vermont than summer concert tours. We'd begun to lay down some roots in Portland, which admittedly would never run as deep as a five-hundred-year-old burr oak's. That tree will always be Pam's true north in the same way that Vermont will probably always feel like home to our family. But that didn't mean we might not, eventually, feel at home somewhere else.

I hoped Pam and the kids shared that sentiment because we had a plane to catch, and there were plenty of hidden corners in our house where somebody could hole up and try to run out the clock. Thankfully, everyone piled into the rental van on time with their bags packed, ready, if not to go home, then at least back to Oregon. Subsequent annual returns to Vermont have been just as joyous, with thankfully less suspense at the departure gate. Along the way, I've sensed in the kids an air of resilience that wasn't there before and would not be present now if we hadn't been forced to craft a new life in a place where we didn't know a soul.

At the same time, there's no denying that the early days in Oregon were lonely and hard. Each moment seemed suffused with a lingering sense of loss for which I alone was responsible. Granted, moving to another place is not a unique challenge, and our kids will have far fewer transitions in their childhood than my wife and I had in ours. But just because someone else has experienced a greater pain doesn't make yours hurt any less, as palliative care reminds me every day. We could have stayed in Vermont except that I felt called to something else.

Intermixed with my guilt is a profound sense of gratitude, both for how far I've come as a person and much more so for the family I'm blessed to have. The suffocating silence that so often envelops child sexual abuse—as it did in my case—is ultimately an inability to express what you need. Survivors are trained to believe that you're not supposed to ask for anything, and even if you dare to, you still don't deserve whatever that is: true love, protection, being believed.

But I did need something to be whole—something big—and not only was I able to express that, the people closest to me were willing to hear it. My chosen and created family acted contrary to their own well-being out of love for me, whereas in my childhood, others acted in their own self-interest under the guise of love. That was not my wife and children's violation to atone for, but through a generosity I'd never known—as exemplified most of all by Noah's hug the night he learned the reasons we might have to leave our forever home—they made it theirs to redeem.

— Kharma: Part two —

Kharma had been diagnosed soon after my family's return to Oregon, and on the day of her planned discharge, I went in to work early. There were so many moving parts—pain control during the long drive south, hospice meeting the family at their home, ongoing post-op care for her brother—that I needed to be certain we'd covered every last detail. I was sitting at my desk, trying to identify anything we might have missed, when my pager went off. When I pressed the button, three words appeared: *Kharma just died.*

That's what we'd all been preparing for, but it wasn't supposed to happen now. Not here. Not this way. Not at all, actually, in that just universe which somehow I'm still talking about, despite all the evidence to the contrary.

Without even thinking, I headed straight up to the oncology floor. Going there wasn't particularly noble or noteworthy because it's what docs—especially palliative care docs—are supposed to do. It's the "without even thinking" part that was significant, at least for me. I had no formal task to accomplish, especially given the wealth of other skilled and compassionate folks involved in Kharma's care, who were trying to console her parents. The danger, once again, was redundancy, which at that moment I didn't really care if I contributed to.

As I walked onto the oncology floor, the first people I saw were Tim and Erin. They were standing outside a closed office door, appearing dazed. Only minutes before, Kharma had been thrashing in her bed from a sudden spike in her pain. The nurse had given her more medication and pulled the drapes to darken the room, but nothing succeeded in calming her until Erin started singing softly:

> *You are my sunshine, my only sunshine*
> *You make me happy when skies are gray*
> *You'll never know dear, how much I love you*
> *Please don't take my sunshine away.*

Gradually, Kharma's eyes closed, and her brow softened, and it seemed to Tim and Erin that her spirit was leaving.

"It's okay, baby," Erin whispered. "Time to go with Levi."

With that permission, Kharma died. And when the nurse opened the curtains to let a sliver of light in, the room was flooded with what Erin and Tim describe as "the biggest, brightest sunbeam" they'd ever seen.

Having refused to leave the hospital without all of their children, Tim and Erin now had no choice. The only thing left was signing some paperwork locked in that office, at which point they would start their long journey home through a steady stream of rain, the sky already having begun to darken.

At the start of my career, I would have imagined what a noble physician would do and then tried to act like that, remaining emotionally buffered until I found a safe place to grieve alone. Now, though, I didn't think, analyze, or observe. Even without soul calluses to protect me—*especially* without them—I walked straight up to Tim and Erin and embraced them in the same three-way hug we'd shared the first time.

"I'm so sorry," I think I said, through the tears.

We stood there for a long while in the hallway of the cancer floor. I didn't search for words to say because I knew I wouldn't find any, but I also didn't let go. I just cried along with them, grateful that, in that moment, we could prop each other up so that nobody fell.

Only later, as I headed back to the team office for our morning rounds, did it occur to me that I'd been fully present in that moment. That was good news for the care I was providing—as well as my own personal development—but bad news when it came to productivity. It turns out that soul calluses are a huge help in getting work done in a highly emotional environment, which you definitely notice when you don't have them anymore.

By the time I reached our office, the rest of the team had heard about Kharma. Knowing how much I'd come to care about her and her family, they forgot about rounds and asked how I was doing.

"I'm really going to need you guys today," I said, "because I don't think I'm going to be at my best."

I can't even imagine admitting such a thing or asking for what I did where I used to work. And that morning, I received a level of support I could never have dreamed of. The rest of the team—whom I'd long since recognized as my people—sat with me, silently, for a completely unproductive and equally necessary few minutes, honoring Kharma's memory as well as my sorrow and generously allowing me to draw us back together when I was finally able to continue.

What is (or at least should be) part of palliative care, though, isn't necessarily a part of every other specialty. An intensive care fellow named Alia Broman happened to be spending time with us to learn more about communication and clarification of goals. She took care of the sickest patients and, over the past few months, had lost quite a few. But she never got the chance to mourn because there was always another critically ill patient who needed help.

Fortunately, in palliative care, we often have time to slow down and feel. (And if we don't have the time, we make it.) Organically and unintentionally, my obvious grief about Kharma opened up a rich avenue of sharing, of how we try to make sense of the death of a child and the grief the parents will carry forever. And how we keep going in the midst of loss. Rounds could wait a little while longer.

"I've never heard an attending say what you just said," Alia observed at the end of our critically important tangent. "About not being at their best because a patient died."

That was quite a statement coming from someone in their tenth year of training (if you count medical school). But I probably shouldn't have been surprised, having come from a place where expressions of need were not always welcomed. I was just grateful that Alia had joined us that morning so she could see that she wasn't alone in feeling as she did and how important it was to have places (and people) to share that pain with.

#

I don't often write letters to surviving parents. Some things are impossible to put into words, and even then, a letter seems a rather formal way of doing so. Especially one that's typewritten, which is necessary since my handwriting is illegible even by doctor standards. But with Tim and Erin living hours away, I not only couldn't attend Kharma's funeral, I doubted we'd ever meet again.

So I sat down at my computer the next morning, which I knew would be awful for Tim and Erin (even if I couldn't comprehend just how awful). The tender image of Erin singing to Kharma as she was dying will always stay with me, but as I typed my letter, it was the first verse of "You Are My Sunshine"—not the familiar refrain—that kept going through my head:

> *The other night dear, as I lay sleeping*
> *I dreamed I held you in my arms*
> *But when I awoke, dear, I was mistaken*
> *So I hung my head and cried*

Trying to offer some small measure of comfort, I told them what amazing parents they were, for standing by all their kids and bravely reassuring Kharma that it was okay to go. I also shared what I'd said to the team the previous morning about not being at my best, which I still wasn't. I described how that had led to a long discussion about grief and self-care and the patients who touch our lives and whom we'll never forget. And how deeply that had impacted an intensive care fellow who will take care of literally thousands of critically ill children over the course of her career.

"All because of Kharma," I wrote. "I thought you might like to know that."

I was grateful for the chance to express what I thought and felt, especially in a form that parents could return to when they were tempted to doubt how hard they'd worked to care for and protect their child. Over many conversations with bereaved parents, I've learned that grief and self-blame swim in the same circles and sometimes are hard to tell apart. Kharma definitely understood that her cancer was incurable, but Tim and Erin had never told her that she was going to die. Which left them to wonder, in the weeks following her death, if not knowing what was happening to her body—and not having the chance to say goodbye on her own terms—might have made Kharma even more scared.

Thankfully, months later, they came upon a sketch Kharma had drawn in the hospital, of her and Levi together again. And they both had wings.

It's probably not a coincidence that, soon after I mailed the letter to Tim and Erin, I started writing this book, which, when you think about it, is really just one long letter of remembrance and gratitude addressed to many patients at once. Nicky, Lily, Thomas, Amelia, Ethan, Grace, Hope, Rider, Harry, Trey, Collin, Emerson, Ella, and Kharma—not to mention Jon, of course, and especially Christopher—deserve to be remembered for who they were (or in Hannah, Tony, Benjamin, and Cora's cases, still are) and the many lives they touched, mine most definitely included. And their parents deserve reassurance that the world will never forget the child they loved so dearly.

"My fear isn't that he'll die—because he already did," Collin's mother, Deb, told me, five years after his death. "Now it's just Bill and me talking about him, and my worry will be that it'll be like he never existed. That he never happened."

But he did happen, as I'm reminded every time I glance at the black-and-white photo hanging on my office wall of him playing the drums on oxygen. Now you know Collin, too, and after that, he is—like every other kid in this book—impossible to forget.

In addition to sharing their stories with the world, this book has also helped me write my own story. At that cocktail party in Boston when I blurted out that I didn't want anyone else to hurt the way I did when I was a kid, I was only starting to understand what drew me to pediatric palliative care. Knowing from personal experience that kids can be wounded drove me to at least try to lessen their pain. That same experience conferred upon me the soul calluses that initially provided some measure of protection from the emotional toll of the work.

Before we go down the "woe is me/brave soul that I am" rabbit hole, though, let's be clear: I'm not selfless enough for that to keep me doing the work, even when my soul calluses were intact. (After all, just because you can take a punch doesn't mean you should go looking for a fight.) Something else was driving me, which I was only able to identify by writing this book.

"Which brings me back to my initial question," Dave had asked me, years ago. "Why palliative care?"

"Because," I would answer him now, if I had another chance, "were it not for this work, I wouldn't know how brave and honest and wise and generous human beings can be."

I was raised to believe that children should act like Exhibit A at dinner parties and to overlook the contradictions of a Bizarro World. My patients, though, showed me that being a kid doesn't mean doing what you're told; it means battling for what you know in your heart is important and true. And occasionally crying yourself to sleep at night, when everybody else would rather believe children don't ever go through what you're going through, before dusting yourself off the next day to fight even harder. Asking for what you need while forgiving people when they can't give it to you, as long as their heart is in the right place. And definitely defying predictions, especially the self-fulfilling kind.

Meanwhile, their parents dare to plan ahead for the day their hearts will break. Or, in order to shield their babies from suffering, hold them for their entire lives. Or send their teenager off to Europe to follow his dreams, hoping—but definitely not praying—that he'll survive long enough that, upon his return, they can get him from the airport to the hospital in time.

Along the way, they say stuff that doesn't make any sense to people who want to believe that children never die. Like, "This is the best, hardest thing we've ever done," as Dave and Julie described yet another sleepless night of rocking Ella. And, as Daniel and Miriam recalled being able hold their daughter, Lily, for only a few minutes: "We're the luckiest unlucky people in the world."

You'd think that, after all the heartbreak they'd been through, after their child died, they'd stay as far away from hospitals and doctors as possible. But instead, they return to the site of their greatest pain in order to cuddle critically ill babies most people are afraid to even touch. They pump breast milk that, in a more merciful world, would nourish their own baby, then ship it off to a distant state for an adopted kid they've never even met. They stand before a sea of white and tell doctors who'd forecast their child's demise that they shouldn't believe everything they were taught in medical school. And they testify before legislators and create educational videos so that other parents in the same situation won't feel as alone as they once did.

Emerging from a Bizarro World where people did things no one ever should—like saying they love you and then committing unspeakable acts—somehow I found my way to a place where people do things I never dreamed a human being even *could*. In the process, it wouldn't at all be an exaggeration to say that those kids and their parents healed my soul. Because of them, I began to trust my own sense of what was good and meaningful and true. That journey involved a blend of home runs ("Hold them for their entire lives") and strike outs ("Hang in there") which my patients and their parents alternately valued and forgave because they trusted that my heart was in the right place, giving me the strength to do the same. And when they said I'd made a difference in their lives, I—who'd long been burdened by a sense of inefficacy in a world I could neither control nor even understand—dared to (mostly) believe them.

But the most profound way they healed my soul was through their honesty and courage, which pierced my previously impenetrable soul calluses. Once I started to feel again, I had no choice but to confront the trauma of my own childhood and also to enter into—vicariously, to be clear, but also proximately—the suffering of the patients and families I was caring for.

Along the way, many times I wondered whether the return of sensation was such a good thing. My therapist thought it long overdue, but when your heart is breaking, it's hard to take the long view. More than once, I thought of the pastoral care adage about not taking away someone's crutch, however unhealthy it might be. My soul calluses certainly weren't healthy, but they had prevented me from falling over the course of my entire life.

Thankfully, sadness wasn't the only feeling that trickled and then eventually flooded into my now porous soul. So did joy and wonder and love. And in the most gracious of ironies, even as I was struggling to reframe impossible decisions for families in need, it was actually my patients and their parents who were reframing hope for *me*.

I so wish I'd never been abused, but I was. Eventually I dusted myself off and, thanks to a lot of therapy and soul-searching, harbored hopes for a perfect rest-of-life, only to watch that dream—after Christopher died and the hospital started flaying me open—fade like the Vermont shore in the distance as the Lake Champlain ferry pulled away from the dock. There was many a day that I didn't know what was left to hope for, and even if I'd come up with something, doubted whether I'd have the strength to try.

But on those days I also witnessed a degree of courage and devotion that, before I started practicing pediatric palliative care, I hadn't thought possible. Before I met Collin, it never occurred to me that someone with CF-riddled lungs could maintain a double-bass punk beat on the drums. Before I knew Daniel, I never thought a parent would even consider making—let alone masterfully handcraft—their child's coffin.

By showing me that goodness not only exists alongside the evil I learned of far too early, but in far greater measure, my patients and their exquisitely brave parents restored the balance of my universe. By piercing my soul calluses, they took away my crutch, yet somehow I didn't fall. Their courage inspired me so I could stand on my own.

Even though I won't ever be half as brave as Collin and Daniel—or any of the other kids or parents described in this book—I now know that people like them exist. They give me the courage to hope that the emotions I once again can feel won't drown me. That I can trust my sense of right and wrong. That I'll be able to let go of the dreams that didn't come true while cherishing those that did, especially my amazing family and the chance to do the work I feel called to. And, most of all, that I might make some measure of difference in this world, like by another kid not hurting the way I once did.

References

— Chapter 1: —
In the beginning

a formal fellowship: Palliative care was first recognized as a medical specialty in 2006, and since 2012, a one-year fellowship after the completion of residency has been required for board certification. In that interval, however, experienced palliative care clinicians were permitted to "grandfather in" based on work experience and passing the board certification exam, which is the route I took.

harmful cellular byproducts: The technical name for these are glycosaminoglycans.

untreatable: Since Nicky died, enzyme replacement therapy for Hunter's has become possible (DAH Whiteman and A Kimura, "Development of idursulfase therapy for mucopolysaccharidosis type II [Hunter Syndrome]: The past, present and the future," *Drug Design, Development and Therapy* 11 (2017): 2467–2480), and gene therapy could soon be possible (P Zapolnik and A Pyrkosz, "Gene therapy for Mucopolysaccharidosis Type II: A review of the current possibilities," *International Journal of Molecular Sciences* 22 (2021): 5490).

get the DNR: See JA Billings, "Getting the DNR," *Journal of Palliative Medicine* 15 (2012): 1288–1290. The abbreviation itself can be misleading because it implies that a patient can actually be resuscitated if doctors just try. In reality, though, only one out of six hospitalized adults who undergo CPR will survive, and the odds are much worse for those who receive CPR outside the hospital (A Zhu and J Zhang, "Meta-analysis of outcomes of the 2005 and 2010 cardiopulmonary resuscitation guidelines for adults with in-hospital cardiac arrest," *American Journal of Emergency Medicine* 34 (2016):1133–1139). It seems more honest to acknowledge that all physicians can do is *attempt* resuscitation, which is why in the remainder of this book the term Do Not Attempt Resuscitation (DNAR) will be used.

Episcopal: The Anglican Communion encompasses forty-two provinces around the world, including the Episcopal Church of the USA.

Garden of Gethsemane: Cf. Matthew 26:36–56.

the cumulative grief would be devastating: N Remen, R May, D Young, and W Berland, "The wounded healer," *Saybrook Review* 5 (1985): 84–93.

— Chapter 2: —
A very good life

some ethics consult requests aren't "ethical" at all: B Lo, *Resolving Ethical Dilemmas: A Guide for Clinicians*, 5th ed. (Philadelphia: Wolters Kluwer Health/Lippincott Williams & Wilkins, 2013).

couldn't comprehend the medical situation, let alone render a decision based on her goals and values: Technically, this would be termed a lack of decision-making capacity.

NG tubes are among the least comfortable interventions hospitalized patients undergo: AJ Singer, PB Richman, R LaVefre, *et al.*, "Comparison of patient and practitioner assessments of pain from commonly performed emergency department procedures," *Academic Emergency Medicine* 4 (1997): 404–405.

what her mother would want: In technical terms, this is referred to as "substituted judgment."

less responsive: Physiologically, this is caused by the kidneys not having enough fluid to filter out toxins that have built up (including urea), which leads to uremia that in turn causes depressed consciousness. Here it is important to recognize that people who don't eat or drink don't die from starvation (a term with profound negative connotations) but rather from dehydration. This is significant because the primary way that dehydration causes suffering is through a sensation of thirst, caused by having a very dry mouth. If the inside of the mouth is kept moist—which is a staple of quality hospice care—thirst and discomfort can be ameliorated.

still small voice: This is a reference to 1 Kings 19:11–13, where God spoke to Elijah, not by earthquake or fire but in a "still small voice."

imposter syndrome: This is not uncommon in medicine, even among physicians at advanced career stages. See KA LaDonna, S Ginsburg, and C Watling, "'Rising to the level of your incompetence': What physicians' self-assessment of their performance reveals about the imposter syndrome in medicine," *Academic Medicine* 93 (2018): 763–768.

— Chapter 3: —
Why is this so important to you?

most deaths in children's hospitals occur in the ICU: A Trowbridge, JK Walter, E McConathey, W Morrison, and C Feudtner, "Modes of death within a children's hospital," *Pediatrics* 142 (2018): e20174182.

Tony, as I'll call him, an eight-year-old with bright red hair: A more academic analysis of this case can be found at RC Macauley and LJ Fritzler, "Parental refusal of pain management:

A potentially unrecognized form of medical neglect," *Palliative Medicine and Care* 1 (2014): 5–11.

strong medications for pain and anxiety: Normally this includes an opioid like morphine, as well as the family of drugs that includes Valium.

Pediatric ethics consultations are comparatively rare: B Carter *et al.*, "Why are there so few ethics consults in children's hospitals?", *HEC Forum* 30 (2018): 91–102.

almost non-existent risk of addiction: See NL Schechter, CB Berde, and M Yaster, *Pain in Infants, Children, and Adolescents*, 2nd ed. (Philadelphia: Lippincott Williams & Wilkins, 2003).

as the Supreme Court famously said: In *Prince v. Massachusetts*, 321 U.S. 158 (1944).

my feelings of anger: I can now recognize this is as a classic example of counter-transference, which occurs when a clinician projects their own unresolved conflicts onto a patient. This phenomenon is increasingly recognized in the practice of palliative care. See LB Rosenberg *et al.*, "The meaning of together: Exploring transference and countertransference in palliative care settings," *Journal of Palliative Medicine* 24 (2021): 1598–1602.

humble inquiry: EH Schein, *Humble Inquiry: The gentle art of asking instead of telling* (Oakland, CA: Berrett-Koehler, 2013).

Over 80 percent of Americans believe in God: Z Hrynowski, "How many Americans believe in God?", available at https://news.gallup.com/poll/268205/americans-believe-god.aspx (accessed September 23, 2023).

patients generally want physicians to be aware of their spiritual beliefs: CD MacLean *et al.*, "Patient preference for physician discussion and practice of spirituality," *Journal of General Internal Medicine* 18 (2003): 38–43.

less than two-thirds of physicians believe in God: FA Curlin *et al.*, "Religious characteristics of U.S. physicians: A national survey," *Journal of General Internal Medicine* 20 (2005): 629–634.

we only inquire about spirituality about one-third of the time: M Best, P Butow, and I Olver, "Doctors discussing religion and spirituality: A systematic literature review," *Palliative Medicine* 30 (2016): 327–337.

he could somehow save the people he loved: Explanatory theories of the nature and mechanism of atonement abound—including the satisfaction theory, the ransom theory, and *Christus victor*—and are outside the scope of this narrative. For a succinct and balanced analysis, see DL Migliore, *Faith Seeking Understanding: An introduction to Christian theology* (Grand Rapids, MI: Eerdmans, 2004), chapter 8.

when that layer begins to regenerate, it causes an exquisite, painful sensation that's referred to as neuropathic pain: S Yao *et al.*, "Pain during the acute phase of Guillain-Barré Syndrome," *Medicine* 97 (2018): e11995.

subsequent painful stimuli to hurt even worse: Studies have shown that even when a child was so young that they don't consciously recall the pain they experienced, those early exposures reset their pain threshold and lead to increased suffering later in life. See A Taddio, *et al.*, "Inadequate pain management during routine childhood immunizations: The nerve of it," *Clinical Therapeutics* 31 (2009): S152–167; and GA Walco, RC Cassidy, and NL Schechter, "Pain, hurt, and harm: The ethics of pain control in infants and children," *New England Journal of Medicine* 331 (1994): 541–544.

increased risk of anxiety: NL Schechter, CB Berde, and M Yaster, *Pain in Infants, Children, and Adolescents*, 2nd ed. (Philadelphia: Lippincott Williams & Wilkins, 2003): 892.

posttraumatic stress disorder: GJ Asmundson, MJ Coons, S Taylor, and J Katz, "PTSD and the experience of pain: Research and clinical implications of shared vulnerability and mutual maintenance models," *Canadian Journal of Psychiatry* 47 (2002): 930–937; and TJ Sharp and AG Harvey, "Chronic pain and posttraumatic stress disorder: Mutual maintenance?" *Clinical Psychology Reviews* 21 (2001): 857–877.

medical neglect: Defined by federal law as any "failure to act on the part of a parent or caretaker, which results in death, serious physical or emotional harm, sexual abuse or exploitation, or an act or failure to act which presents an imminent risk of serious harm" (Child Abuse Prevention and Treatment Act. 42 USC 5101 et seq; 42 USC 5116 et seq.).

American Academy of Pediatrics recommendations on how to respond to possible medical neglect: AAP Committee on Child Abuse and Neglect, "Recognizing and responding to medical neglect," *Pediatrics* 120 (2007): 1385–1389.

studies have shown that it reduces the risk of suicide attempts in psychiatric patients: RD Gibbons, K Hur, CH Brown, and JJ Mann, "Gabapentin and suicide attempts," *Pharmacoepidemiological Drug Safety* 19 (2010): 1241–1247.

nobody else: And, frankly, it kind of freaks me out to think that, if this book gets published one day, anyone who happens to pick it up will know something so intimate about me, which nearly all my friends have no clue about. I want to believe that simply naming my pain is a step toward healing; right from the beginning, there have been way too many secrets in my life.

upperclass: Based on annual income, I'm in the top 10 percent of Americans, which means upper class. In a world where millionaires like to call themselves "upper-middle" class because it sounds better, I think it's important to be honest. See R Frank, "Most millionaires say they're middle class" (available at https://www.cnbc.com/2015/05/06/naires-say-theyre-middle-class.html; accessed September 23, 2023)

Bizarro World: The Bizarro World of Htrae ("Earth" spelled backward), created by DC Comics in the 1960s, is inhabited by weirdly inverted versions of characters in the Superman saga. Society there is ruled by the Bizarro Code: "Us do opposite of all Earthly things! Us hate beauty! Us love ugliness! Is big crime to make anything perfect on Bizarro World!" Many know the concept best from the "Bizarro Jerry" episode of *Seinfeld* (https://en.wikipedia.org/wiki/The_Bizarro_Jerry), although it is also referenced several times by characters on *Buffy the Vampire Slayer*.

dissociation: This is a common symptom in survivors of sexual abuse. See JS Kirby, JA Chu, and DL Dill, "Correlates of dissociative symptomatology in patients with physical and sexual abuse histories," *Comprehensive Psychiatry* 34 (1993): 258–263.

greater power and eloquence: Many powerful examples can be found at https://1in6.org/get-information/books-films/mens-stories-memoirs/

not substantiate the accusation of neglect: Though definitely disheartening, it probably shouldn't have been surprising that DCF did not "substantiate" the report of medical neglect. Each year, state departments of children and families receive over three million reports of child abuse and neglect. Only one out of six reports is ultimately "substantiated." (U.S. Department of Health and Human Services, "Child Maltreatment 2021," available at https://www.acf.hhs.gov/sites/default/files/documents/cb/cm2021.pdf; accessed September 23, 2023)

suffering as inherently redemptive: See further K Lebacqz, "Redemptive suffering redeemed: A Protestant view of suffering," in RM Green and NJ Palpant, eds., *Suffering and Bioethics* (New York: Oxford University Press, 2014): 262–274.

make it less shitty: In our conversations leading up to this book, Khanti—ever gracious—wanted to make sure that what I took very much as a compliment didn't come across as minimizing. He said, "In reality, you took a really shitty situation, and you provided context, hope, and compassion. You gave us relativity and context when we found ourselves in a tiny unexpected bubble of uncertainty with seemingly no air to breathe."

***Nonviolent Communication*:** MB Rosenberg, *Nonviolent Communication: A language of life*, 3rd ed. (Encinitas, CA: PuddleDancer Press, 2015).

— Chapter 4: —
When hello means goodbye

When hello means goodbye: The title of this chapter is drawn from a book by the same name by Paul Kirk and Pat Schwiebert (Grief Watch, 2012).

missing a band of nerve fibers that joins the two hemispheres: The technical name for this is "agenesis of the corpus callosum."

a hole in the muscular wall that separated the two sides of her heart: The technical name for this is a ventricular septal defect (VSD).

inheriting a version from my wife or me that we didn't exhibit: The technical term for this is "variable expression."

the Neonatal Resuscitation Protocol at the time: American Heart Association and American Academy of Pediatrics, "2005 AHA guidelines for cardiopulmonary resuscitation and emergency cardiovascular care of pediatric and neonatal patients: Neonatal resuscitation guidelines," *Pediatrics* 117 (2006): e1029–1038.

absence of the brain: The technical term for absence of both cerebral hemispheres (along with a large part of the skull) is anencephaly.

a full moon: DA Thompson and SL Adams, "The full moon and ED patient volumes: Unearthing a myth," *American Journal of Emergency Medicine* 14 (1996):161–164.

Friday the 13th or a particular sign of the zodiac, either: J Schuld, et al., "Popular belief meets surgical reality: Impact of lunar phases, Friday the 13th and zodiac signs on emergency operations and intraoperative blood loss," *World Journal of Surgery* 35 (2011):1945–1949.

from even more studies: K Grind, "Hospitals really believe bad things happen on a full moon," *Wall Street Journal* (October 17, 2016).

a small risk, though, of inducing a miscarriage: While it was long thought that amniocentesis caused miscarriage in 1 out of 100 pregnancies, newer studies reveal the risk to be significantly lower (1 in 300–500 pregnancies). See LJ Salmon et al, "Risk of miscarriage following amniocentesis and chorionic villus sampling:

Systematic review of literature and updated meta-analysis," *Ultrasound in Obstetrics and Gynecology* 54 (2019): 442–451.

he wept at the grave of Lazarus: John 11:1–44.

a trendy spiritual exercise: D Giffels, *Furnishing Eternity: A father, a son, a coffin, and a measure of life* (New York: Scribner, 2018).

a risk of uterine rupture along the previous C-section incision: Recent studies suggest a risk of approximately 0.5 percent. See K Motomura *et al.*, "Incidence and outcomes of uterine rupture among women with prior caesarian section: WHO Multicountry Survey of Maternal and Newborn Health," *Scientific Reports* 7 (2017): 44093.

one of out of every forty births in the US is via C-section "by maternal request": American College of Obstetricians and Gynecologists, "Cesarean delivery on maternal request," ACOG Committee Opinion No. 761, *Obstetrics and Gynecology* 133 (2019): e73–77.

If wanting to minimize the amount of maternity leave you take is a good enough reason for a C-section, how can wanting to hold your living baby not be?: A few years after Lily's birth, the American College of Obstetrics and Gynecology acknowledged that "there may be scenarios for which intrapartum fetal monitoring, timed delivery, or cesarean delivery for fetal indications may be valid parts of a perinatal palliative comfort care birth plan. For example, intrapartum fetal monitoring and cesarean delivery may reasonably be requested by a well-informed patient who wishes to have a live birth or desires a religious ceremony involving a liveborn neonate." (RS Miller, JJ Cummings, R Macauley, and SJ Ralston, "Perinatal palliative care," ACOG Committee Opinion 786, *Obstetrics and Gynecology* 134 (2019): e84–89)

Prematurity of even a few weeks substantially increases the risk of respiratory, neurologic, and infectious complications: RW Loftin *et al.*, "Late preterm birth," *Reviews in Obstetrics and Gynecology* 3 (2010): 10–19.

more likely to attend patient funerals than other specialties: Studies have shown that being female and in practice for many years also increase the likelihood of attending patient funerals (K Kim *et al.*, "Bereavement practices employed by hospitals and medical practitioners toward attending funeral of patients: A systematic review," *Medicine* 98 (2019): e16692).

***The Great Divorce*:** London: Geoffrey Bles, 1945.

I'd just gotten home: This section is adapted from R Macauley, "Turn of phrase," *Journal of Palliative Medicine* 18 (2015): 197–199.

twenty-three weeks as of that night: When the triplets were born, twenty-three weeks was taken to be the cusp of viability. Subsequent studies have shown that twenty-two-weekers have over a 20 percent chance of surviving with maximal treatment (MA Rysavy *et al.*, "Between-hospital variation in treatment and outcomes in extremely preterm infants," *New England Journal of Medicine* 372 (2015): 1801–1811). Admittedly, two-thirds of the babies in this study were singletons and most survivors had moderate-to-severe neurodevelopmental impairment.

online database: The National Institute of Child Health and Human Development (NICHD) Neonatal Research Network: Extremely Preterm Birth Outcome Data (https://www1.nichd.nih.gov/epbo-calculator/Pages/epbo_case.aspx).

life review: RM Keall, JM Clayton, and PN Butow, "Therapeutic life review in palliative care: A systematic review of quantitative evaluations," *Journal of Pain and Symptom Management* 49 (2015): 747–761.

dignity therapy: GN Thompson and HM Chochinov, "Dignity-based approaches in the care of terminally ill patients," *Current Opinions in Supportive and Palliative Care* 2 (2008): 49–53.

— Chapter 5: —
When the "right" answer isn't

circulating blood through their body: The technical term for this is extracorporeal membrane oxygenation—or ECMO—where a pump circulates blood through an artificial lung, essentially functioning as a patient's heart and lungs.

a committee at Harvard coined the term: Ad Hoc Committee of the Harvard Medical School to Examine the Definition of Brain Death, "A definition of irreversible coma," *JAMA* 205 (1968): 337–340.

newspaper articles that proclaimed "life-support" was removed from a brain-dead patient: N Merchant, "Family: Brain-dead Texas woman off life support," Associated Press (January 26, 2014).

Uniform Determination of Death Act: The Uniform Determination of Death Act—on which nearly every state law is based—clearly states that "an individual who has sustained either (1) irreversible cessation of circulatory and respiratory functions, or (2) irreversible cessation of all functions of the entire brain, including the brain stem, is dead."

dead donor rule: JA Robertson, "The dead donor rule," *Hastings Center Report* 29 (1999): 6–14.

had written scholarly articles about it: SE Bliss and RC Macauley, "The least bad option: Unilateral extubation after declaration of death by neurological criteria," *Journal of Clinical Ethics* 26 (2015): 260–265.

doesn't allow physicians to declare a patient brain dead: New Jersey Declaration of Death Act, Pub. L. No. 6A, 26 Stat. 5 (1991).

generally believe that as long as the heart and lungs are functioning, a patient is still alive: JD Bleich, *Bioethical Dilemmas: A Jewish perspective* (Hoboken, NJ: KTAV Publishing, 1998).

New York's law: New York State Department of Health, Guidelines for determining brain death (2011). (https://www.health.ny.gov/professionals/hospital_administrator/letters/2011/brain_death_guidelines.pdf)

parents might never accept the diagnosis: This concern would be personified, years later, by Jahi McMath, a teenager who was declared brain dead in California. Her parents transported her to New Jersey where she was legally deemed alive again, even though her condition hadn't changed. See LO Gostin, "Legal and ethical responsibilities following brain death: The McMath and Munoz cases," *JAMA* 311 (2014): 903–904.

formal brain death examination: There are some risks associated with the examination, related to lower blood oxygen levels. Some commentators thus argue that consent is required before proceeding. See BM Lee *et al.*, "Can a parent refuse the brain death examination?" *Pediatrics* 145 (2020): e20192340.

even patients who have been declared dead by neurological criteria maintain some hormonal function: AD Shewmon, "The brain and somatic integration: Insights into the standard biological rationale for equating 'brain death' with death," *Journal of Medicine and Philosophy* 26 (2001): 457–478.

arguing that the entire brain doesn't need to stop functioning for a patient to be declared dead: RD Truog *et al.*, "Brain death at fifty: Exploring consensus, controversy, and contexts," *Hastings Center Report* 48 (2018): S2–5.

safety coffins: M Cascella, "Taphophobia and 'life preserving coffins' in the nineteenth century," *History of Psychiatry* 27 (2016): 345–349.

Justice is one of the four core principles of bioethics: TL Beauchamp and JF Childress, *Principles of Biomedical Ethics*, 8th ed. (New York: Oxford University Press, 2019).

pretty much the only thing the Episcopal church I attended had in common with evangelicalism was the letter "e" at the start of their names: It is important to note that there is an evangelical strain within Episcopalianism. The so-called "low church" prioritizes scripture over the other primary sources of revelation (i.e., tradition and reason), and represents much of the global Anglican communion, especially in Africa.

— Chapter 6: —
The finite miracle of modern medicine

My Most Hated Disease: Neuroblastoma's competition includes Duchenne Muscular Dystrophy, mostly because if you get it and happen to have an older brother, there's a fifty-fifty chance he has it, too. Not only are you going to watch him decline before your eyes, but you get to do so knowing that all that stuff is going to happen to you, too. Cystic fibrosis is also in the running, mostly because of Collin (Chapter 9).

even stronger opioids: The news media makes a big deal about the potency of opioids, stressing just how much more potent drugs like Dilaudid and fentanyl are than morphine (roughly 6 and 100 times, respectively). For the most part, though, you can achieve the same effect from any opioid, depending on how much you give. In that respect, opioids are like coins: morphine is a penny, Dilaudid a nickel, and fentanyl a dollar coin. You can make a dollar out of any of them, but it just takes a whole lot more pennies.

filling the rapport bucket: The business guru Stephen Covey similarly refers to making a deposit in an "emotional bank account," which refers to "the amount of trust that's been built up in a relationship." See SR Covey, *The 7 Habits of Highly Effective People: Powerful Lessons in Personal Change* (New York: Free Press, 2004): 189.

fire a warning shot: JL Old, "Communicating bad news to your patients," *Family Practice Management* 18 (2011): 31–35.

total pain: C Saunders, "The symptomatic treatment of incurable malignant disease," *Prescribers' Journal* 4 (1964): 68–73.

Pain is whatever the experiencing person says it is, existing whenever the experiencing person says it does: M McCaffery and A Beebe, *Pain: Clinical manual for nursing practice* (St. Louis, MO: Mosby, 1989).

doctors frequently overestimating how long patients have left to live: NA Christakis and TJ Iwashyna, "Attitude and self-reported practice regarding prognostication in a national sample of internists," *Archives of Internal Medicine* 158 (1998): 2389–2395.

This study found that physicians overestimate the life expectancy of hospice patients by a factor of five. (In other words, take your doctor's prediction of how long you have left to live and divide it by five to get the right answer.) In addition, the longer the physician had treated the patient, the more extreme the overestimation, likely reflecting the human tendency not to admit that something bad was going to happen to someone you've come to care deeply about.

most hospice patients die within three weeks of enrolling: Medicare Payment Advisory Commission, "Hospice services," available at https://www.medpac.gov/wp-content/uploads/2023/03/Ch10_Mar23_MedPAC_Report_To_Congress_SEC.pdf (accessed September 30, 2023).

an intermediate level of hospice services: Normally, a hospice agency is paid a *per diem* fee to provide for essentially all of a terminally ill patient's care needs. But state pediatric waivers authorize a limited number of services over a more prolonged period of time. These services include enhanced care coordination, family/caregiver training, expressive therapies (such as art, music, and play therapy, and child life services), short-term skilled respite to give family a chance to rest, and grief support.

weren't expected to live into adulthood: The technical qualification is a median life expectancy of twenty-one years or less. See J Keim-Malpass, TG Hart, and JR Miller, "Coverage of palliative and hospice care for pediatric patients with a life-limiting illness: A policy brief," *Journal of Pediatric Health Care* 27 (2013): 511–516.

For example, it took California—whose advocates were highly organized and well-funded—nearly a decade: The Children's Hospice and Palliative Care Coalition (https://coalitionccc.org/) was instrumental in getting their waiver passed. For its impact, see LC Lindley, "The effective of pediatric palliative care policy on hospice utilization among California Medicaid beneficiaries," *Journal of Pain and Symptom Management* 52 (2016): 688–694.

Less than 1 percent of hospice patients are kids: LC Lindley, B Mark, and SD Lee, "Providing hospice care to children and young adults: A descriptive study of end-of-life organizations," *Journal of Hospice and Palliative Nursing* 11 (2009): 315–323.

adult hospice actually saves money: Z Obermeyer *et al.*, "Association between the Medicare hospice benefit and health care utilization and costs for patients with poor-prognosis cancer," *JAMA* 312 (2014): 1888–1896.

patients in the last six months of life: Some patients stay on hospice for more than six months, as long as their physician still believes they are likely to die within the next six months. As noted earlier, prognostication is an uncertain science.

By the end of the year, our tiny state had its very own Medicaid-funded pediatric palliative care program: See https://www.healthvermont.gov/children-youth-families/children-special-health-needs/palliative-care (accessed September 30, 2023).

What else do you hope for?: C Feudtner, "The breadth of hopes," *New England Journal of Medicine* 361 (2009): 2306–2307.

One study: J Kamihara *et al.*, "Parental hope for children with advanced cancer," *Pediatrics* 145 (2015): 868–874.

Broadway: A narrated, visual version of this experience can be found at https://tinyurl.com/MacauleyTedX, starting at minute 17.

creemees: This is the uniquely Vermont term for soft serve ice cream.

— Chapter 7: —
Never, never giving you up

retinopathy of prematurity: A severe eye condition affecting premature babies, especially those requiring supplemental oxygen (which can be toxic to developing blood vessels in the retina). This is the cause of Stevie Wonder's blindness. He was born six weeks premature, at a time when oxygen toxicity wasn't yet recognized.

***Crucial Conversations* and *Difficult Conversations*:** K Patterson, J Grenny, R McMillan, and A Switzler, *Crucial Conversations: Tools for Talking When Stakes Are High*, 2nd ed. (New York: McGraw-Hill, 2011); and D Stone, B Patton, and S Heen, *Difficult Conversations: How to Discuss What Matters Most*, rev. ed. (New York: Penguin, 2023).

Revolutionary treatments have subsequently been discovered: RS Finkel *et al.*, "Nusinersen versus sham control in infantile-onset spinal muscular atrophy," *New England Journal of Medicine* 377 (2017): 1723–1732; and MA Waldrop *et al.*, "Gene therapy for spinal muscular atrophy: Safety and early outcomes," *Pediatrics* 146 (2020): e20200729.

exorbitant cost: Nusinersin typically costs $750,000 for one year of treatment, while gene therapy is a one-time intervention at a price of over $3 million.

surgical feeding tube: There are two types of feeding tubes: temporary ones that run through the mouth or nose into the stomach and more permanent ones that are surgically implanted through the abdominal wall (known as gastrostomy or simply "G" tubes).

tracheostomy: Short-term mechanical ventilation can be accomplished through an endotracheal tube, which goes through the mouth into the windpipe. Over time, though, this can cause irritation and erosion of the trachea and vocal cords. Longer-term ventilation requires a tracheostomy, which also offers the possibility of speaking.

compassionate extubation: Removing a patient's breathing tube with the expectation that they won't survive off the ventilator. Previously, this was known as "withdrawing life-sustaining therapy" (which was felt to be too negative) and then "terminal extubation" (which falsely implied that removing the breathing tube—rather than the underlying disease—caused the patient's death).

This is my child, whom I love, and with whom I am well pleased: Matthew 3:17.

— Chapter 8: —
Return of sensation

or at least some of them: While Medicare is a federal program, Medicaid is a joint federal/state program. As such, every state establishes the income threshold for children to qualify for

Medicaid, which ranges from 142 percent of the federal poverty level—currently about $30,000 per year for a family of four—in some states to over 300 percent in others. (Kaiser Family Foundation, "Medicaid and CHIP income eligibility levels for children as a present of the federal poverty level," https://www.kff.org/health-reform/state-indicator/medicaid-and-chip-income-eligibility-limits-for-children-as-a-percent-of-the-federal-poverty-level, accessed September 30, 2023). Put another way, in some states, a family of four can earn $42,000 per year and be considered too rich to qualify for Medicaid.

a fraction of what Medicare (which covers the elderly) does: 72 percent, to be precise. See "Medicaid-to-Medicare fee index," (2019), available at https://www.kff.org/medicaid/state-indicator/medicaid-to-medicare-fee-index/, accessed September 30, 2023.

wondering if I would be up to the academic expectations: I was right to be concerned, especially when my renowned tutor responded to my first paper—which was by far the best I'd ever written, such that my college profs might well have bronzed it—by saying, "If this is the quality of your work, then you don't belong at Oxford, and you certainly don't deserve to be studying with me." Fortunately, I was able to up my game over the course of that year, learning an immense amount along the way.

that book: RC Macauley, *Ethics in Palliative Care: A Complete Guide* (New York: Oxford University Press, 2018).

surgeons over there aren't even referred to as "Doctor": This custom dates back to the 1500s when surgeons were trained in barber shops, not universities, and thus (unlike physicians) had no formal qualifications. See I Loudon, "Why are (male) surgeons still as addressed as Mr?", *BMJ* 321 (2000): 1589–1591.

of the risk of burnout in modern medicine, with palliative care among the highest risk specialties: A recent study showed that 62 percent of palliative care clinicians reported burnout, even higher than other stressful specialties like oncology. See AH Kamal *et al.*, "Prevalence and predictors of burnout among

hospice and palliative care clinicians in the U.S.," *Journal of Pain and Symptom Management* 51 (2016): 690–696.
shepherd leaves his flock: Luke 15:3–7.
the one she dropped: Luke 15:8–10.

— Chapter 9: —
Battalions of sorrows

only half of CF patients who receive a lung transplant are still alive ten years later: AL Stephenson *et al.*, "Clinical and demographic factors associated with post-lung transplantation survival in individuals with cystic fibrosis," *Journal of Heart and Lung Transplantation* 34 (2015): 1139–1145.
***The Private Worlds of Dying Children*:** Princeton, NJ: Princeton University Press, 1980.
more recent study: U Kreicbergs, U Valdimarsdóttir, E Onelöv, J Henter, and G Steineck, "Talking about death with children who have severe malignant disease," *New England Journal of Medicine* 351 (2004): 1175–1186.
late thirties: Since then, gene therapies have started to hold out the hope for cure (see S Sutharsan *et al.*, "Efficacy and safety of elexacaftor plus tezacaftor plus ivacaftor versus tezacaftor plus ivacaftor in people with cystic fibrosis homozygous for F508del-CFTR: A 24-week, multicentre, randomised, double-blind, active-controlled, phase 3b trial," *Lancet Respiratory Medicine* 10 (2022): 267–277), with current life expectancy of young children with CF predicted to be fifty-six years of age. That's one of the reasons that Collin's older sister Jillian is not only still alive but is actually getting better.
***Buffy the Vampire Slayer and Philosophy: Fear and Trembling in Sunnydale*:** JB South and W Irwin, eds. (Chicago, IL: Open Court, 2003).
cognitive part of their brain: Also known as the pre-frontal cortex.
feeling part of their brain: Also known as the limbic system or what some call the "lizard brain."

- **studies have shown that patients are more likely to decline a procedure when the risks are framed in the negative:** MF Haward, RO Murphy, and JM Lorenz, "Message framing and perinatal decisions," *Pediatrics* 122 (2008): 109–118.
- **affects only 2 percent of patients with CF who undergo lung transplant:** EM Lowery *et al.*, "Increased risk of PTLD in lung transplant recipients with cystic fibrosis," *Journal of Cystic Fibrosis* 16 (2017): 727–734.
- **Only about one in five patients with it survives:** P Savage and J Waxman, "Post-transplantation lymphoproliferative disease," *QJM* 90 (1997): 497–503.
- ***wish* and *wonder*:** Rather than saying that you're sorry for what a patient or family is going through—which can be misinterpreted as either pity or apology—in palliative care, we often say that we *wish* that the patient weren't facing what they are. Similarly, *wonder* invites a patient to imagine what a different course of treatment would look like without feeling pressured to commit to it. As in, "I wonder what it would feel like if we focused entirely on your comfort."
- **on TV, most patients not only survive CPR, they typically emerge rejuvenated and refreshed:** SJ Diem, JD Lantos, and JA Tulsky, "Cardiopulmonary resuscitation on television: Miracles and misinformation," *New England Journal of Medicine* 334 (1996): 1578–1582.
- **only about 15 percent of hospitalized patients who undergo CPR ever leave the hospital:** A Zhu and J Zhang, "Meta-analysis of outcomes of the 2005 and 2010 cardiopulmonary resuscitation guidelines for adults with in-hospital cardiac arrest," *American Journal of Emergency Medicine* 34 (2016):1133–1139.
- **prolonging his death:** Terminal irreversible illness was the one situation where, from the earliest days of CPR becoming a procedure that was automatically performed unless the patient refused it, the American Medical Association said it shouldn't be provided. See American Medical Association, "Standards for

cardiopulmonary resuscitation (CPR) and emergency cardiac care (ECC)," *JAMA* 227 (1974): 833–868.

sedating him: The technical term is "proportional sedation" (formerly "palliative sedation"), which refers to depressing a patient's level of consciousness so that they are no longer able to experience suffering that has been deemed refractory and intolerable. In the most severe cases, deep sedation is maintained until the patient dies naturally.

— Chapter 10: —
Back when I was in medical school

on call: This term can refer to many things, including being available by pager in case a need arises. For residents, it has historically referred to nights spent in the hospital sandwiched between full work days. For instance, if a resident is on call every other night, that means they come in early in the morning, work through the day, assume responsibility that night for all the other residents' patients, return that responsibility the following morning when those well-rested residents return, and then work another normal day. Then they get one evening off before starting the cycle all over again.

long-needed reforms: The new rules limited interns to no more than sixteen consecutive hours of patient care, with an additional four hours permitted for activities related to patient safety, education, and effective transitions. Six years later, the limit was relaxed to permit interns to work twenty-four consecutive hours on patient care with the same additional four for related activities.

patient safety: Limits on resident work hours showed a reduction in negative patient outcomes, including mortality. KG Volpp *et al.*, "Mortality among patients in VA hospitals in the first 2 years following ACGME resident duty hour reform," *JAMA* 298 (2007): 984–992.

intestinal blockage: Technically, they had "duodenal atresia," where a section of the small intestine is discontinuous, akin to a washed-out bridge that once connected two segments of a road.

to raise them with a mongoloid: JM Gustafson, "Mongolism, parental desires, and the right to life," Perspectives in Biology and Medicine 16 (1973): 529-557.

surveys revealing a large majority of pediatric surgeons (and nearly half of pediatricians) willing to honor the parents' refusal: A Shaw et al., "Ethical issues in pediatric surgery: A national survey of pediatricians and pediatric surgeons," *Pediatrics* 60 (1977): 588–599; and ID Todres *et al.*, "Pediatricians' attitudes affecting decision-making in defective newborns," *Pediatrics* 60 (1977): 197–201.

even to the point of becoming TV stars: N Randle, "'Our ticket to acceptance': Actor with Down's Syndrome on 'Life Goes On' has become role model for many," *LA Times* (December 20, 1990).

triathletes: K Streeter, "Chris Nikic, you are an Ironman. And your journey is remarkable," *New York Times* (November 16, 2020).

next most common trisomies: C Irving et al., "Changes in fetal prevalence and outcome for trisomies 13 and 18: A population-based study over 23 years," *Journal of Maternal-Fetal & Neonatal Medicine* 24 (2011): 137–141.

Expectant women were often told that their child (if born) would experience a life of suffering, or would be a "vegetable.": A Janvier, B Farlow, and BS Wilfond, "The experience of families with children with trisomy 13 and 18 in social networks," *Pediatrics* 130 (2012): 293–298.

ventricular septal defect (or VSD) in her heart: Each side of the heart has an upper chamber (the "atrium") and a a lower chamber (the "ventricle"). Normally, a septum divides the right from the left, but when there is a hole in that septum, blood flows from the higher pressure left side to the lower pressure right side. That isn't usually a problem with the atria, which are mostly holding chambers. But if a ventricular septal defect is large like Cora's, significant amounts of blood can shift from the left ventricle—which is stronger because it needs to force blood through the rest of the body—to the right, leading to overcirculation to the lungs.

median life expectancy in the US was around three days: Survival is usually reported as median life expectancy—meaning that, by that time, half of children with that condition will have died—rather than average life expectancy, which can be skewed high by a few patients who survive for an unusually long period of time. See S Root and JC Carey, "Survival in trisomy 18," *American Journal of Medical Genetics* 49 (1994): 170–174; NB Embleton *et al.*, "Natural history of Trisomy 18," *Archives of Diseases in Children Fetal and Neonatal Edition* 75 (1996): F38–F41.

one outlier study: SA Rasmussen *et al.*, "Population-based analyses of mortality in trisomy 13 and trisomy 18," *Pediatrics* 111 (2003): 777–784.

recent Japanese study: T Kosho *et al.*, "Neonatal management of trisomy 18: Clinical details of 24 patients receiving intensive treatment," *American Journal of Medical Genetics* 140 (2006): 937–944.

a thirty-four-year-old woman with T18: "Stacy's story" (https://trisomy.org/blog/stories/stacy-lynn-vanherreweghe).

this moving reflection: L Fenton, "Trisomy 13 and 18 and quality of life: Treading 'softly'," *American Journal of Medical Genetics Part A* 155 (2011): 1527–1528.

the real-life inspiration for Hawkeye Pierce: "Sail on John Davis, the real Hawkeye Pierce" (http://www.buffettnews.com/forum/viewtopic.php?t=88189).

trenchant commentary: TK Koogler, BM Wilfond, and LF Ross, "Lethal language, lethal decisions," *Hastings Center Report* 33 (2003): 37–42.

those guidelines had been revised: American Academy of Pediatrics, *Textbook of Neonatal Resuscitation, 6th ed.* (Elk Grove Village, IL: American Academy of Pediatrics, 2011). This revision was released in the interval between Lily's birth and Cora's.

recent survey: MP McGraw and JM Perlman, "Attitudes of neonatologists toward delivery room management of confirmed trisomy 18: Potential factors influencing a changing dynamic," *Pediatrics* 121 (2008): 1106–1110.

postoperative mortality for kids with T18 was nearly triple that of other children: MH Ma, W He, and OJ Benavidez, "Congenital heart surgical admissions in patients with Trisomy 13 and 18: Frequency, morbidity, and mortality," *Pediatric Cardiology* 40 (2019): 595–601.

only 8 percent of physicians would recommend repairing a VSD for a patient with T18, with an additional 30 percent being willing to do so if the parents "want everything done.": AR Yates *et al.*, "Pediatric sub-specialist controversies in the treatment of congenital heart disease in trisomy 13 or 18," *Journal of Genetic Counseling* 20 (2011): 495–509.

quote studies: E.g., J Maeda *et al.*, "The impact of cardiac surgery in patients with trisomy 18 and trisomy 13 in Japan," *American Journal of Medical Genetics Part A* 155 (2011): 2641–2646.

article from their small hometown newspaper: S Vondrasek, "'Little Cora' brings joy, and challenges: Randolph Center baby has rare condition," *The Herald* (November 7, 2013). (https://www.ourherald.com/articles/little-cora-brings-joy-and-challenge/)

identically titled articles and lectures: For example, E Digitale, "Compatible with life? Doctors and families grapple with what's next when a severe genetic disorder is diagnosed during pregnancy," *Stanford Medicine* (Fall 2018). (https://stanmed.stanford.edu/2018fall/genetic-disorders-incompatible-life-options.html)

definitive analysis of improved T18 outcomes: KE Nelson *et al.*, "Survival and surgical interventions for children with Trisomy 13 and 18," *JAMA* 316 (2016): 420–428.

editorial by arguably the foremost pediatric bioethicist in the country: JD Lantos, "Trisomy 13 and 18—Treatment decisions in a stable gray zone," *JAMA* 316 (2016): 396–398.

got back into therapy: Thank you Elizabeth, David, and especially Chris.

— Chapter 11: —
The very best of friends

intraosseous needle: As a last resort if an IV can't be placed, a large-bore "IO" needle can be rammed into a bone (usually the tibia) in order to infuse fluids or medications.

A recent study had found that the longer CPR goes on, the better the chance of getting the heart beating again: ZD Goldberger *et al.*, "Duration of resuscitation efforts and survival after in-hospital cardiac arrest: An observational study," *Lancet* 380 (2012): 1473–1481.

sudden and unexpected death is more likely to cause "complicated grief": MK Shear, "Grief and mourning gone awry: Pathway and course of complicated grief," *Dialogues in Clinical Neuroscience* 14 (2012): 119–128.

Free Will Defense: See A Plantinga, *God, Freedom, and Evil* (Grand Rapids, MI: Eerdmans, 1977) and R Swinburne (who happens to have been my tutor at Oxford), *Providence and the Problem of Evil* (Oxford: Oxford University Press, 1998).

actually coined by Marilyn Monroe: See https://www.goodreads.com/quotes/12379-i-believe-that-everything-happens-for-a-reason-people-change (accessed December 7, 2023).

real theologians like Kate Bowler have properly skewered: See her *Everything Happens For a Reason: And other lies I've loved* (New York: Random House, 2018).

***My God, my God*:** This quotation is from Psalm 22, which Jesus repeated on the cross (Matthew 27:46).

divine *pathos*: The technical term for this is "anthropopathy," referring to the human feelings that God experiences. See especially chapter 15 of AJ Heschel, *The Prophets* (New York: Harper, 1962).

O Lord, how long shall I cry for help, and thou wilt not hear?: Habakkuk 1:2.

in the suffering of Christ, God himself suffers: J Möeltmann, *The Crucified God* (New York: Fortress, 1973): 47.

— Chapter 12: —
Doing to and doing for

rare: Affecting between 1 in 20,000 and 200,000 live births. See L Nalysnyk *et al.*, "Gaucher disease epidemiology and natural history: A comprehensive review of the literature," *Hematology* 22 (2017): 65–73.

the absence of one particular enzyme leads to the buildup of toxic substances: The enzyme is called glucocerebrosidase, which normally breaks down substances called glycolipids into glucose and lipid components. Without that enzyme, glycolipids build up within cellular structures called lysosomes—which is why Gaucher's is classified as a lysosomal storage disease—causing damage to internal organs.

small town in Vermont: Wyoming is the only state with a lower population, which means that a small town in Vermont is *really* small.

Courageous Parents Network: https://courageousparentsnetwork.org/

many pediatric palliative care teams offer them: EC Kaye *et al.*, "Pediatric palliative care in the community," *CA: A Cancer Journal for Clinicians* 65 (2015): 316–333.

distinction between doing something for someone and doing it to them: KG Cloyes *et al.*, "'A true human interaction': Comparison of family caregiver and hospice nurse perspectives on needs of family hospice caregivers," *Journal of Hospice and Palliative Care Nursing* 16 (2014): 282–290.

"It's nice to know you care.": M Konner, *Becoming a Doctor: A Journey of Initiation in Medical School* (New York: Penguin, 1988): 21.

medical decisions should be made in the child's best interest: LF Ross and AH Swota, "The best interest standard: Same name but different roles in pediatric bioethics and child rights frameworks," *Perspectives in Biology and Medicine* 60 (2017): 186–197.

studies show takes two basic forms: DL Hill *et al.*, "Changes over time in good-parent beliefs among parents of children with serious illness: A two-year cohort study," *Journal of Pain and Symptom Management* 58 (2019): 190–197.

a glowing article about palliative care in *The New Yorker*: A Gawande, "Letting go: What should medicine do when it can't save your life," *New Yorker* (July 26, 2010).

bestselling book: *Being Mortal: Medicine and what matters at the end* (New York: Metropolitan, 2014).

some universities even have combined sections of ethics and palliative care: One example is the University of Pittsburgh (https://dom.pitt.edu/dgim/SPC/).

distinct approaches can be complementary: BS Carter and LD Wocial, "Ethics and palliative care: Which consultant and when?" *American Journal of Hospice and Palliative Care* 29 (2012): 146–150.

the politics of the university are so intense because the stakes are so low: FR Shapiro, ed., *The Yale Book of Quotations* (New Haven: Yale University Press, 2006): 670. This is a more colloquial version of what has become known as Sayre's Law: "In any dispute, the intensity of feeling is inversely proportional to the value of the issues at stake."

pediatrics both genetic (think: Lily, Collin, Cora, and Emerson) and neuromuscular (think: Rider) conditions are more common: See C Feudtner *et al.*, "Pediatric palliative care patients: A prospective multicenter cohort study," *Pediatrics* 127 (2011): 1094–1101.

Faith's Lodge: www.faithslodge.org

autosomal recessive: More detailed explanation of autosomal recessive conditions is found on p. 18

about how protecting your child is a huge part of being a good parent: Sarah and Steve's description—plus some beautiful photos of Emerson—can be found at https://courageousparentsnetwork.org/videos/we-were-actively-protecting-her-from-things-that-wouldnt-be-right-for-her/.

— Chapter 13: —
My people

only about one-third of Americans have completed an advance directive: KN Yadav *et al.*, "Approximately one in three US adults completes any type of advance directive for end-of-life care," *Health Affairs* 36 (2017): 1244–1251.

eleven seconds before interrupting them: NS Ospina *et al.*, "Eliciting the patient's agenda: Secondary analysis of recorded clinical encounters," *Journal of General Internal Medicine* 34 (2019): 36–40.

most of the history of Western medicine: Essentially from Hippocrates in the fifth century B.C.E. until the beginning of the twentieth century.

that's one of the most important elements that patients consider when making a medical decision: AD Gurmankin *et al.*, "The role of physicians' recommendations in medical treatment decisions," *Medical Decision Making* 22 (2002): 262–271.

concern about infringing on patient autonomy: RM Veatch, "Models for ethical medicine in a revolutionary age: What physician-patient roles foster the most ethical relationship?" *Hastings Center Report* 2 (1972): 5–7.

a middle road: It probably wasn't a coincidence that I chose that image since Anglicanism is often referred to as the *via media* (or "middle way"), initially referring to its moderating position between the "extremes" of Puritanism and Roman Catholicism. See R Hooker, *The Laws of Ecclesiastical Polity (1594)* (Cambridge: Belknap Press of Harvard University Press, 1977).

Abbie Hoffman: He was the epitome of a radical: an anarchist revolutionary who co-founded the Youth International Party ("Yippies") and was also a leading proponent of the Flower Power movement. It's safe to say this is the first time I've ever been compared to him.

the rich young ruler: Luke 18:18–30.

healing a crippled woman on the Sabbath: Luke 13:10–17.

greatest in the kingdom of heaven: Matthew 18:4.

Truly I tell you, whoever does not receive the kingdom of God as a little child will never enter it: Luke 18:17.

Hope for the best and prepare for the worst: This is a common saying in pediatric palliative care (see JD Lotz *et al.*, "'Hope for the best, prepare for the worst': A qualitative interview study on parents' needs and fears in pediatric advance care planning," *Palliative Medicine* 31 (2017): 764–771, but a wise colleague and friend has actually expanded on this to something that describes palliative care even better: "Hope for the best, attend to the present, celebrate success, and prepare for the rest."

— Chapter 14: —
Irrigation and debridement

Gospel of Thomas: MW Meyer, trans., 2nd rev. ed. (New York: HarperOne, 2004).

friends in places from Texas to Tennessee: Thank you Todd, Jeff, and Justin.

cool enough to have their own TV show: *Portlandia* (IFC Original Productions, 2011–2018).

Oregon ranks among the top ten states in total number of microbreweries, while Vermont tops the list on a per capita basis: "Number of craft breweries in the United States in 2018, by state" (https://www.statista.com/statistics/726518/number-craft-breweries-state/); and K Norton, "Vermont leads nation in breweries and beer production per capita," *VT Digger* (https://vtdigger.org/2019/01/14/vermont-leads-nation-breweries-per-capita/).

AMEN protocol: RS Cooper, A Ferguson, JN Bodurtha, and TJ Smith, "AMEN in challenging conversations: Bridging the gaps between faith, hope, and medicine," *Journal of Oncology Practice* 10 (2014): e191–e195.

the things that people need to say before they die: I Byock, *The Four Things That Matter Most: A Book about living* (New York, NY: Atria Books, 2014).

— Chapter 15: —
Redemption

in no particular order, contrary to what the textbooks say: The classic stages of grief—denial, anger, bargaining, grief, and acceptance—set forth in Elisabeth Kübler-Ross's *On Death and Dying* (New York: Scribner, 1969) don't always work out that neatly in real life.

what I wanted to say: Available at https://tinyurl.com/UVMMedGrad2018, beginning at 27:30.

WWMD: A variation on the abbreviation for "What Would Jesus Do?" that is popular among Christian bracelet-wearers.

intensive care fellow: A fellow is a doctor who's already completed their residency and is pursuing additional subspecialty training. To become a Pediatric ICU physician, for instance, one has to complete three years of pediatric residency and then another three years of critical care fellowship.

what episode of *BtVS* was the best: It's a tie, by the way, between "The body" and "Hush," with an honorable mention going to "Once more, with feeling."

Abbreviations and medical terms

BtVS Buffy the Vampire Slayer
CF Cystic Fibrosis
DCF Department of Children and Families
DNI Do Not Intubate
DNAR Do Not Attempt Resuscitation
DNR Do Not Resuscitate
Gastrostomy Also known as a G-tube, which is surgically implanted through the abdominal wall into the stomach, to deliver nutrition, hydration, and medication. More stable than an NG tube.
GBS Guillain-Barré Syndrome
HPCCV Hospice and Palliative Care Council of Vermont
NICU Neonatal Intensive Care Unit
NG tube Nasogastric tube, which is slipped through the nose down into the stomach to deliver nutrition, hydration, and medication. Generally a temporary measure as it is susceptible to being dislodged.

PACT Pediatric Advanced Care Team (a common name for a pediatric palliative care team)

PICU Pediatric Intensive Care Unit

PTLD Post-transplant lymphoproliferative disorder

SOFT Support Organization for Trisomy 18, 13 and Related Disorders

T18 Trisomy 18

Tracheostomy A small hole in the neck with a short tube that directly enters the windpipe (trachea) below the vocal cords, offering the possibility of speaking. This is used to effect long-term ventilation, as it is more stable and comfortable than an endotracheal tube, which goes through the mouth down into the windpipe.

Trisomy Possessing three copies of a particular chromosome rather than the standard pair

UDDA Uniform Determination of Death Act

VSD Ventricular septal defect or a hole in the wall separating the left and right lower chambers of the heart.

Acknowledgments

The idea for writing this book came to me as I was reading Sunita Puri's beautiful *That Good Night*, which tells the stories of adults she cared for as a palliative care physician. I kept thinking how different pediatric palliative care is, and a few unforgettable patients came to mind. The next day, more did, so I started making a list. Feeling like there was something important that needed to be said, I reached out to the parents of those kids and asked if it would be okay if I tried to write about their child.

That led to some incredibly tender reminiscences over Zoom as I prepared to write each chapter and then another round to review what I'd written and correct anything I'd gotten wrong. There was many an evening or weekend when, after a tearful conversation with parents I might not have been in touch with for years, during which we shared our memories as well as our grief, that I felt more emotionally exhausted—and also fulfilled—than after a full day of work at the hospital.

To those parents: thank you for trusting me to tell a part of your child's story. And to their children: thank you for teaching me what it means to really be a kid and, in the process, healing wounds I thought I'd carry forever.

Writing this book wasn't easy, but getting it published turned out to be even harder.

"Oh, that's *definitely* going to be a bestseller," a friend of mine said, the sarcasm palpable, when I told him I was writing a book about pediatric palliative care.

As he proceeded to offer unsolicited ideas for the marketing campaign—including one that involved embedding a tiny box of Kleenex in the back cover in some macabre cross-promotion—I pointed out that some patients do get better. Tony survived unbearable pain and Benjamin fully recovered, neither ever aware of how much they taught me. Cora continues on her mission to educate and inspire, as each day, her median life expectancy becomes an ever-smaller blip in the rearview mirror. And Hannah, who started my pediatric journey over three decades ago, not only is the inspiration for the second-largest handicap-accessible "boundless playground" in the country—named in her honor—but also went on to become a licensed clinical social worker.*

My friend had a point, though: most people think palliative care is about dying. Which explains the TNTC** rejections I received from agents and editors.

I've experienced a lot of rejection in my writing life, but always before it was merely personal. This was different, because it wasn't my story I was telling. So I kept trying, and whenever I was tempted to throw in the towel, I'd always come back to something Collin's mother, Deb, said to me.

As with all the other parents mentioned here, I'd told her at the outset that, if at any point she didn't want me to include her child in this book, she just had to say the word. Channeling the first rule

---

* I know that because, as I was completing the final revision of this manuscript, I realized that, even all these years later, I remembered her full name. A little creative Googling allowed us to reconnect. After having been FP (Fisher-Price) friends back then, it seems fitting that we're FB (Facebook) friends now.

** That's the medical abbreviation, usually applied to cells seen under a microscope, for "too numerous to count."

of medicine to "first, do no harm," I made it clear that my primary goal—amid all the lofty aspirations of readers learning more about pediatric palliative care and the incredibly brave children and parents I encounter every day—was not to make anything worse.

"You know," Deb replied, "the worst thing that could ever happen to me happened to me: my son died. The second worst thing that could happen is that the world forgets him. So if your book makes that less likely, then it has to be a good thing."

From that point on, any rejection felt like an agent or editor was saying that Collin and the other kids in this book weren't worth remembering. I couldn't let that happen.

So I called in every conceivable connection and favor, which all came to naught until a very fortuitous conversation with my friend and fellow Vermont College of Fine Arts alum, the accomplished poet Annie Lighthart. Hearing me describe my book, she asked to read it. And having read it, she asked if it would be okay if she introduced me to her publisher, Eric Muhr.

Questions don't come any easier than that.

I can't begin to express my gratitude to Eric and the good folks at Chehalem Press for recognizing that palliative care is more about living than dying and bringing the inspiring stories of these kids and their parents to the world.

It's hard to describe the deep appreciation I feel for the dear friends who read the early manuscript and offered invaluable suggestions: Will Kennedy, Blyth Lord, and Elisha Waldman (whose book *This Narrow Space* you really should read if you haven't already). Robin Oliveira—who has been so generous with her counsel and encouragement since my first day as a student at Vermont College of Fine Arts, back when she was a graduate assistant there—sent practically page-by-page emails of effusive praise as she worked her way through the manuscript, providing desperately needed encouragement during a particularly rejection-filled period. Chris Adrian, Richard Hain, and Dick Schmidt read revised versions, offering crucial feedback and encouragement. Paula Vanderford read the penultimate version and offered a fresh perspective (not to mention catching a ton of typos that

I, having become so familiar with the text over time, could no longer see).

As should be clear from the examples in this book, palliative care is inherently a team sport, and I'm so thankful for the amazing members of the PACT team at the University of Vermont and especially the Bridges team at Oregon Health & Science University, both past and present: Shelly Field, Hannah Holiman, Monica Holland, Guy Keplinger, Natalie Lanocha, Anat LeBlanc, Jen Levi, Melanie Madigan, Maija Mikkelsen, Kathy Perko, Tyler Tate, Sara Taub, Greg Thomas, Julie Thomas, Paula Vanderford, Frances Way, Zack Wheat, and Lindsay Wooster-Halberg. Were it not for the stalwart support of my chair, Dana Braner, and the generosity of the Cambia Health Foundation, this work wouldn't be possible.

So many people have been instrumental in teaching me about palliative care and supporting me (both personally and professionally) in my work in the field. As mentors, I am fortunate to count Ira Byock, Diane Meier, Joanne Wolfe, and most especially the Rev. Bob Ficks (my priest mentor and dear friend) and Dr. Bob Orr. And Justin Baker, Sally Bliss, Chris Collura, Jacob Dahlke, Jeff Klick, Kevin Madden, Lexy Morvant, Dave Nowels, Todd Pearson, Tom Strouse, and Martha Twaddle are colleagues and friends who've been there for me every step of the way.

I've spent a lot of hours in therapy, where I benefited immensely from the wisdom and compassion of David Boedy, Elizabeth Seward, and especially Chris Greene, who marked the beginning of my journey toward self-understanding and somehow managed—after not seeing me for over fifteen years—to know what words I needed to hear and how to say them. Over coffee, on the eve of my move to Oregon, he introduced me to the quote from the Gospel of Thomas that both encapsulated the reasons for my taking a huge leap of faith and offered a holy challenge for all the choices left to make.

My deepest thanks, as always, goes to my amazing wife and kids. Catie has been my partner-in-crime in everything from Burning Man to hikes on the Long Trail, and saved this book by coming up with a far better title than I ever could; Noah's hug made me feel more loved than I ever had before; Lucy's songs got me through the hardest days;

and Charley's curious and adventurous spirit consistently inspires me. Pam gave up—at least temporarily—something she treasured, in order for me to get what I needed. I've done quite a few things in my life and weathered more than a storm here and there, but the home I always return to—and am blessed to take refuge in—is my core identity: husband to Pam, father to Catie, Noah, Lucy, and Charlotte.

In conclusion, I should note how interesting it is, after all the therapy and conversations and even writing a book about it, that healing is an ongoing process. Even now, with the Bizarro World left behind long ago, I still doubt my memory. Not just about smaller details, which I'm so grateful to the parents of the kids in this book for correcting and clarifying when I went astray. But the big stuff, too, like my recollection of the last time I saw Collin and the belief that I'd given him the Giles action figure that for years had sat upon my desk.

In the incredibly tender and honest conversations I had with his parents, Bill and Deb, as I prepared to write the chapter about him, that moment never came up. Even in the original draft, I didn't include it, largely (I now realize) out of fear that I might have merely wanted to give that to him but might not have had the courage to actually do so.

Yet it felt really important to me—sacred, even—not only to include it in the book but to claim the truth of that moment and of my memory.

"Do you remember," I tentatively said to Bill over Zoom, as we debriefed the first draft, "Collin's last day in the hospital, when I stopped by?"

Bill nodded, tears yet again welling up in his yes.

"I really wanted to give him something," I continued, not brave enough to come right out and ask.

But then a bright smile spread across Bill's face, as he reached up for something on the shelf above his computer, outside the field of his webcam.

"Do you mean this?" he asked, holding a six-inch, plastic version of Giles, bedecked in a striped dress shirt, silk tie, and tailored metallic gray three-piece suit, holding in one hand a double-headed battle axe and in the other what curiously resembles a physician's classic "little black bag."

"Yes," I replied, confident that Bill knew what that action figure had symbolized to Collin, even if he had no way of knowing (until now) what the memory of that moment signifies to me. "That's exactly what I meant."

If you want to help

As this book makes clear, pediatric palliative care is a labor-intensive and poorly reimbursed specialty. To provide the care that kids with serious illness both desperately need and absolutely deserve, not only must there be institutional commitment but also philanthropic support. As noted on the back cover, all proceeds from this book go to support the pediatric palliative care program here at Oregon Health & Science University, with a portion donated to Darkness to Light (an incredible organization dedicated to ending child sexual abuse).

If you would like to do more to support kids like the ones described in this book, there are many ways to do so:

1. Donate to a pediatric palliative care program in your area, which won't be difficult to locate, as nearly all academic medical centers—especially those with children's hospitals—have one. Alternatively, our program in Oregon is always immensely grateful for any support and encouragement that comes our way (www.ohsufoundation.org, directed to the Bridges Pediatric Palliative Care program).
2. Donate to a local hospice agency, directing the funds to pediatric-specific initiatives.

3. Support one of the remarkable advocacy organizations out there, raising awareness about the needs of kids with serious illness (such as at CourageousParentsNetwork.org).
4. Volunteer with a local hospice or palliative care program, offering your time and heart to kids and families facing incredible challenges.
5. Donate to Darkness to Light (www.D2L.org). I often say that my greatest wish is to be out of a job, because that would mean no kid is suffering and in need of palliative care. I yearn, too, for a world where Darkness to Light can close up shop because there's no more child sexual abuse. Until that day dawns, though, their mission is crucial.

A wide range of resources and materials can be found at my website (www.RobertMacauley.com). Please feel free to contact me there with comments, feedback, or any general questions—I would love to hear from you!

Author biography

Robert Macauley, MD is one of only a few hundred pediatricians in the United States who is board certified in hospice and palliative medicine. After simultaneously attending both medical school and divinity school at Yale, he completed pediatric residency at Johns Hopkins. For over a decade he directed both the Department of Clinical Ethics as well as the Pediatric Palliative Care Team at the University of Vermont. He is now Cambia Health Foundation Endowed Chair in Pediatric Palliative Care at Oregon Health and Science University.

He has held leadership roles in a wide variety of national organizations, including serving on the Board of Directors of the American Academy of Hospice and Palliative Medicine (AAHPM) and as Chair of both the American Academy of Pediatrics (AAP) Committee on Bioethics, as well as the American Board of Internal Medicine (ABIM) Hospice and Palliative Medicine Test Writing Committee.

He is also an accomplished writer. Having earned an MFA in Fiction from Vermont College of Fine Arts—where he was awarded the Founders Scholarship—he is the author of the definitive textbook in his field (*Ethics in Palliative Care: A Complete Guide,* Oxford University Press, 2018), as well as over fifty peer-reviewed articles and editorials in the academic literature, in journals such as *Pediatrics*, *Journal of Palliative Medicine*, and *Journal of Medical Ethics*. He was awarded Honorable Mention in the Writer's Digest Short Story competition and has published poetry in journals such as *The Red Wheelbarrow*.

In addition to his medical work, Dr. Macauley is also an Episcopal priest, having served parishes in Maryland, Connecticut, New York, Vermont, and Oregon.

www.ingramcontent.com/pod-product-compliance
Lightning Source LLC
Chambersburg PA
CBHW031722230426
43669CB00007B/206